The Diabetes Carbohydrate and Fat Gram Guide

Second Edition

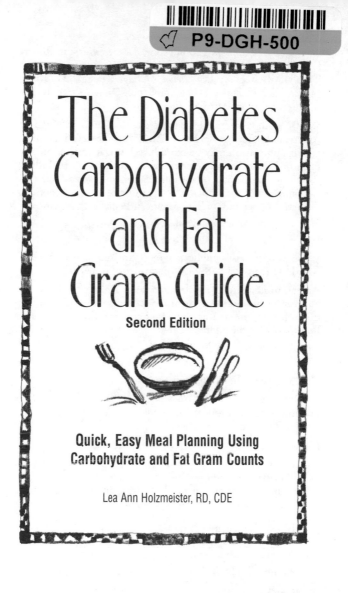

Quick, Easy Meal Planning Using Carbohydrate and Fat Gram Counts

Lea Ann Holzmeister, RD, CDE

Director, Book Publishing, John Fedor; *Book Acquisitions,* Robert J. Anthony; *Editor,* Aime M. Ballard; *Production Director,* Carolyn R. Segree; *Production Manager,* Peggy M. Rote; *Composition,* Harlowe Typography, Inc.; *Cover Design,* Renée Boudreau; *Printer,* Port City Press.

Printed in the United States of America
7 9 10 8 6

⊗ The paper in this publication meets the requirements of the ANSI Standard Z39.48-1992 (permanence of paper).

American Diabetes Association titles may be purchased for business or promotional use or for special sales. For information, please write to Lee Romano Sequeira, Special Sales & Promotions, at the address below.

American Diabetes Association
1701 North Beauregard Street, Alexandria, Virginia 22311

The American Dietetic Association
216 West Jackson Boulevard, Chicago, Illinois 60606

Portions of the data in the first edition were obtained from ESHA Research, Salem, OR.

Library of Congress Cataloging-in-Publication Data

Holzmeister, Lea Ann.
    The diabetes carbohydrate and fat gram guide : quick, easy meal planning using carbohydrate and fat gram counts / Lea Ann Holzmeister.—2nd ed.
      p. cm.
    ISBN 1-58040-050-7 (pbk. : alk. paper)
      1. Diabetes—Diet therapy. 2. Food exchange lists. 3. Food—Carbohydrate content—Tables. 4. Food—Fat content—Tables. I. Title.

RC662 .H66 2000
616.4'620654—dc21   00-025293

The suggestions and information contained in this publication are generally consistent with the *Clinical Practice Recommendations* and other policies of the American Diabetes Association and The American Dietetic Association, but they do not represent the policy or position of the Associations or any of their boards or committees. Reasonable steps have been taken to ensure the accuracy of the information presented. However, the Associations cannot ensure the safety or efficacy of any product or service described in this publication. Individuals are advised to consult a physician or other appropriate health care professional before undertaking any diet or exercise program or taking any medication referred to in this publication. Professionals must use and apply their own professional judgment, experience, and training and should not rely solely on the information contained in this publication before prescribing any diet, exercise, or medication. The Associations—their officers, directors, employees, volunteers, and members—assume no responsibility or liability for personal or other injury, loss, or damage that may result from the suggestions or information in this publication.

Dedication

To Jeff, Erin, Adam, and Emily

Contents

vii   Preface

viii   Acknowledgments

ix   Introduction

1   Appetizers and Dips

7   Beverages

22   Bread Products and Baked Goods

54   Candy

64   Cereals

82   Cheese and Cheese Products

96   Combination Foods and Frozen Entrees

148   Desserts

187   Eggs and Egg Dishes

190   Ethnic Foods

211   Fast Foods

284   Fats, Oils, and Salad Dressings

302   Fruits and Fruit Juices

307   Grains, Noodles, and Rice

317   Legumes

325   Meats, Fish, and Poultry

349   Milk and Yogurt

362   Nuts, Seeds, and Nut/Seed Products

370   Sauces, Condiments, and Gravies

398   Snack Foods

430   Soups and Stews

446   Vegetables and Vegetable Juices

463   Vegetarian Foods

Preface to the Second Edition

Since the *Diabetes Carbohydrate and Fat Gram Guide* was first published, many new food products have been introduced and fast-food restaurants have revised their menus. This second edition includes over 1,200 new listings, as well as three additional nutrient facts. Because of your comments and many people's desire to monitor their intake of more than just carbohydrates and fat, we have added carbohydrate, fiber, and protein counts for each food.

America is becoming increasingly multicultural, and diabetes is taking a toll on minority populations. With this in mind, over 300 ethnic foods have been added to this edition. A new chapter lists foods/ingredients found in Alaska Native, Chinese-American, Filipino-American, Hmong, Jewish, Mexican-American, Navajo, and Plains Indian cooking. Many familiar ethnic foods—some of which we may not even think of as ethnic—can also be found in other sections of the book according to the type of product. For example, many prepared Mexican-, Chinese-, and Italian-American dishes can be found in the chapter Combination Foods and Frozen Entrees.

To prepare this new edition, we contacted food companies and fast-food franchises to obtain current nutrition information and product listings, scanned grocery store shelves for the newest foods and most up-to-date nutrition facts, and compiled ethnic food data from the American Diabetes Association and The American Dietetic Association's Ethnic and Regional Food Practice Series. The result is a more complete resource for anyone who is concerned about nutrition.

Acknowledgments

Thanks to Richard Ziriax for his expert technical support and collaboration.

Thanks to Madelyn L. Wheeler, MS, RD, FADA, CDE, and Patti Bazel Geil, MS, RD, CDE, for their valuable review comments.

Introduction

Since its discovery hundreds of years ago, diabetes has been linked with what people eat. What people with diabetes are advised to eat and how they plan their meals has changed over the years. The latest American Diabetes Association (ADA) *Nutrition Recommendations and Principles for People With Diabetes Mellitus* (published each year in January in Supplement 1 of the journal *Diabetes Care*) emphasizes individuality and flexibility, which are essential for helping people with diabetes follow a healthy eating plan.

Many people with diabetes use some type of meal planning system to help them meet their individual nutrition goals. Just as there is no one diet that is right for everyone with diabetes, there is also no one meal planning approach that meets everyone's needs.

It is important to know your own nutrition goals. A registered dietitian (RD) can help you determine your individual nutrition goals and develop a meal plan based on your food preferences, lifestyle, blood glucose and blood lipid (fat) levels, overall health, and abilities. Your doctor may be able to recommend a dietitian. Or call The American Dietetic Association at 1-800-366-1655 for a referral to a local dietitian.

Types of Meal Planning Approaches

Four types of meal planning approaches are described in this book: carbohydrate counting, fat gram counting, food exchange system, and calorie counting. The advantages and disadvantages of each are discussed, and information about where to learn more is provided.

It is important to select a meal planning approach that you are comfortable using and that will work toward achieving your goals. You do not have to use the same approach your entire life. As your individual nutrition goals change, so may your meal planning approach. Before switching though, it is a good idea to consult with your dietitian.

Carbohydrate Counting

Carbohydrate counting has been used for many years in Europe and is becoming increasingly popular in the United States. The three main nutrients in the foods we eat are carbohydrate, protein, and fat. The carbohydrate in foods affects your blood glucose level more than protein or fat. In carbohydrate counting, you count only carbohydrate.

To use carbohydrate counting, you must know your total carbohydrate allotment for the day. Your dietitian can help you determine this. Together, you and your dietitian will make a carbohydrate counting meal plan based on your usual food intake, lifestyle, diabetes medications, and physical activity. Once you have your carbohydrate counting meal plan, you'll need to become familiar with the carbohydrate content in foods. Carbohydrate is found in many foods, such as grains, vegetables, fruits, milk, and table sugar. It is important to count all carbohydrate regardless of its source.

The two main types of carbohydrate are sugars and starches. According to ADA's nutrition recommendations, it is more important to eat the same amount of carbohydrate at meals and snacks each day than to focus on the type of carbohydrate eaten. Research has shown that sugars do not raise blood glucose any more than starches. This means that you can eat foods that contain sugar as long as you count them as part of your total carbohydrate allotment for the day. Keep in mind that foods high in sugar are often high in fat and calories and low in vitamins and minerals, so they contribute little to the overall healthfulness of your diet.

Carbohydrate counting can provide some advantages over other meal planning approaches. Some people feel that focusing on only one nutrient makes this system easier. With the focus on carbohydrate, food and insulin can be matched more precisely. Matching food and insulin increases flexibility in meal and snack times. This can be particularly helpful when your appetite varies or your schedule changes. Also, insulin can be matched to carbohydrate eaten at specific times during the day. For example, some people need more insulin at breakfast for each gram of carbohydrate eaten. Thus, carbohydrate counting may be most appropriate for people with type 1 diabetes who take insulin.

One disadvantage of carbohydrate counting is that when you focus only on carbohydrate, it is easy to lose sight of the overall nutritional quality of foods. For example, counting the carbohydrate in ice cream but ignoring its fat content may lead you to eat it more often. Too much fat in the diet increases your risk of heart disease, cancer, and weight gain. If you pay no attention to the overall nutritional quality of foods, you may end up eating a diet that is too high in fat or protein.

To learn more about carbohydrate counting, contact your dietitian. The American Diabetes Association and The American Dietetic Association have jointly published three instructional booklets on carbohydrate counting: *Carbohydrate Counting: Getting Started, Carbohydrate Counting: Moving On,* and *Carbohydrate Counting: Using Carbohydrate/Insulin Ratios.* You can obtain these booklets from your dietitian.

Fat Gram Counting

Fat gram counting has been around since the 1980s, when it was introduced as a tool to teach low-fat eating to reduce the risk of cancer. Since that time, it has also been used for teaching heart-healthy eating for heart disease and reduced-calorie eating for weight reduction. Fat gram counting may be particularly useful for people with type 2 diabetes who are overweight. Fat provides two and a half times as many calories per gram as carbohydrate or protein.

The first step in using fat gram counting is to establish a daily calorie requirement based on your height, weight, activity level, and weight goal. Your dietitian can help you determine this. Then, based on your nutrition goals, a daily fat gram goal will be determined. In fat gram counting, you keep a record of the foods you eat and their fat content.

There are some advantages to fat gram counting. It is simple, and it allows a considerable amount of flexibility and control over your food choices. With fat gram counting, you will usually improve the overall quality of your food choices, because you will tend to select lower fat foods, such as fruits, vegetables, grains, and low-fat dairy products. Like carbohydrate counting, you are focusing on only one nutrient. This can be especially appealing when weight loss is the primary goal and other approaches have not worked.

One disadvantage of fat gram counting is that it does not take into consideration foods that may affect your blood glucose. Therefore, your blood glucose values may be inconsistent.

To learn more about fat gram counting, contact your dietitian. Your local American Heart Association may also have additional information on fat gram counting programs.

Food Exchange System

For many years, the food exchange system has been used as a meal planning approach for people with diabetes, regardless of the type of diabetes and how it is treated. This system groups foods with similar nutritional value into lists with the goal of helping people with diabetes eat consistent amounts of nutrients. Each food has approximately the same number of calories, carbohydrate, protein, and fat as the other foods on the same list. Any food on a list can be traded or "exchanged" for any other food on the same list.

To use the exchange system, you need an individualized meal plan that tells you how many exchanges from each list to select for meals and snacks. Your dietitian can help you design your individualized meal plan and teach you how to use this system.

The American Diabetes Association and The American Dietetic Association's *Exchange Lists for Meal Planning* booklet groups food into three broad groups: the carbohydrate group, the meat and meat substitutes group, and the fat group.

The carbohydrate group includes five lists: the starch list, the fruit list, the milk list, the other carbohydrates list, and the vegetable list. The meat and meat substitutes group includes four lists: the very lean list, the lean list, the medium-fat list, and the high-fat list. The fat group includes a monounsaturated fats list, a polyunsaturated fats list, and a saturated fats list. In addition to these lists, there is a free foods list, a combination foods list, and a fast foods list.

One advantage of the food exchange system is its emphasis on more than one nutrient and the importance of the overall nutritional content of foods. This system also encourages consistency in the timing and amount of your meals and snacks.

People desiring to lose weight might find this approach useful for learning the caloric and fat values of foods. Food exchanges can also be used as a reference for those using carbohydrate counting. Each serving of a food in the carbohydrate group counts as 15 grams of carbohydrate.

One disadvantage of this system is the level of understanding needed to grasp the concept of "exchanging" foods. It also requires learning where a food that is not listed fits. To learn more about the food exchange system for meal planning, contact your dietitian.

Calorie Counting

Calorie counting has been used for many years as a way to achieve weight loss, weight gain, or weight maintenance. This approach is most appropriate for people who are overweight and do not take insulin. Even modest weight loss improves blood glucose levels.

To use calorie counting, you and your dietitian establish a calorie goal that will help you achieve your weight goal. Your weight goal will be based on your current weight, height, and activity level. If you desire to lose weight, your calorie goal will be set lower than your usual intake of calories. If you wish to maintain your current weight, your calorie goal will be set at a calorie level similar to your current intake of calories.

You keep records of the foods you eat and their calorie content. A periodic comparison of your food records and weekly weight can give you feedback on how you are progressing toward your weight goal. These records can also help you identify problem areas. For example, you might realize after reviewing your records that you tend to overeat when away from home. Knowing this information will help you and your dietitian develop strategies for changing this behavior.

The main advantage of calorie counting is the expanded choice of foods, which gives you more flexibility in what you eat. You decide whether and how a food might fit into your meal plan. For example, say your daily calorie goal is 1,500 calories, and a food you want to eat contains 600 calories. You can eat that food as long as you plan what other foods you'll eat that day to add up to the remaining 900 calories. Your serving size, too, is based on how you want to "spend" your calories. You might decide you can work in only half a serving of pasta salad, or you might choose to have a double serving of pasta salad.

One disadvantage of calorie counting might be the amount of time involved in keeping records and calculating the calorie content of foods. Also, because this approach does not guide you toward making nutritionally balanced choices, you may end up with a high-fat diet or one low in essential vitamins and minerals. Your dietitian can provide you with basic nutrition guidelines by which to select your foods to ensure that you meet your nutrition goals as well.

Estimating Serving Sizes

The success of any meal planning approach depends on how accurately you estimate your serving sizes. Therefore, it is essential to train your eyes to do this. Equip your kitchen with measuring spoons, measuring cups, and a food scale. Use these tools to measure and weigh foods consistently for 2 weeks or until you have trained your eyes to recognize what a cup of pasta looks like on your plate or where a cup of milk fills your favorite glass.

Without some practice, it is surprisingly easy to mistakenly pour yourself one cup instead of a half cup of juice. A cup of juice has twice the carbohydrate and calories as a half cup of juice. This might tip you over your calorie or carbohydrate goal. If you did this with two to three foods each day, it could spoil your efforts at weight loss and blood glucose control.

Of course, it is not practical to measure servings when you eat out in a restaurant, but training your eyes will help. Fortunately, the serving sizes of fast foods are fairly standardized among restaurants, i.e., a taco at any Taco Bell restaurant is likely to be the same size.

How Food Counts Can Work For You

The meal planning approach you select will determine what you will "count" in your diet. But using a meal planning approach to guide your food choices is only a starting point. To reach your individual goals (e.g., blood glucose, blood lipids, weight, general health), you need to respond every day to blood glucose changes and periodically to other indicators of your progress (e.g., blood lipid levels, weight gain or loss).

Food Counts and Blood Glucose

Making the connection between what you eat and how it affects your blood glucose level can be a very powerful step toward achieving your blood glucose goals. Once you have recorded your food intake and blood glucose values, you can learn to analyze the data to see how individual foods and meals affect your blood glucose. You can then try adjusting food intake, physical activity, and diabetes medications.

Food Counts and Blood Lipids

Counting total fat and saturated fat in your diet while keeping tabs on your blood lipid levels (total cholesterol, HDL [high-density lipoprotein] cholesterol, LDL [low-density lipoprotein] cholesterol, and triglycerides) allows you to determine whether your meal plan is helping you to achieve your blood lipid goals. Suppose you have been advised to follow a diet with less than 70 grams of fat and less than 25 grams of saturated fat per day in an attempt to reduce your total cholesterol from 250 to 200 mg/dl. By comparing your food records of fat and saturated fat intake to your blood lipid levels over time, you can determine how close you are coming to your blood lipid goals.

Using This Book of Food Counts

This book is intended to be a comprehensive listing of both generic and brand name foods that are available nationally. The nutrition information in this 2nd edition comes from several sources, including the U.S. Department of Agriculture, Agricultural Research Service, 1999 USDA Nutrient Database for Standard Reference, Release 13; the American Diabetes Association and The American Dietetic Association's *Exchange Lists for Meal Planning* nutrient database; a variety of food-processing companies and fast-food franchises; and Nutrition Facts from food labels.

Foods are listed alphabetically by food category and manufacturer. Nutrient information for foods from mixes (e.g., puddings and cakes) reflect values after the food has been prepared according to package directions.

This book lists the calories, carbohydrate, fat, saturated fat, cholesterol, sodium, fiber, and protein of many foods. These particular nutrients were selected because they are the most commonly monitored by people with diabetes (see Table 1).

The nutrient values you use will depend on your meal planning approach. You may need one, two, or even more of the values to figure out how a food fits in your plan.

Values have been rounded to the nearest calorie, gram (g), or milligram (mg) per serving (a gram is a unit of mass and weight in the metric system; an ounce is about 30 grams). The serving sizes listed in this book are those most commonly

TABLE 1. American Diabetes Association Nutrient Recommendations

Calories: Most adults require 1,800 to 2,500 calories per day. However, your calorie needs are best determined by your dietitian.

Carbohydrate: Carbohydrates raise your blood glucose level. You might get 50% or more of your daily calories from carbohydrates. Your dietitian can help you determine how much carbohydrate you need in a day.

Fat: Fat contributes to weight gain. Most people need no more than 30% of their daily calories from fat. People who are over-weight should consider reducing their intake of fat. Your dietitian can help you determine what percentage of your daily calories should come from fat.

Saturated Fat: Saturated fat can raise your blood cholesterol level. Most people should get no more than 10% of their daily calories from saturated fat.

Cholesterol: Cholesterol found in foods from animal sources can raise your blood cholesterol level. Limit cholesterol in your diet to 300 milligrams or less daily.

Sodium: Sodium has been linked to high blood pressure (hypertension). People with normal blood pressure should get no more than 2,400 to 3,000 milligrams of sodium per day. People with moderately high blood pressure are advised to get 2,400 milligrams or less of sodium per day, and people with high blood pressure and kidney disease are advised to get 2,000 milligrams or less of sodium per day.

Fiber: Daily consumption of 20–35 grams of dietary fiber from both soluble and insoluble fibers from a wide variety of food sources is recommended. Dietay fiber may be helpful in the treatment and prevention of constipation and several

TABLE 1. American Diabetes Association Nutrient Recommendations (*Continued*)

gastrointestinal disorders. Soluble fiber has a beneficial effect on serum lipids and provides satiety value to your diet.

Protein: Most adults, including people with diabetes, require approximately 10–20% of their calories from protein. Those with initial signs of diabetes-induced kidney disease may benefit from restricting protein to 10% of daily calories.

---

used. Similar foods will have the same serving sizes. The serving size may be very different from the amount you serve yourself or eat. If your serving size is different, ask your dietitian to help you recalculate the numbers.

The exchange values of foods have been calculated using the "rounding off method" (Wheeler ML, Franz M, Barrier PH, Holler H, Cronmiller N, Delahanty LM: Macronutrient and energy database for the 1995 Exchange Lists for Meal Planning: A rationale for clinical practice decisions. *J Am Diet Assoc* 96:1167–1170, 1996). Table 2 shows the amount of nutrients in one serving from each list.

Some of the foods in this book have a nutrient claim, such as "reduced-fat" or "low-calorie," as part of their name. These claims have standard meanings set by the Food and Drug Administration (FDA). Some of these terms and their meanings are listed in Table 3.

TABLE 2. Nutrient Content of Exchange Lists

Groups/Lists	Carb. (g)	Prot. (g)	Fat (g)	Cal.
Carbohydrate Group				
Starch List	15	3	1 or less	80
Fruit List	15	0	0	60
Milk List				
Skim/Low-Fat	12	8	0–3	90
Reduced-Fat	12	8	5	120
Whole	12	8	8	150
Other Carbohydrates List	15	varies	varies	varies
Vegetable List	5	2	0	25
Meat and Meat Substitutes Group				
Very Lean List	0	7	0–1	35
Lean List	0	7	3	55
Medium-Fat List	0	7	5	75
High-Fat List	0	7	8	100
Fat Group				
Monounsaturated Fats List	0	0	5	45
Polyunsaturated Fats List	0	0	5	45
Saturated Fats List	0	0	5	45
Free Foods List	5 or less	varies	varies	less than 20
Combination Foods List	varies	varies	varies	varies
Fast Foods List	varies	varies	varies	varies

Adapted from the American Diabetes Association and The American Dietetic Association: *Exchange Lists for Meal Planning.* Alexandria, VA, 1995, p. 3.

TABLE 3. Nutrient Claims on Food Labels

Term	Meaning
Calorie-Free	Less than 5 calories per serving
Cholesterol-Free	Less than 2 mg of cholesterol per serving and 2 g or less of saturated fat per serving
Extra Lean	Less than 5 g of fat, 2 g of saturated fat, and 95 mg of cholesterol per serving
Fat-Free	Less than 0.5 g of fat per serving
Lean	Less than 10 g of fat, 4.5 g of saturated fat, and 95 mg of cholesterol per serving
Light or Lite	33.3% fewer calories or 50% less fat per serving than comparison food
Low-Calorie	40 calories or less per serving
Low-Cholesterol	20 mg or less of cholesterol per serving and 2 g or less of saturated fat per serving
Low-Fat	3 g or less of fat per serving
Low-Saturated Fat	1 g or less of saturated fat per serving and 15% or less of calories from saturated fat
Low-Sodium	140 mg or less of sodium per serving
Reduced	25% less per serving than comparison food
Saturated Fat-free	Less than 0.5 g of saturated fat per serving
Sodium-Free	Less than 5 mg of sodium per serving
Sugar-Free	Less than 0.5 g of sugar per serving

APPETIZERS AND DIPS

Products	Cal.	Carb. (g)	Fat (g)	Sat. Fat (g)	Chol. (mg)	Sod. (mg)	Fib. (g)	Prot. (g)	Servings/Exchanges
Dip, Jalapeño Pepper Bean (2 Tbsp)	46	6	2	<1	0	382	2	2	1/2 strch
Mushrooms, Stuffed w/Meat (2)	113	8	7	2	6	279	<1	4	1/2 carb., 1 fat
BREAKSTONE									
Dip, Bacon & Onion Sour Cream (2 Tbsp)	60	2	5	3	20	180	0	2	1 fat
Dip, Fat Free Creamy Salsa (2 Tbsp)	20	3	0	0	<5	240	0	1	free
Dip, Fat Free French Onion (2 Tbsp)	25	4	0	0	<5	260	0	2	free
Dip, Fat Free Ranch (2 Tbsp)	25	4	0	0	<5	330	0	2	free
Dip, French Onion Sour Cream (2 Tbsp)	50	2	5	3	20	160	0	1	1 fat
Dip, Toasted Onion Sour Cream (2 Tbsp)	50	2	5	3	20	170	0	1	1 fat
CHUN KING									
Egg Rolls, Chicken (1)	190	22	9	5	20	650	2	6	1 1/2 carb., 2 fat
Egg Rolls, Shrimp (1)	180	24	7	3	15	490	2	5	1 1/2 carb., 1 fat

APPETIZERS AND DIPS

Products	Cal.	Carb. (g)	Fat (g)	Sat. Fat (g)	Chol. (mg)	Sod. (mg)	Fib. (g)	Prot. (g)	Servings/Exchanges
Mini Egg Rolls, Chicken (6)	210	25	9	3	8	650	2	6	2 carb., 1 fat
Mini Egg Rolls, Pork & Shrimp (6)	210	27	9	3	15	540	2	6	2 carb., 2 fat
Mini Egg Rolls, Shrimp (6)	190	28	9	2	10	730	2	5	2 carb., 2 fat
FRITO-LAY									
Dip, French Onion (2 Tbsp)	60	4	5	3	15	230	0	1	1 fat
Dip, Fritos Bean (2 Tbsp)	40	6	1	<1	0	140	0	2	1/2 carb.
Dip, Fritos Chili Cheese (2 Tbsp)	45	3	3	1	<5	310	0	1	1 fat
Dip, Fritos Hot Bean (2 Tbsp)	40	5	1	0	0	170	1	2	1/2 strch
Dip, Jalapeño & Cheddar Cheese (2 Tbsp)	50	4	4	1	5	300	0	1	1 fat
Dip, Mild Cheddar Cheese (2 Tbsp)	60	3	4	2	5	330	0	1	1 fat
Fritos Texas-Style Chili Hearty Topping (1/4 cup)	50	8	2	<1	10	330	1	2	1/2 carb.
Fritos Ultimate Taco Hearty Topping (1/4 cup)	50	8	2	<1	10	330	1	2	1/2 carb.
KNUDSEN									
Dip, Fat Free Creamy Salsa (2 Tbsp)	20	3	0	0	<5	240	0	1	free

Dip, Fat Free French Onion (2 Tbsp)	25	4	0	0	<5	260	0	2	free
Dip, Fat Free Ranch (2 Tbsp)	25	4	0	0	<5	330	0	2	free
KRAFT									
Dip, Avocado (2 Tbsp)	60	4	4	3	0	240	0	1	1 fat
Dip, Bacon & Horseradish (2 Tbsp)	60	3	5	3	0	220	0	1	1 fat
Dip, Clam (2 Tbsp)	60	3	4	3	0	250	0	1	1 fat
Dip, Fat Free French Onion (2 Tbsp)	25	4	0	0	<5	330	0	2	free
Dip, Fat Free Ranch (2 Tbsp)	25	4	0	0	<5	330	0	2	free
Dip, Fat Free Salsa (2 Tbsp)	20	3	0	0	<5	240	0	1	free
Dip, French Onion (2 Tbsp)	60	4	4	3	0	230	0	1	1 fat
Dip, Green Onion (2 Tbsp)	60	4	4	3	0	190	0	1	1 fat
Dip, Jalapeño (2 Tbsp)	60	3	4	3	0	260	0	1	1 fat
Dip, Premium Bacon & Horseradish (2 Tbsp)	60	2	5	3	15	240	0	2	1 fat
Dip, Premium Bacon & Onion (2 Tbsp)	60	2	5	3	20	180	0	2	1 fat
Dip, Premium Clam (2 Tbsp)	50	1	4	3	20	180	0	1	1 fat
Dip, Premium Creamy Onion (2 Tbsp)	45	2	4	3	15	160	0	1	1 fat

APPETIZERS AND DIPS

Products	Cal.	Carb. (g)	Fat (g)	Sat. Fat (g)	Chol. (mg)	Sod. (mg)	Fib. (g)	Prot. (g)	Servings/Exchanges
Dip, Premium French Onion (2 Tbsp)	45	2	4	3	15	160	0	<1	1 fat
Dip, Ranch (2 Tbsp)	60	3	5	3	0	210	0	1	1 fat
LA CHOY									
Egg Rolls, Chicken (1)	210	15	9	5	15	550	4	6	1 carb., 2 fat
Egg Rolls, Pork (1)	220	24	11	3	10	390	2	5	1 1/2 carb., 1 fat
Egg Rolls, Shrimp (1)	180	25	7	2	15	490	2	5	1 1/2 carb., 1 fat
Egg Rolls, Sweet & Sour Chicken (1)	220	29	9	2	15	350	2	5	2 carb., 2 fat
Mini Egg Rolls, Chicken (6)	210	25	9	3	15	650	2	6	1 1/2 carb., 2 fat
Mini Egg Rolls, Chinese-Style Vegetables w/Lobster (6)	190	27	7	2	5	440	2	5	2 carb., 1 fat
Mini Egg Rolls, Pork & Shrimp (5)	210	27	9	3	15	540	2	5	2 carb., 2 fat
Mini Egg Rolls, Shrimp (5)	190	29	5	2	10	730	2	5	2 carb., 1 fat
MARIE'S									
Dip, Bacon Ranch (2 Tbsp)	150	3	16	2	15	200	0	1	3 fat

Dip, Fiesta Bean (2 Tbsp)	140	2	14	2	10	160	<1	<1	3 fat
Dip, Homestyle Ranch (2 Tbsp)	150	3	15	2	15	140	0	0	3 fat
Dip, Parmesan Garlic (2 Tbsp)	140	2	14	2	10	140	<1	<1	3 fat
Dip, Spinach (2 Tbsp)	140	3	14	2	10	200	0	0	3 fat
Dip, Sun-Dried Tomato (2 Tbsp)	140	2	14	2	15	135	<1	<1	3 fat
OLD EL PASO									
Dip, Black Bean (2 Tbsp)	25	5	0	0	0	280	1	1	free
Dip, Cheese 'n Salsa, Low Fat (2 Tbsp)	30	3	2	1	5	240	0	0	1 fat
Dip, Cheese 'n Salsa, Mild/Medium (2 Tbsp)	40	3	3	1	<5	300	0	<1	1 fat
Dip, Chunky Salsa, Mild/Medium (2 Tbsp)	15	3	0	0	0	230	<1	1	free
Dip, Jalapeño (2 Tbsp)	30	4	1	0	<5	125	2	1	free
PROGRESSO									
Artichoke Hearts, In Brine (2)	30	6	0	0	0	240	1	2	1 vegetable
Cherry Peppers, Drained (2)	30	6	0	0	0	500	0	0	1 vegetable
Eggplant Appetizer (2 Tbsp)	25	2	2	0	0	130	2	0	1 vegetable
Fried Peppers, Drained (2 Tbsp)	60	3	5	<1	0	60	1	0	1 fat

APPETIZERS AND DIPS

Products	Cal.	Carb. (g)	Fat (g)	Sat. Fat (g)	Chol. (mg)	Sod. (mg)	Fib. (g)	Prot. (g)	Servings/Exchanges
Olive Salad, Drained (2 Tbsp)	25	1	3	0	0	360	<1	0	1 fat
Olives, Oil-Cured (6)	80	3	6	<1	0	330	1	0	1 fat
Pepper Salad, Drained (2 Tbsp)	15	1	1	0	0	160	<1	0	1/2 fat
Peppers, Hot Cherry (2 Tbsp)	25	2	2	0	0	30	1	0	free
Peppers, Roasted (2)	10	1	0	0	0	55	0	0	free
Peppers, Sweet Fried w/Onion (2 Tbsp)	20	2	2	0	0	130	1	0	free
Tuscan Peppers, Drained (3)	10	1	0	0	0	450	0	0	free
TOSTITOS									
Beef Fiesta Nacho Topping (1/4 cup)	120	6	8	3	10	500	<2	4	1/2 carb., 2 fat
Chicken Quesadilla Topping (1/4 cup)	90	6	6	2	10	600	<2	4	1/2 carb., 1 fat
Salsa Con Queso (1/4 cup)	80	10	5	2	<10	560	<2	2	1/2 carb., 1 fat
Salsa Con Queso, Low-Fat (1/4 cup)	70	8	3	2	<10	560	<2	2	1/2 carb., 1 fat
Salsa, Mild/Medium/Hot (1/4 cup)	30	6	0	0	0	520	2	2	1 vegetable
Salsa, Restaurant Style (1/4 cup)	30	6	0	0	0	420	<2	<2	1 vegetable
Salsa, Ultimate Garden (1/4 cup)	30	6	0	0	0	460	2	2	1 vegetable

BEVERAGES

Products	Cal.	Carb. (g)	Fat (g)	Sat. Fat (g)	Chol. (mg)	Sod. (mg)	Fib. (g)	Prot. (g)	Servings/Exchanges
Beer, Alcoholic Beverage (12 oz)	146	13	0	0	0	18	<1	1	3 fat
Beer, Light (12 oz)	99	5	0	0	0	11	0	<1	2 fat
Club Soda (12 oz)	0	0	0	0	0	75	0	0	free
Coffee, Brewed (8 oz)	5	<1	<1	<1	0	5	0	<1	free
Coffee, Cappuccino Mix & Water (6 oz)	61	11	2	2	0	104	0	<1	1 carb.
Coffee, Demitasse (8 oz)	5	<1	0	<1	0	5	0	<1	free
Coffee, Espresso (8 oz)	5	<1	0	<1	0	5	0	<1	free
Coffee, Instant, Prepared (8 oz)	5	<1	<1	<1	0	7	0	<1	free
Cola-Type Soda (12 oz)	152	39	<1	0	0	15	0	0	2 1/2 carb.
Cream Soda (12 oz)	189	49	0	0	0	45	0	0	3 carb.
Diet Cola/Coke w/Aspartame (12 oz)	4	<1	0	0	0	21	0	<1	free
Fruit Drink Powder & Water, Low-Calorie (8 oz)	43	11	0	0	0	50	0	0	1/2 carb.

BEVERAGES

Products	Cal.	Carb. (g)	Fat (g)	Sat. Fat (g)	Chol. (mg)	Sod. (mg)	Fib. (g)	Prot. (g)	Servings/Exchanges
Fruit Punch Drink, Canned (8 oz)	119	30	<1	<1	0	56	<1	0	2 carb.
Ginger Ale (12 oz)	124	32	0	0	0	26	0	0	2 carb.
Grape Soda (12 oz)	160	42	0	0	0	56	0	0	3 carb.
Lemon-Lime Soda (12 oz)	147	38	0	0	0	41	0	0	2 1/2 carb.
Lemonade, Frozen Concentrate & Water (8 oz)	99	26	<1	<1	0	7	<1	<1	2 carb.
Orange Soda (12 oz)	179	46	0	0	0	45	0	0	3 carb.
Root Beer (12 oz)	152	39	0	0	0	48	0	0	2 1/2 carb.
Tea, Brewed (8 oz)	2	<1	<1	<1	0	7	0	0	free
Tonic Water, Sugar-Free (12 oz)	0	<1	0	0	0	57	0	0	free
Tonic Water/Quinine Water (12 oz)	124	32	0	0	0	15	0	0	2 carb.
Wine, Dry Dessert (4 oz)	149	5	0	0	0	11	0	0	1 fat
Wine, Medium White (4 oz)	80	<1	0	0	0	6	0	<1	2 fat
Wine, Nonalcoholic, Light or Regular (8 oz)	15	3	0	0	0	18	0	<1	free
Wine, Red (4 oz)	85	2	0	0	0	6	0	<1	2 fat

ALL SPORT

Blue Ice (8 oz)	70	20	0	0	55	0	0	1 carb.
Cherry Slam (8 oz)	70	20	0	0	55	0	0	1 carb.
Fruit Punch (8 oz)	70	20	0	0	55	0	0	1 carb.
Lemon-Lime (8 oz)	70	20	0	0	55	0	0	1 carb.
Orange (8 oz)	70	20	0	0	55	0	0	1 carb.
Raspberry Burst (8 oz)	70	20	0	0	80	0	0	1 carb.

CAPRI SUN

Natural Juice Drink, Maui Punch (9.6 oz)	100	27	0	0	20	0	0	2 carb.
Natural Juice Drink, Orange (9.6 oz)	100	25	0	0	20	0	0	1 1/2 carb.
Natural Juice Drink, Pacific Cooler (9.6 oz)	100	26	0	0	20	0	0	2 carb.
Natural Juice Drink, Red Berry (9.6 oz)	100	26	0	0	20	0	0	2 carb.
Natural Juice Drink, Safari Punch (9.6 oz)	100	25	0	0	20	0	0	2 carb.
Natural Juice Drink, Strawberry Cool (9.6 oz)	90	25	0	0	20	0	0	2 carb.
Natural Juice Drink, Wild Cherry (9.6 oz)	110	30	0	0	20	0	0	2 carb.

BEVERAGES

Products	Cal.	Carb. (g)	Fat (g)	Sat. Fat (g)	Chol. (mg)	Sod. (mg)	Fib. (g)	Prot. (g)	Servings/Exchanges
COCA-COLA									
Cherry Coke (8 oz)	104	28	0	0	0	4	0	0	2 carb.
Citra (8 oz)	91	25	0	0	0	16	0	0	1 1/2 carb.
Coca-Cola Classic (8 oz)	97	27	0	0	0	9	0	0	2 carb.
Diet Coke (8 oz)	1	<1	0	0	0	4	0	0	free
Fanta Grape (8 oz)	117	31	0	0	0	9	0	0	2 carb.
Fanta Orange (8 oz)	118	32	0	0	0	9	0	0	2 carb.
Fresca (8 oz)	2	<1	0	0	0	1	0	0	free
Minute-Maid Orange (8 oz)	118	32	0	0	0	0	0	0	2 carb.
Sprite (8 oz)	96	26	0	0	0	23	0	0	2 carb.
Surge (8 oz)	116	31	0	0	0	3	0	0	2 carb.
TAB (8 oz)	<1	<1	0	0	0	4	0	0	free
COUNTRY TIME									
Iced Tea Drink w/Sugar (8 oz)	70	17	0	0	0	0	0	0	1 carb.

Lem'N Berry Sippers, Cranberry-Raspberry (8 oz)	90	21	0	0	0	0	0	0	1 1/2 carb.
Lem'N Berry Sippers, Raspberry Lemonade (8 oz)	90	21	0	0	0	0	0	0	1 1/2 carb.
Lem'N Berry Sippers, Sugar-Free (8 oz)	5	0	0	0	0	0	0	0	free
Lemonade Drink (8 oz)	70	17	0	0	0	15	0	0	1 carb.
Lemonade Drink, Sugar-Free, Low-Calorie (8 oz)	5	0	0	0	0	0	0	0	free

CRYSTAL LIGHT

Cranberry Breeze Drink (8 oz)	5	0	0	0	0	20	0	0	free
Iced Lemon Tea Drink (8 oz)	5	0	0	0	0	40	0	0	free
Lemonade Drink, Sugar Free (8 oz)	5	0	0	0	0	20	0	0	free

FRUITOPIA

Berry Lemonade (8 oz)	106	28	0	0	0	77	0	0	2 carb.
Fruit Integration (8 oz)	111	29	0	0	0	78	0	0	2 carb.
Kiwiberry Ruckus (8 oz)	109	29	0	0	0	77	0	0	2 carb.
Peachberry Quencher (8 oz)	113	30	0	0	0	78	0	0	2 carb.
Strawberry Passion Awareness (8 oz)	114	30	0	0	0	78	0	0	2 carb.
The Grape Beyond (8 oz)	118	31	0	0	0	79	0	0	2 carb.

BEVERAGES

Products	Cal.	Carb. (g)	Fat (g)	Sat. Fat (g)	Chol. (mg)	Sod. (mg)	Fib. (g)	Prot. (g)	Servings/Exchanges
Tremendously Tangerine (8 oz)	109	29	0	0	0	78	0	0	2 carb.
Tropical Temptation (8 oz)	107	29	0	0	0	79	0	0	2 carb.
FRUITWORKS									
Apple Raspberry (12 oz)	160	42	0	0	0	110	0	0	3 carb.
Guava Berry (12 oz)	170	46	0	0	0	80	0	0	3 carb.
Tangerine Citrus (12 oz)	150	42	0	0	0	80	0	0	3 carb.
GATORADE									
Frost Sports Drink (8 oz)	50	14	0	0	0	110	0	0	1 carb.
Sports Drink (8 oz)	50	14	0	0	0	110	0	0	1 carb.
GENERAL FOODS									
Coffee, International Café Francais (8 oz)	60	7	4	1	0	95	0	<1	1/2 carb., 1 fat
Coffee, International Café French Vanilla (8 oz)	60	10	3	<1	0	55	0	<1	1/2 carb., 1/2 fat
Coffee, International Café Hazelnut Belgian (8 oz)	70	12	2	<1	0	60	0	<1	1 carb.
Coffee, International Café Kahlua (8 oz)	60	10	2	<1	0	55	0	<1	1/2 carb.

Coffee, International Café Vienna (8 oz)	70	11	3	<1	0	110	<1	<1	1 carb.
Coffee, International French Vanilla, Sugar-Free (8 oz)	25	5	0	0	0	65	0	0	free
Coffee, International Italian Cappuccino (8 oz)	60	10	2	<1	0	50	0	<1	1/2 carb.
Coffee, International Orange Cappuccino (8 oz)	70	11	2	<1	0	100	<1	<1	1 carb.
Coffee, International Suisse Mocha (8 oz)	60	9	2	<1	0	35	0	<1	1/2 carb., 1/2 fat
Coffee, International Suisse Mocha, Sugar-Free (8 oz)	25	5	0	0	0	35	<1	0	1/2 fat
Flavored Teas, English Breakfast Crème (8 oz)	70	13	2	<1	13	65	0	0	1 carb.
Flavored Teas, English Raspberry Crème (8 oz)	70	13	2	<1	0	65	0	0	1 cart.
Flavored Teas, Island Orange Crème (8 oz)	70	13	2	<1	0	65	0	0	1 carb.
HI-C									
Fruit Punch (8 oz)	120	33	0	0	0	140	0	0	2 carb.
KOOL-AID									
Bursts Soft Drink, Cherry (6.7 oz)	100	25	0	0	0	30	0	0	2 carb.
Cherry Drink, Sugar-Free, Low-Calorie (8 oz)	5	0	0	0	0	5	0	0	free

BEVERAGES

Products	Cal.	Carb. (g)	Fat (g)	Sat. Fat (g)	Chol. (mg)	Sod. (mg)	Fib. (g)	Prot. (g)	Servings/Exchanges
Cherry Drink w/Sugar (8 oz)	60	16	0	0	0	0	0	0	1 carb.
Splash Soft Drink, Blue Raspberry (8 oz)	120	30	0	0	0	35	0	0	2 carb.
MAXWELL HOUSE									
Coffee, Iced Cappuccino (8 oz)	180	27	5	3	20	125	<1	8	2 carb., 1 fat
Coffee, Mocha Cappuccino (8 oz)	100	17	3	1	0	65	0	2	1 carb., 1/2 fat
Coffee, Mocha Cappuccino, Sugar-Free (8 oz)	60	7	3	1	0	80	<1	1	1/2 carb., 1 fat
Coffee, Vanilla Cappuccino (8 oz)	90	19	1	0	0	65	0	1	1 carb.
Coffee, Vanilla Cappuccino, Sugar-Free (8 oz)	60	7	3	<1	0	85	0	<1	1/2 carb., 1 fat
MINUTE MAID									
Concord Punch (8 oz)	115	30	0	0	0	21	NA	0	2 carb.
Cranberry Apple Raspberry Blend (8 oz)	123	33	0	0	0	24	0	0	2 carb.
Fruit Punch (8 oz)	113	30	0	0	0	21	0	0	2 carb.
NESTEA									
Cool From Nestea (8 oz)	82	22	0	0	0	68	0	0	1 1/2 carb.
Diet Cool From Nestea (8 oz)	1	<1	0	0	0	31	0	0	free

Iced Tea, Diet Lemon (8 oz)	2	<1	0	0	0	0	25	0	0	free
Iced Tea, Lemon-Sweetened (8 oz)	77	21	0	0	0	0	23	0	0	1 1/2 carb.
Iced Tea, Peach (8 oz)	78	21	0	0	0	0	23	0	0	1 1/2 carb.
Iced Tea, Raspberry (8 oz)	78	21	0	0	0	0	23	0	0	1 1/2 carb.
Iced Tea, Sweet (8 oz)	63	17	0	0	0	0	24	0	0	1 carb.
Iced Tea, Unsweetened (8 oz)	2	<1	0	0	0	0	25	0	0	free
NEW YORK SELTZER										
Black Cherry (8 oz)	90	22	0	0	0	0	15	0	0	1 1/2 carb.
Black Cherry, Diet (8 oz)	2	0	0	0	0	0	15	0	0	free
Iced Tea, Lemon Sparkling (8 oz)	90	21	0	0	0	0	50	0	0	1 1/2 carb.
Iced Tea, Raspberry Sparkling (8 oz)	100	21	0	0	0	0	50	0	0	1 1/2 carb.
Peach (8 oz)	90	22	0	0	0	0	15	0	0	1 1/2 carb.
Raspberry (8 oz)	90	22	0	0	0	0	15	0	0	1 1/2 carb.
Raspberry, Diet (8 oz)	2	0	0	0	0	0	15	0	0	free
OCEAN SPRAY										
Cran-blueberry Drink (8 oz)	160	41	0	0	0	0	35	0	0	3 carb.

BEVERAGES

Products	Cal.	Carb. (g)	Fat (g)	Sat. Fat (g)	Chol. (mg)	Sod. (mg)	Fib. (g)	Prot. (g)	Servings/Exchanges
Cran-raspberry Drink (8 oz)	140	36	0	0	0	35	0	0	2 1/2 carb.
Cranberry Juice Cocktail (8 oz)	140	34	0	0	0	35	0	0	2 carb.
Cranberry Juice Cocktail Reduced-Calorie (8 oz)	50	13	0	0	0	35	0	0	1 carb.
Fruit Punch (8 oz)	130	32	0	0	0	35	0	0	2 carb.
Lightstyle Cranberry Juice Cocktail (8 oz)	40	10	0	0	0	75	0	0	1/2 carb.
Lightstyle Cran Grape (8 oz)	40	9	0	0	0	75	0	0	1/2 carb.
Mauna La'i Island Grove (8 oz)	130	32	0	0	0	35	0	0	2 carb.
Ruby Red Grapefruit Juice Drink (8 oz)	130	33	0	0	0	35	0	0	2 carb.
PEPSI COLA									
Diet Pepsi (12 oz)	0	0	0	0	0	35	0	0	free
Mountain Dew (12 oz)	170	46	0	0	0	70	0	0	3 carb.
Pepsi One (12 oz)	1	0	0	0	0	45	0	0	free
Regular Pepsi (12 oz)	150	41	0	0	0	35	0	0	3 carb.
Storm (12 oz)	140	39	0	0	0	35	0	0	2 1/2 carb.

Storm Light (12 oz)	0	<1	0	0	0	35	0	0	free
Wild Cherry Pepsi (12 oz)	160	43	0	0	0	35	0	0	3 carb.
POWERADE									
Artic Shatter (8 oz)	72	19	0	0	0	53	0	0	1 carb.
Dark Downburst (8 oz)	72	19	0	0	0	53	0	0	1 carb.
Fruit Punch (8 oz)	74	19	0	0	0	53	0	0	1 carb.
Green Squall (8 oz)	72	19	0	0	0	53	0	0	1 carb.
Jagged Ice (8 oz)	73	19	0	0	0	53	0	0	1 carb.
Lemon-Lime (8 oz)	72	19	0	0	0	53	0	0	1 carb.
Mountain Blast (8 oz)	71	19	0	0	0	53	0	0	1 carb.
Orange Tangerine (8 oz)	71	19	0	0	0	53	0	0	1 carb
ROSS									
Glucerna, Chocolate (8 oz)	220	22	11	1	<5	210	2	10	1/2 carb., 1 low-fat milk, 1 fat
Glucerna, Vanilla (8 oz)	220	22	11	1	<5	210	2	10	1/2 carb., 1 low-fat milk, 1 fat
SEVEN UP									
7-Up (12 oz)	150	21	0	0	0	75	0	0	2 1/2 carb.

BEVERAGES

Products	Cal.	Carb. (g)	Fat (g)	Sat. Fat (g)	Chol. (mg)	Sod. (mg)	Fib. (g)	Prot. (g)	Servings/Exchanges
SLICE									
Grape (12 oz)	190	51	0	0	0	70	0	0	3 1/2 carb.
Lemon-Lime (12 oz)	150	40	0	0	0	55	0	0	2 1/2 carb.
Lemon-Lime, Diet (12 oz)	0	1	0	0	0	35	0	0	free
Orange (12 oz)	170	46	0	0	0	55	0	0	3 carb.
SNAPPLE									
Bali Blast Juice Drink (8 oz)	110	28	0	0	0	10	0	0	2 carb.
Cranberry Raspberry Juice Drink (8 oz)	120	29	0	0	0	10	0	0	2 carb.
Elements, Earth-Grape Cranberry Fruit Drink (8 oz)	130	34	0	0	0	10	0	0	2 carb.
Elements, Fire-Dragonfruit Fruit Drink (8 oz)	120	29	0	0	0	10	0	0	2 carb.
Elements, Lightning-Ginseng Black Tea (8 oz)	90	22	0	0	0	10	0	0	1 1/2 carb.
Elements, Moon-Green Tea (8 oz)	80	19	0	0	0	10	0	0	1 carb.
Elements, Rain-Agave Cactus Fruit Drink (8 oz)	120	29	0	0	0	10	0	0	2 carb.
Elements, Sun-Starfruit Orange Fruit Drink (8 oz)	120	29	0	0	0	10	0	0	2 carb.

Hydro Fruit Punch (8 oz)	90	22	0	0	0	40	0	0	1 1/2 carb.
Hydro Lemon Lime (8 oz)	100	24	0	0	0	40	0	0	1 1/2 carb.
Hydro Orange Tangerine (8 oz)	100	24	0	0	0	40	0	0	1 1/2 carb.
Lemonade (8 oz)	120	30	0	0	0	10	0	0	2 carb.
Mango Madness Juice Drink (8 oz)	110	29	0	0	0	10	0	0	2 carb.
Orangeade Juice Drink (8 oz)	120	29	0	0	0	10	0	0	2 carb.
Pink Lemonade (8 oz)	120	29	0	0	0	10	0	0	2 carb.
Pink Lemonade, Diet (8 oz)	20	4	0	0	0	10	0	0	free
Summer Peach Juice Drink (8 oz)	120	30	0	0	0	10	0	0	2 carb.
Sun Tea (8 oz)	90	23	0	0	0	10	0	0	1 1/2 carb.
Sun Tea, Diet (8 oz)	0	1	0	0	0	10	0	0	free
Tea, Ginseng (8 oz)	80	20	0	0	0	10	0	0	1 carb.
Tea, Green (8 oz)	100	25	0	0	0	10	0	0	1 1/2 carb.
Tea, Just Plain, Unsweetened (8 oz)	0	0	0	0	0	10	0	0	free
Tea, Lemon (8 oz)	100	25	0	0	0	10	0	0	1 1/2 carb.
Tea, Lemon, Diet (8 oz)	0	1	0	0	0	10	0	0	free

BEVERAGES

Products	Cal.	Carb. (g)	Fat (g)	Sat. Fat (g)	Chol. (mg)	Sod. (mg)	Fib. (g)	Prot. (g)	Servings/Exchanges
Tea, Lemonade Iced (8 oz)	110	28	0	0	0	10	0	0	2 carb.
Tea, Mint (8 oz)	110	27	0	0	0	10	0	0	2 carb.
Tea, Peach, Diet (8 oz)	0	1	0	0	0	10	0	0	free
Tea, Raspberry (8 oz)	100	26	0	0	0	10	0	0	2 carb.
Tea, Sweetened (8 oz)	120	31	0	0	0	10	0	0	1 carb.
WhipperSnapple, Orange Dream (10 oz)	150	36	0	0	0	60	0	0	2 1/2 carb.
WhipperSnapple, Peach Mango (10 oz)	150	39	0	0	0	60	0	0	2 1/2 carb.
WhipperSnapple, Power Citrus (10 oz)	150	39	0	0	0	60	0	0	2 1/2 carb.
WhipperSnapple, Wild Cherry (10 oz)	150	39	0	0	0	60	0	0	2 1/2 carb.
SUNNY DELIGHT									
Orange Drink/Ade (8 oz)	130	32	0	0	0	130	0	0	2 carb.
TANG									
Mango Drink Mix (8 oz)	100	25	0	0	0	0	0	0	1 1/2 carb.
Orange Drink (8 oz)	90	23	0	0	0	0	0	0	1 1/2 carb.

Orange Drink, Sugar-Free (8 oz)	5	0	0	0	0	0	0	0	free

TROPICANA

Apple Raspberry Blackberry Twister (8 oz)	120	31	0	0	0	20	0	<1	2 carb.
Orange Cranberry Twister (8 oz)	120	30	0	0	0	45	0	<1	2 carb.
Orange Strawberry Banana Twister (8 oz)	130	32	0	0	0	45	<1	0	2 carb.
Pink Grapefruit Twister, Light (8 oz)	40	9	0	0	0	100	<1	0	1/2 carb.
Strawberry Kiwi Twister (8 oz)	130	33	0	0	0	20	0	0	2 carb.
Tropical Strawberry Twister, Light (8 oz)	40	10	0	0	0	100	<1	0	1/2 carb.

BREAD PRODUCTS AND BAKED GOODS

Products	Cal.	Carb. (g)	Fat (g)	Sat. Fat (g)	Chol. (mg)	Sod. (mg)	Fib. (g)	Prot. (g)	Servings/Exchanges
Bagel (1/2)	98	19	<1	<1	0	190	<1	4	1 strch
Bagel, Cinnamon Raisin (1)	195	39	1	<1	0	229	2	7	2 1/2 strch
Baklava (2 x 2-inch piece)	333	29	23	9	36	291	2	5	2 carb., 4 fat
Biscuit (1, 2 1/2-inch)	127	17	6	<1	0	368	<1	2	1 strch, 1 fat
Bread, Banana (1 slice)	203	33	7	2	26	119	<1	3	2 carb., 1 fat
Bread, Buckwheat (1 slice)	71	13	1	<1	<1	100	<1	2	1 strch
Bread, Butter Croissant (1)	231	26	12	7	43	424	2	5	2 strch, 2 fat
Bread, Cheese (1 slice)	71	12	1	<1	2	144	<1	2	1 strch
Bread, Corn (2-oz piece)	152	25	4	<1	23	375	1	4	1 strch, 1 fat
Bread, Cracked Wheat (1 slice)	65	12	1	<1	0	135	1	2	1 strch
Bread, Date Nut (1 slice)	217	30	10	2	28	140	<1	3	2 carb., 2 fat
Bread, French (1 slice)	69	13	<1	<1	0	152	<1	2	1 strch
Bread, Fruit, No Nuts (1 slice)	150	23	6	2	22	109	<1	2	1 1/2 carb., 1 fat

Bread, Indian Fry (5-inch)	296	48	9	2	0	626	2	6	3 strch, 2 fat
Bread, Italian (1 slice)	81	15	1	<1	0	175	<1	3	1 strch
Bread, Mixed-Grain (1 slice)	65	12	<1		0	127	2	3	1 strch
Bread, Oat Bran (1 slice)	71	12	1	<1	0	122	1	3	1 strch
Bread, Oatmeal (1 slice)	72	13	1		0	162	1	2	1 strch
Bread, Pita (1/2, 6-inch)	83	17	<1	<1	0	161	<1	3	1 strch
Bread, Pita, Whole-Wheat (1)	170	35	2	<1	0	239	5	6	2 strch
Bread, Potato (1 slice)	69	13	<1	<1	<1	143	<1	2	1 strch
Bread, Pumpernickel (1 slice)	80	15	1	<1	0	215	2	3	1 strch
Bread, Raisin (1 slice)	71	14	1	<1	0	101	1	2	1 strch
Bread, Rye (1 slice)	83	16	1	<1	0	211	2	3	1 strch
Bread, Sourdough (1 slice)	69	13	<1	<1	0	152	<1	2	1 strch
Bread, Sweet Potato (1 slice)	72	13	2	<1	14	228	<1	2	1 strch
Bread, Triticale (1 slice)	63	12	<1	<1	0	136	2	2	1 strch
Bread, Vienna (1 slice)	69	13	<1	<1	0	152	<1	2	1 strch
Bread, Wheat Bran (1 slice)	89	17	1	<1	0	175	1	3	1 strch

BREAD PRODUCTS & BAKED GOODS

Products	Cal.	Carb. (g)	Fat (g)	Sat. Fat (g)	Chol. (mg)	Sod. (mg)	Fib. (g)	Prot. (g)	Servings/Exchanges
Bread, White (1 slice)	67	12	<1	<1	0	134	2	2	1 strch
Bread, White, Reduced-Calorie (2 slices)	96	20	1	<1	0	208	4	4	1 strch
Bread, Whole-Wheat (1 slice)	70	13	1	<1	0	149	2	3	1 strch
Bread Sticks, Crisp (2, 4-inch)	82	14	2	<1	0	131	<1	2	1 strch
Bread Stuffing (1/3 cup)	117	14	6	1	0	359	2	2	1 strch, 1 fat
Bread Stuffing, Homemade (1/3 cup)	129	17	6	1	0	353	2	3	1 strch, 1 fat
Bun, Hamburger (1/2)	61	11	1	<1	0	120	<1	2	1 strch
Bun, Hot Dog (1/2)	61	11	1	<1	0	120	<1	2	1 strch
Cream Puff w/Custard Filling (1)	335	30	20	5	174	375	<1	9	2 carb., 4 fat
Crepe/French Pancake (1)	239	22	13	4	163	274	<1	9	1 1/2 strch, 3 fat
Croissant, Cheese (1)	236	27	12	6	37	316	2	5	2 strch, 2 fat
Croutons (1 cup)	122	22	2	<1	0	209	<1	4	1 strch, 1 fat
Danish Pastry, Cinnamon (1)	349	47	17	4	28	326	<1	5	3 carb., 3 fat
Danish Pastry, Fruit-Filled (1)	335	45	16	3	19	333	NA	5	3 carb., 3 fat

Food								
Dinner Roll/Bun, French (1)	105	19	2	<1	0	231	1	3	1 strch
Dinner Roll/Bun, Wheat (1)	98	16	2	<1	0	122	1	3	1 strch
Doughnut, Cake (1)	198	23	11	2	18	257	<1	2	1 1/2 carb., 2 fat
Doughnut, Cake, w/Chocolate Icing (1)	204	21	13	4	25	184	<1	2	1 1/2 carb., 3 fat
Doughnut, Cake, Sugared/Glazed (1)	192	23	10	2	14	181	<1	2	1 1/2 carb., 2 fat
Doughnut, Custard-Filled w/Icing (1)	261	34	13	6	21	125	1	3	2 carb., 3 fat
Doughnut, Yeast, Creme-Filled (1)	307	26	21	6	20	263	<1	5	2 carb., 4 fat
Doughnut, Yeast, Glazed (1)	242	27	13	4	4	205	1	4	2 carb., 2 fat
Doughnut, Yeast, Jelly-Filled (1)	289	33	16	4	22	190	<1	5	1 1/2 carb., 2 fat
Dumpling, Plain (medium)	42	7	1	<1	1	105	<1	1	1/2 strch
Egg Bread/Challah (1 slice)	115	19	2	<1	20	197	<1	4	1 strch
Eclair, Chocolate w/Custard Filling (1)	262	24	16	4	127	337	<1	6	1 1/2 carb., 3 fat
English Muffin (1/2)	67	13	<1	<1	0	132	<1	2	1 strch
French Toast, Frozen (1 slice)	126	19	4	1	48	292	<1	4	1 strch, 1 fat
French Toast, Homemade w/2% Milk (1 slice)	149	16	7	2	75	311	<1	5	1 strch, 1 fat
Muffin (1)	133	19	5	1	18	210	1	3	1 strch, 1 fat

BREAD PRODUCTS & BAKED GOODS

Products	Cal.	Carb. (g)	Fat (g)	Sat. Fat (g)	Chol. (mg)	Sod. (mg)	Fib. (g)	Prot. (g)	Servings/Exchanges
Muffin, Cheese (1)	184	23	8	3	30	274	<1	5	1 1/2 strch, 2 fat
Muffin, Chocolate Chip (1)	190	27	9	3	25	186	1	4	2 strch, 2 fat
Muffin, Cranberry Nut (1)	164	25	5	2	39	326	<1	4	1 1/2 strch, 1 fat
Muffin, Oat Bran (1)	154	28	4	<1	0	224	3	4	2 strch. 1 fat
Muffin, Pumpkin w/Raisins & Nuts (1)	181	34	4	<1	26	154	1	3	2 strch, 1 fat
Muffin, Wheat Bran (1)	161	24	7	2	19	335	2	4	1 1/2 strch, 1 fat
Muffin, Whole-Wheat (1)	142	20	6	2	21	283	3	4	1 strch, 1 fat
Muffin, Zucchini w/Nuts (1)	210	26	11	2	37	169	<1	3	2 strch, 2 fat
Pancakes, From Mix (2)	166	22	6	2	54	384	1	6	1 strch, 1 fat
Pannetone or Italian Sweetbread (1 slice)	86	15	2	1	19	96	<1	2	1 strch
Popover, Homemade w/Whole Milk (1)	90	11	3	1	47	81	<1	4	1 strch, 1 fat
Pretzel, Soft (2 oz)	190	38	2	<1	2	772	<1	5	2 1/2 strch
Roll, Plain (1)	85	14	2	<1	0	148	<1	2	1 strch
Roll, Submarine/Hoagie (1, 5 oz)	392	75	4	<1	0	783	4	12	5 strch

Roll, Whole-Wheat (1)	75	15	1	<1	0	167	2	3	1 strch
Scone (1, 1 1/2 oz)	150	19	7	2	51	246	<1	4	1 strch, 1 fat
Scone, Whole-Wheat (1)	145	18	7	2	50	174	3	5	1 strch, 1 fat
Sweet Roll, Cheese (1)	238	29	12	4	40	236	<1	5	2 strch, 2 fat
Sweet Roll, Cinnamon Raisin (1)	145	20	7	2	40	149	1	4	1 carb., 1 fat
Sweet Roll, Cinnamon w/Raisins & Nuts, Homemade (1)	196	30	7	2	13	185	1	4	2 carb., 1 fat
Taco Shells (2)	122	16	6	<1	0	95	2	2	1 strch, 1 fat
Tortilla, Corn (1, 6-inch)	56	12	<1	<1	0	40	1	1	1 strch
Tortilla, Flour (1, 7-inch)	114	20	3	<1	0	167	1	3	1 strch
Tortilla, Flour (1, 10 1/2-inch)	185	32	4	1	0	272	2	5	2 strch, 1 fat
Tortilla, Whole-Wheat (1)	73	20	<1	<1	0	171	2	3	1 strch
Waffles, Blueberry (1, 4-inch)	97	16	3	<1	18	272	<1	3	1 strch, 1 fat
Waffles, From Mix (1, 4 1/2-inch)	145	17	7	1	35	256	<1	4	1 strch, 1 fat
Waffles, Homemade (1)	218	25	11	2	52	383	1	6	1 1/2 strch, 2 fat
Waffles, Low-Fat (1, 4 1/2-inch)	80	17	<1	<1	0	270	<1	3	1 strch

BREAD PRODUCTS & BAKED GOODS

Products	Cal.	Carb. (g)	Fat (g)	Sat. Fat (g)	Chol. (mg)	Sod. (mg)	Fib. (g)	Prot. (g)	Servings/Exchanges
AUNT FANNY'S									
Honey Bun, Applesauce (1)	330	43	17	4	0	300	1	6	3 carb., 3 fat
Honey Bun, Banana Cream (1)	350	32	18	4	0	290	2	5	2 carb., 3 fat
Honey Bun, Iced Honey (1)	350	32	18	4	0	290	2	5	2 carb., 3 fat
Honey Bun, Raspberry-Filled (1)	350	45	17	5	0	290	2	5	3 carb., 3 fat
Honey Bun, Regular (1)	360	41	20	5	0	300	2	5	3 carb., 3 fat
Honey Bun, Vanilla Creme (1)	350	32	18	4	0	290	2	5	2 carb., 3 fat
AUNT JEMIMA									
French Toast (2 pieces)	240	35	7	2	95	310	8	10	2 carb., 1 fat
French Toast, Cinnamon (2 pieces)	240	35	7	2	30	330	8	10	2 carb., 1 fat
Microwave Pancakes, Blueberry (3)	210	40	4	<1	20	670	2	6	2 1/2 strch, 1 fat
Microwave Pancakes, Buttermilk (3)	210	40	4	1	20	600	2	6	2 strch, 1 fat
Microwave Pancakes, Homestyle(3)	210	40	4	<1	20	560	8	6	2 1/2 strch, 1 fat
Microwave Pancakes, Low Fat (3)	150	30	2	0	<5	530	8	5	2 strch

Microwave Waffles, Blueberry (2)	210	34	6	2	<5	470	1	5	2 strch, 1 fat
Microwave Waffles, Buttermilk (2)	200	33	6	2	<5	550	1	5	2 strch, 1 fat
Microwave Waffles, Homestyle (2)	200	32	6	2	<5	440	1	5	2 strch, 1 fat
Microwave Waffles, Low Fat (2)	160	32	2	<1	0	540	1	5	2 strch
Pancake/Waffle Mix, Buckwheat (1/4 cup)	120	22	1	0	0	560	4	5	1 1/2 strch
Pancake/Waffle Mix, Buttermilk (1/3 cup)	190	31	2	<1	10	480	2	6	2 strch
Pancake/Waffle Mix, Original (1/3 cup)	150	28	<1	0	0	620	1	4	2 strch
Pancake/Waffle Mix, Whole Wheat (1/4 cup)	130	28	<1	0	0	560	3	6	2 strch
Pancake/Waffle Mix, Regular (1/3 cup)	190	39	2	<1	15	470	1	6	2 1/2 strch
Pancakes From Mix, Reduced Calorie Buttermilk (1/3 cup)	140	30	2	<1	15	510	5	8	2 strch
Waffles, Cinnamon (2)	180	28	6	2	10	470	1	4	2 strch, 1 fat
Waffles, Blueberry (2)	190	28	7	2	10	530	1	4	2 strch, 1 fat
Waffles, Buttermilk (2)	170	27	6	2	10	410	1	4	2 strch, 1 fat
Waffles, Original (2)	170	28	6	1	6	590	1	4	2 strch, 1 fat
Waffles, Raisin (2)	200	36	4	NA	5	530	NA	5	2 1/2 strch, 1 fat

BREAD PRODUCTS & BAKED GOODS

Products	Cal.	Carb. (g)	Fat (g)	Sat. Fat (g)	Chol. (mg)	Sod. (mg)	Fib. (g)	Prot. (g)	Servings/Exchanges
Waffles, Whole-Grain (2)	170	24	7	1	0	450	2	5	1 1/2 strch, 1 fat
BALLARD									
Extra Light Oven-Ready Biscuit Dough (1)	50	10	<1	<1	0	165	<1	1	1/2 strch
Extra Light Oven-Ready Biscuit Dough, Buttermilk (1)	50	10	<1	<1	0	165	<1	1	1/2 strch
BETTY CROCKER/GENERAL MILLS									
Muffin Mix, Apple Cinnamon, Prepared (1)	130	23	4	1	0	200	NA	1	1 1/2 strch, 1 fat
Muffin Mix, Banana Nut, Prepared (1)	130	22	4	1	0	230	NA	2	1 1/2 strch, 1 fat
Muffin Mix, Blueberry, Prepared (1)	120	24	3	<1	0	210	NA	1	1 1/2 carb., 1 fat
Muffin Mix, Golden Corn, Prepared (1)	110	24	1	0	0	210	NA	2	1 1/2 strch
Muffin Mix, Lemon Poppyseed, Prepared (1)	120	24	2	<1	0	180	NA	1	1 1/2 strch
Muffin Mix, Low Fat Blueberry, Prepared (1)	110	26	0	0	0	190	NA	2	2 strch
Waffle Mix, Belgian, Prepared (1)	370	47	17	9	130	1020	1	8	3 strch, 3 fat

ENTENMANN'S

Buns, Fat-Free Cholesterol-Free Apple (1)	150	33	0	0	0	140	1	3	2 carb.
Buns, Fat-Free Cholesterol-Free Blueberry Cheez (1)	140	31	0	0	0	150	1	4	2 carb.
Buns, Fat-Free Cholesterol-Free Cinnamon Raisin (1)	160	36	0	0	0	125	1	3	2 1/2 carb.
Buns, Fat-Free Cholesterol-Free Pineapple Cheez (1)	140	30	0	0	0	150	<1	4	2 carb.
Buns, Fat-Free Cholesterol-Free Raspberry Cheez (1)	160	36	0	0	0	135	1	4	2 1/2 carb.
Coffee Cake, Cheese Topped (1/9)	190	26	8	3	30	180	1	3	2 strch, 2 fat
Coffee Cake, Fat-Free Cheese-Filled Crumb (1/9)	130	29	0	0	0	230	1	4	2 strch
Coffee Cake, New York Crumb (1/10)	250	33	12	3	15	200	1	4	2 strch, 2 fat
Danish, Cheese Crumb (1/8)	200	25	9	4	40	190	<1	4	1 1/2 strch, 2 fat
Danish Pastry Ring, Pecan (1/6)	250	25	15	3	30	160	1	3	1 1/2 carb., 3 fat
Danish Pastry Twist, Raspberry (1/8)	220	27	11	4	20	170	<1	3	2 carb., 2 fat

BREAD PRODUCTS & BAKED GOODS

Products	Cal.	Carb. (g)	Fat (g)	Sat. Fat (g)	Chol. (mg)	Sod. (mg)	Fib. (g)	Prot. (g)	Servings/Exchanges
Donuts, Glazed 50% Less Fat (1)	190	34	5	2	15	240	<1	2	2 carb., 1 fat
Donuts, Glazed Popems (1)	270	35	13	3	15	290	0	3	2 carb., 3 fat
Donuts, Rich Frosted Popettes (3)	280	26	18	5	15	220	1	3	2 carb., 4 fat
Donuts, Rich Frosted Variety (1)	310	34	19	5	15	170	2	3	2 carb., 4 fat
Donuts, Soft Powdered Cinnamon Popettes (3)	240	24	15	4	15	220	<1	2	1 1/2 carb., 3 fat
Eclairs, Chocolate (1)	250	44	9	2	70	220	0	3	3 carb., 1 fat
Muffins, Blueberry (1)	160	24	7	2	40	210	<1	2	1 1/2 carb., 1 fat
Muffins, Fat-Free Cholesterol-Free Blueberry (1)	120	26	0	0	0	220	<1	2	2 carb.
Pastry, Apple Puffs (1)	260	36	12	3	0	220	1	2	2 1/2 carb., 2 fat
Pastry, Fat-Free Cholesterol-Free Apricot (1 slice)	150	34	0	0	0	110	<1	3	2 carb.
Pastry, Fat-Free Cholesterol-Free Black Forest (1 slice)	130	32	0	0	0	115	2	3	2 carb.
Pastry, Fat-Free Cholesterol-Free Cinnamon Apple Twist (1 slice)	150	35	0	0	0	110	<1	3	2 carb.

Pastry, Fat-Free Cholesterol-Free LemonTwist (1/8)	130	29	0	0	0	190	1	2	2 carb.
Pastry, Fat-Free Cholesterol-Free Raspberry Cheez (1 slice)	140	32	0	0	0	110	1	3	2 carb.
Pastry, Fat-Free Cholesterol-Free RaspberryTwist (1/8)	140	32	0	0	0	180	1	2	2 carb.
Popems, Glazed (4)	240	31	12	3	15	230	1	2	2 carb., 2 fat
Popems, Devil's Food Chocolate (4)	260	32	15	4	10	150	2	2	2 carb., 3 fat
Rolls, Cinnamon (1/2 roll)	170	35	3	<1	0	240	2	3	2 carb., 1 fat
GOLD MEDAL/GENERAL MILLS									
Biscuit Mix, Baking Powder, Prepared (1)	160	25	5	1	0	460	<1	4	1 1/2 strch, 1 fat
Biscuit Mix, Buttermilk, Prepared (1)	170	24	8	3	0	420	<1	3	1 1/2 strch, 2 fat
Biscuit Mix, Cinnamon Raisin, Prepared (1)	260	41	9	3	0	560	1	4	3 strch, 1 fat
Biscuit Mix, Prepared (1)	160	22	7	2	0	420	<1	3	1 1/2 strch, 1 fat
Honey Corn Bread Mix, Prepared (1 slice)	140	26	3	1	10	290	0	2	2 strch, 1 fat
Muffin Mix, Blueberry, Prepared (1)	260	44	7	2	10	320	<1	3	3 strch, 1 fat
Muffin Mix, Corn Bread, Prepared (1)	140	25	4	1	5	290	<1	2	1 1/2 strch, 1 fat

BREAD PRODUCTS & BAKED GOODS

Products	Cal.	Carb. (g)	Fat (g)	Sat. Fat (g)	Chol. (mg)	Sod. (mg)	Fib. (g)	Prot. (g)	Servings/Exchanges
Muffin Mix, Raisin Bran, Prepared (1)	270	46	8	2	10	450	2	3	3 strch, 2 fat
Pancake Mix, Buttermilk, Prepared (2)	200	36	5	0	20	300	0	4	1 strch, 1 fat
GRANDS (see also Pillsbury)									
Refrigerated Biscuits, Buttermilk (1)	200	23	10	3	0	573	1	4	1 1/2 strch, 2 fat
Refrigerated Biscuits, Homestyle (1)	190	24	9	2	0	595	1	4	1 1/2 strch, 2 fat
Refrigerated Biscuits, Southern (1)	200	23	10	3	0	573	1	4	1 1/2 strch, 2 fat
HEALTH VALLEY									
Fat-Free Healthy Scones, Apple Kiwi (1)	80	15	0	0	0	160	7	7	1 strch
Fat-Free Healthy Scones, Cinnamon Raisin (1)	80	15	0	0	0	160	7	7	1 strch
Fat-Free Healthy Scones, Cranberry Orange (1)	80	15	0	0	0	160	7	7	1 strch
Fat-Free Healthy Scones, Mountain Blueberry (1)	80	15	0	0	0	160	7	7	1 strch
Fat-Free Healthy Scones, Pineapple Raisin (1)	80	15	0	0	0	160	7	7	1 strch
HUNGRY JACK (see also Pillsbury)									
Biscuit Dough, Flaky (1)	81	14	5	1	0	350	0	2	1 strch, 1 fat

Item								
Microwave Pancakes, Blueberry (2)	155	30	2	<1	5	370	<1	3	2 strch
Microwave Pancakes, Buttermilk (2)	162	31	3	<1	5	390	<1	3	3 strch, 1 fat
Microwave Pancakes, Mini Buttermilk (11)	170	32	3	<1	6	400	<1	4	2 strch, 1 fat
Microwave Pancakes, Original (3)	162	31	3	<1	5	365	<1	3	2 strch, 1 fat
KELLOGG'S									
Corn Flake Crumbs (2 Tbsp.)	40	9	0	0	0	80	0	1	1/2 strch
Croutettes Stuffing Mix (1 cup)	120	25	0	0	0	460	0	5	1 1/2 strch
Pop-Tarts Pastry, Apple Cinnamon (1)	210	37	6	1	0	180	1	2	2 1/2 carb., 1 fat
Pop-Tarts Pastry, Blueberry (1)	200	37	5	1	0	190	1	2	2 1/2 carb., 1 fat
Pop-Tarts Pastry, Brown Sugar Cinnamon (1)	210	35	6	1	0	190	1	3	2 carb., 1 fat
Pop-Tarts Pastry, Cherry (1)	200	37	5	1	0	180	1	2	2 1/2 carb., 1 fat
Pop-Tarts Pastry, Cherry, Frosted (1)	200	38	5	1	0	170	1	2	2 1/2 carb., 1 fat
Pop-Tarts Pastry, Chocolate Fudge, Frosted (1)	200	37	5	1	0	220	1	3	2 1/2 carb., 1 fat
Pop-Tarts Pastry, Chocolate Vanilla Creme, Frosted (1)	200	37	5	1	0	220	1	3	2 1/2 carb., 1 fat
Pop-Tarts Pastry, Grape, Frosted (1)	200	38	5	1	0	170	1	2	2 1/2 carb., 1 fat

BREAD PRODUCTS & BAKED GOODS

Products	Cal.	Carb. (g)	Fat (g)	Sat. Fat (g)	Chol. (mg)	Sod. (mg)	Fib. (g)	Prot. (g)	Servings/Exchanges
Pop-Tarts Pastry, Low Fat Brown Sugar Cinnamon, Frosted (1)	190	39	3	<1	0	230	1	2	2 1/2 strch, 1 fat
Pop-Tarts Pastry, Low Fat Chocolate Fudge, Frosted (1)	190	39	3	<1	0	270	2	3	2 1/2 carb., 1 fat
Pop-Tarts Pastry, Low Fat Strawberry, Frosted (1)	190	39	3	<1	0	210	1	2	2 1/2 carb., 1 fat
Pop-Tarts Pastry, Low Fat Strawberry (1)	190	39	3	<1	0	230	1	2	2 1/2 carb., 1 fat
Pop-Tarts Pastry, Raspberry, Frosted (1)	210	37	5	1	0	170	1	2	2 1/2 carb., 1 fat
Pop-Tarts Pastry, S'mores, Frosted (1)	200	36	6	1	0	200	1	3	2 1/2 carb., 1 fat
Pop-Tarts Pastry, Strawberry (1)	200	37	5	1	0	190	1	2	2 1/2 carb., 1 fat
Pop-Tarts Pastry, Strawberry, Frosted (1)	200	38	5	1	0	170	1	2	2 1/2 carb., 1 fat
Pop-Tarts Pastry, Wild Berry, Frosted (1)	210	39	5	1	0	170	1	2	2 1/2 carb., 1 fat
Pop-Tarts Pastry, Wild Magicburst, Frosted (1)	200	37	6	1	0	180	1	2	2 1/2 carb., 1 fat
Pop-Tarts Pastry, Wild Tropical Blast, Frosted (1)	210	39	5	2	0	170	1	2	2 1/2 carb., 1 fat
Pop-Tarts Pastry, Wild Watermelon, Frosted (1)	210	39	5	1	0	170	1	2	2 1/2 carb., 1 fat

KELLOGG'S EGGO

Pancakes, Buttermilk (3)	270	44	8	2	15	610	1	7	3 strch, 2 fat
Toaster Muffins, Blueberry (1)	120	19	4	<1	15	250	0	3	1 strch, 1 fat
Toaster Muffins, Cinnamon (1)	130	20	5	1	15	270	0	3	1 strch, 1 fat
Toaster Muffins, Strawberry (1)	130	20	5	1	15	260	0	3	1 strch, 1 fat
Waffles, Apple Cinnamon (2)	200	30	7	2	20	400	2	5	2 strch, 1 fat
Waffles, Banana Bread (2)	190	30	6	1	0	280	2	5	2 strch, 1 fat
Waffles, Blueberry (2)	200	30	7	2	20	420	1	5	2 strch, 1 fat
Waffles, Buttermilk (2)	190	28	7	2	20	420	2	5	2 strch, 1 fat
Waffles, Chocolate Chip (2)	200	32	7	2	15	380	1	4	2 strch, 1 fat
Waffles, Cinnamon Toast (2)	290	46	10	3	25	480	1	5	3 strch, 2 fat
Waffles, Golden Oat (2)	140	26	3	<1	0	270	3	5	2 strch, 1 fat
Waffles, Homestyle (2)	190	29	7	2	20	440	2	5	2 strch, 1 fat
Waffles, Low Fat Homestyle (2)	160	31	3	<1	15	300	1	5	2 strch, 1 fat
Waffles, Low Fat Nutri-Grain (2)	140	28	3	<1	0	430	3	5	2 strch, 1 fat
Waffles, Low Fat Nutri-Grain Blueberry (2)	150	30	3	<1	0	420	4	5	2 strch, 1 fat

BREAD PRODUCTS & BAKED GOODS

Products	Cal.	Carb. (g)	Fat (g)	Sat. Fat (g)	Chol. (mg)	Sod. (mg)	Fib. (g)	Prot. (g)	Servings/Exchanges
Waffles, Minis Homestyle (12)	260	38	9	2	25	600	2	7	2 1/2 strch, 2 fat
Waffles, Nut & Honey (2)	220	30	9	2	20	390	2	6	2 strch, 2 fat
Waffles, Nutri-Grain (2)	170	28	5	1	0	420	3	5	2 strch, 1 fat
Waffles, Nutri-Grain Multi-Bran (2)	160	29	5	1	0	360	5	5	2 strch, 1 fat
Waffles, Special K (2)	120	26	0	0	0	280	1	6	2 strch
Waffles, Strawberry (2)	200	30	7	2	20	420	2	5	2 strch, 1 fat
MARIE CALLENDER'S									
Bread, Original Garlic (1 slice)	190	25	8	2	0	290	2	4	1 1/2 strch, 2 fat
Bread, Parmesan Romano Garlic (1 slice)	200	23	10	3	5	430	2	5	1 1/2 strch, 2 fat
MORTON									
Honey Buns (1)	250	35	10	3	0	160	<1	3	2 carb., 2 fat
Mini Honey Buns (1)	160	19	8	2	0	100	1	2	1 carb., 2 fat
NABISCO									
Cake Crumbs, Oreo Base (1/4 cup)	140	23	5	1	0	260	1	2	1 1/2 strch, 1 fat

OLD EL PASO

Item									
Taco Shells, Mini (7)	150	19	7	1	0	130	2	2	1 strch, 2 fat
Taco Shells, Super (2)	170	22	3	1	0	150	2	2	1 1/2 strch, 2 fat
Taco Shells, White Corn (3)	150	19	7	1	0	135	2	2	1 strch, 2 fat
Tortilla, Flour (1)	130	21	4	1	0	290	0	3	1 1/2 strch, 1 fat
Tortillas, Soft Taco (2)	160	26	5	1	0	350	0	3	2 strch, 1 fat
Tostada Shells (3)	150	19	7	1	0	135	2	2	1 strch, 1 fat

ORTEGA

Item									
Taco Shells (2)	140	20	7	1	0	200	2	2	1 strch, 1 fat
Tostada Shells (2)	150	18	8	2	0	190	2	2	1 strch, 2 fat

PANCHO VILLA

Item									
Taco Shells (3)	160	21	7	1	0	0	2	2	1 1/2 strch, 2 fat

PEPPERIDGE FARM

Item									
Biscuits, Garlic & Cheese (1)	170	24	6	3	10	510	2	4	1 1/2 strch, 1 fat
Biscuits, Original Water (6)	72	13	1	<1	4	120	<1	2	1 strch
Bread, 1 1/2-lb Natural Wheat (1 slice)	90	16	2	0	0	170	1	4	1 strch

BREAD PRODUCTS & BAKED GOODS

Products	Cal.	Carb. (g)	Fat (g)	Sat. Fat (g)	Chol. (mg)	Sod. (mg)	Fib. (g)	Prot. (g)	Servings/Exchanges
Bread, 1 1/2-lb Wheat (1 slice)	90	16	2	0	0	190	1	3	1 strch
Bread, 2-lb Family Wheat (1 slice)	70	13	1	0	0	135	1	2	1 strch
Bread, Apple Walnut Swirl (1 slice)	80	14	2	<1	0	120	1	2	1 strch
Bread, Cinnamon (1 slice)	80	14	3	<1	0	115	2	3	1 carb., 1 fat
Bread, Cinnamon Swirl (1 slice)	80	14	3	<1	0	115	2	3	1 strch, 1 fat
Bread, Classic Dark Pumpernickel (1 slice)	80	15	1	<1	0	230	1	3	1 strch
Bread, Cracked Wheat, Thin-Sliced (1 slice)	70	12	1	0	0	140	<1	2	1 strch
Bread, Garlic (1 slice)	160	14	10	3	30	250	1	5	1 strch, 2 fat
Bread, Garlic Parmesan (1)	160	19	7	2	10	260	2	6	1 strch, 1 fat
Bread, Golden Swirl Vermont Maple (1 slice)	90	15	3	1	0	100	<1	2	1 strch, 1 fat
Bread, Hearty Country White (1 slice)	90	19	1	0	0	190	2	3	1 strch
Bread, Hearty Crunchy Oat (1 slice)	100	17	2	0	0	180	2	4	1 strch
Bread, Hearty Honey Wheatberry (1 slice)	100	18	2	0	0	200	2	3	1 strch
Bread, Hearty Russet Potato (1 slice)	90	18	2	<1	3	260	3	4	1 strch

Food									
Bread, Hearty Sesame Wheat (1 slice)	100	17	2	0	0	180	2	4	1 strch
Bread, Hearty Slice 7-Grain (1 slice)	100	18	2	0	0	180	2	3	1 strch
Bread, Hearty White (1 slice)	90	19	1	0	0	190	2	3	1 strch
Bread, Jewish Seeded Rye (1)	80	15	1	<1	0	210	1	3	1 strch
Bread, Jewish Seedless Family Rye (1 slice)	80	15	1	<1	0	210	1	3	1 strch
Bread, Large Family White, Thin-Sliced (1 slice)	80	14	2	0	0	160	0	2	1 strch
Bread, Light-Style Seven-Grain (1 slice)	47	9	<1	0	0	107	2	2	1/2 strch
Bread, Light-Style Sourdough (1 slice)	43	9	<1	0	0	107	1	2	1/2 strch
Bread, Light-Style Wheat (1 slice)	43	9	<1	<1	0	97	2	2	1/2 strch
Bread, Light Vienna (1 slice)	43	9	<1	<1	0	100	2	2	1/2 strch
Bread, Monterey Jack w/Jalapeño Cheese (1 slice)	200	22	10	4	40	280	1	5	1 1/2 strch, 2 fat
Bread, Mozzarella Garlic (1 slice)	200	21	10	5	40	280	1	6	1 1/2 strch, 2 fat
Bread, Oatmeal, Light (1 slice)	47	9	<1	0	0	103	2	2	1/2 strch
Bread, Old-Fashioned Honey Bran (1 slice)	90	17	1	0	0	160	2	3	1 strch
Bread, Onion Rye (1 slice)	80	15	1	<1	0	210	1	3	1 strch
Bread, Party Pumpernickel (3 slices)	110	22	2	0	0	320	4	6	1 1/2 strch

BREAD PRODUCTS & BAKED GOODS

Products	Cal.	Carb. (g)	Fat (g)	Sat. Fat (g)	Chol. (mg)	Sod. (mg)	Fib. (g)	Prot. (g)	Servings/Exchanges
Bread, Party Rye (3 slices)	110	22	2	0	0	410	3	6	1 1/2 strch
Bread, Raisin Cinnamon Swirl (1 slice)	80	14	2	0	0	105	1	3	1 strch
Bread, Raisin w/Cinnamon (1 slice)	80	14	2	0	0	105	1	3	1 strch
Bread, Soft Oatmeal (1 slice)	60	12	<1	0	0	2	0	2	1 strch
Bread, Sourdough Garlic (1 slice)	180	20	9	3	10	220	2	5	1 strch, 2 fat
Bread, Thin-Sliced Dijon Rye (2 slices)	100	18	2	<1	0	340	2	4	1 strch
Bread, Two Cheddar Cheese (1 slice)	210	21	11	5	50	280	1	5	1 1/2 strch, 2 fat
Bread, Very Thin-Sliced White (3 slices)	110	23	2	0	0	270	2	4	1 1/2 strch
Bread, Vienna, Thick-Sliced (1)	70	12	1	0	0	150	<1	3	1 strch
Bread, White Sandwich (2 slices)	65	12	1	<1	0	130	<1	2	1 strch
Bread, White, Thin-Sliced (1 slice)	80	13	2	0	0	135	0	2	1 strch
Bread, 100% Whole-Wheat (1 slice)	90	15	1	0	0	160	2	4	1 strch
Bread, Whole-Wheat, Thin-Sliced (1 slice)	60	11	1	0	0	120	<1	3	1 strch
Breadsticks, Brown & Serve (1)	150	28	2	<1	0	290	1	7	2 strch

Item									
Bun, Multi-Grain Sandwich (1)	150	24	3	<1	0	230	3	6	1 1/2 strch, 1 fat
Bun, Sourdough Sandwich (1)	170	28	4	2	0	290	1	6	2 strch, 1 fat
Buns/Rolls, 5-inch Sandwich Hearty (1)	210	36	5	2	0	346	2	7	2 1/2 strch, 1 fat
Buns/Rolls, Potato Sandwich (1)	160	28	4	<1	0	260	<1	4	2 strch, 1 fat
Croissants, Petite (1)	130	13	8	4	20	180	<1	3	1 strch, 2 fat
Croutons, Caesar Homestyle (1/2 oz)	71	8	3	0	0	183	0	2	1/2 strch, 1 fat
Croutons, Cheddar & Romano Cheese (1/2 oz)	61	8	2	0	0	193	0	2	1/2 strch
Croutons, Cheese & Garlic (1/2 oz)	71	8	3	0	0	162	0	4	1/2 strch, 1 fat
Croutons, Italian Homestyle (1/2 oz)	71	8	3	1	5	132	0	2	1/2 strch, 1 fat
Croutons, Olive Oil & Garlic Homestyle (1/2 oz)	61	10	2	0	0	162	0	2	1/2 strch
Croutons, Onion & Garlic (1/2 oz)	61	10	2	0	0	162	0	2	1/2 strch
Croutons, Seasoned (1/2 oz)	71	8	3	0	0	172	0	2	1/2 strch, 1 fat
Croutons, Sourdough Cheese Homestyle (1/2 oz)	60	8	2	0	5	162	0	2	1/2 strch
Danish, Apple (1)	210	29	9	3	15	190	2	4	2 carb., 2 fat
Danish, Cheese (1)	230	25	11	4	55	230	1	6	1 1/2 strch, 2 fat
Danish, Raspberry (1)	210	29	9	3	15	190	2	4	2 strch, 2 fat

BREAD PRODUCTS & BAKED GOODS

Products	Cal.	Carb. (g)	Fat (g)	Sat. Fat (g)	Chol. (mg)	Sod. (mg)	Fib. (g)	Prot. (g)	Servings/Exchanges
Dinner Rolls, Country-Style Classic (1)	50	7	1	<1	0	77	<1	3	1/2 strch
English Muffins (1)	130	26	1	0	0	250	2	5	2 strch
English Muffins, Cinnamon Raisin (1)	140	28	1	0	0	230	2	5	2 strch
English Muffins, 7-Grain (1)	130	26	1	0	0	230	2	5	2 strch
English Muffins, Sourdough (1)	130	26	1	0	0	250	2	5	2 strch
Finger Dinner Rolls w/Poppy Seed (1)	50	7	2	<1	2	77	<1	2	1/2 strch
Finger Dinner Rolls w/Sesame Seed (1)	50	7	2	<1	<5	8	<1	2	1/2 strch
Muffins, Apple Oatmeal (1)	160	28	4	<1	0	190	3	4	2 strch, 1 fat
Muffins, Blueberry (1)	140	27	3	0	0	190	2	3	2 strch, 1 fat
Muffins, Bran w/Raisins (1)	150	30	3	<1	0	260	4	4	2 strch, 1 fat
Muffins, Corn (1)	150	27	3	0	0	190	1	4	2 strch, 1 fat
Puff Pastry, Apple Dumplings (1)	290	44	11	3	0	160	3	3	3 carb., 2 fat
Puff Pastry, Apple Mini Turnovers (1)	140	15	8	2	0	80	1	2	1 carb., 2 fat
Puff Pastry, Apple Turnovers, Vanilla Icing (1)	380	53	14	3	0	190	2	3	3 1/2 carb., 2 fat

Puff Pastry, Cherry Mini Turnovers (1)	140	16	8	2	0	70	1	2	1 carb., 2 fat
Puff Pastry, Cherry Turnovers, Vanilla Icing (1)	340	51	13	3	0	200	3	4	3 1/2 carb., 2 fat
Rolls, Baked French-Style, Sliced (1)	120	24	2	<1	0	260	1	4	1 1/2 strch
Rolls, Cinnamon (1)	250	33	12	3	15	220	2	4	2 carb., 2 fat
Rolls, Deli Classic Soft Hoagie (1)	200	32	5	3	0	340	2	7	2 strch, 1 fat
Rolls, Dijon Frankfurter (1)	140	23	3	2	0	240	2	6	1 1/2 strch, 1 fat
Rolls, European Bake Shop, French (1)	100	19	1	0	0	230	1	4	1 strch
Rolls, Frankfurter, Top- or Side-Sliced (1)	140	24	3	1	0	270	<1	5	1 1/2 strch, 1 fat
Rolls, Garlic & Cheese (1)	130	16	5	2	15	280	2	6	1 strch, 1 fat
Rolls, Hamburger, Sliced (1)	130	22	3	1	0	230	1	5	1 1/2 strch, 1 fat
Rolls, Heat & Serve Butter Crescent (1)	110	13	5	3	15	160	1	3	1 strch, 1 fat
Rolls, Heat & Serve Golden Twist (1)	110	13	4	2	<5	160	1	2	1 strch, 1 fat
Rolls, Onion Sliced Sandwich (1)	150	26	3	2	0	270	1	5	2 strch, 1 fat
Rolls, Party Enriched (5)	170	26	5	2	10	240	2	7	2 strch, 1 fat
Rolls, Sandwich Sliced w/Sesame Seeds (1)	140	23	3	2	0	240	1	5	1 1/2 strch, 1 fat
Rolls, 7-Grain, French (1)	80	19	2	0	0	270	2	4	1 strch

BREAD PRODUCTS & BAKED GOODS

Products	Cal.	Carb. (g)	Fat (g)	Sat. Fat (g)	Chol. (mg)	Sod. (mg)	Fib. (g)	Prot. (g)	Servings/Exchanges
Stuffing, Corn Bread (1/2 cup)	113	22	1	0	0	320	1	3	1 1/2 strch
Stuffing, Country-Style (1/2 cup)	93	18	1	0	0	253	1	3	1 1/2 strch
Stuffing, Cube (1/2 cup)	93	19	1	0	0	353	1	3	1 strch
Stuffing, Distinctive, Apple Raisin (1/2 cup)	140	27	2	0	0	520	2	4	2 strch
Stuffing, Distinctive, Classic Chicken (1/2 cup)	130	24	2	0	0	490	3	5	1 1/2 strch
Stuffing, Distinctive, Garden Herb (1/2 cup)	150	22	5	1	0	360	2	4	1 1/2 strch, 1 fat
Stuffing, Distinctive, Harvest Vegetable Almond (1/2 cup)	140	23	3	<1	0	300	2	5	1 1/2 strch, 1 fat
Stuffing, Distinctive, Honey Pecan Corn Bread (1/2 cup)	140	23	5	<1	0	400	<1	3	1 1/2 strch, 1 fat
Stuffing, Distinctive, Wild Rice Mushroom (1/2 cup)	130	17	5	1	0	310	2	4	1 strch, 1 fat
Stuffing, Herb-Seasoned (3/4 cup)	170	33	2	0	0	600	3	5	2 strch
Stuffing, Sage & Onion, for Turkeys (1/2 cup)	150	28	2	0	0	520	2	5	2 strch
Turnovers, Apple (1)	330	48	14	3	0	181	6	4	3 carb., 2 fat

Turnovers, Blueberry (1)	340	45	16	3	0	200	6	4	3 carb., 3 fat
Turnovers, Cherry (1)	320	46	13	3	0	190	6	4	3 carb., 2 fat
Turnovers, Peach (1)	340	47	15	3	0	180	6	4	3 carb., 2 fat
Turnovers, Raspberry (1)	330	47	14	3	0	190	6	4	3 carb., 2 fat
PILLSBURY									
Ballard Corn Bread (1/18)	130	23	3	1	25	520	<1	4	1 1/2 strch, 1 fat
Big Country Biscuit Dough, Buttermilk (1)	100	14	4	1	0	360	0	2	1 strch, 1 fat
Big Country Biscuit Dough, Butter-Tastin' (1)	100	13	4	1	0	360	0	2	1 strch, 1 fat
Big Country Biscuit Dough, Scuthern (1)	100	14	4	1	0	360	0	2	1 strch, 1 fat
Biscuit Dough, Country (1)	150	29	2	0	0	540	<1	4	2 strch
Biscuit Dough, Tender Layer Buttermilk (3)	160	27	5	1	0	520	<1	4	2 strch, 1 fat
Bread Machine Mix, Cracked Wheat (1/12)	130	25	2	0	0	260	2	4	1 1/2 strch
Bread Machine Mix, Crusty White (1/12)	130	25	2	0	0	250	2	4	1 1/2 strch
Gingerbread Mix (1/8)	220	40	5	2	0	340	<1	3	2 1/2 carb., 1 fat
Grands Biscuit Dough, Buttermilk (1)	100	12	5	2	0	320	0	2	1 strch, 1 fat fat
Grands Biscuit Dough, Butter-Tastin' (1)	200	24	10	3	0	620	<1	4	1 1/2 strch, 2 fat

BREAD PRODUCTS & BAKED GOODS

Products	Cal.	Carb. (g)	Fat (g)	Sat. Fat (g)	Chol. (mg)	Sod. (mg)	Fib. (g)	Prot. (g)	Servings/Exchanges
Grands Biscuit Dough, Extra Rich (1)	220	25	12	3	0	580	<1	4	1 1/2 strch, 2 fat
Grands Biscuit Dough, Flaky (1)	200	25	9	2	0	580	<1	4	1 1/2 strch, 2 fat
Grands Biscuit Dough, Reduced Fat Buttermilk (1)	190	27	7	2	0	620	<1	4	2 strch, 1 fat
Hungry Jack Biscuit Dough, Butter Tastin Flaky (1)	100	14	5	1	0	350	0	2	1 strch, 1 fat
Hungry Jack Biscuit Dough, Cinnamon & Sugar (1)	110	17	4	1	0	280	<1	2	1 strch, 1 fat
Hungry Jack Biscuit Dough, Flaky Buttermilk (1)	100	14	5	1	0	360	0	2	1 strch, 1 fat
Muffin Mix, Blueberry (1/3 cup)	180	31	5	2	5	190	0	3	2 strch, 1 fat
Muffin Mix, Chocolate Chip (1/3 cup)	190	31	6	3	5	190	<1	3	2 strch, 1 fat
Muffin Mix, Low Fat Blueberry (1/4 cup)	160	34	2	1	0	210	<1	2	2 strch
Quick Bread Mix, Apple Cinnamon (1/12)	180	30	6	1	20	170	1	2	2 strch, 1 fat
Quick Bread Mix, Banana (1/12)	170	26	6	1	35	200	<1	3	2 strch, 1 fat
Quick Bread Mix, Blueberry (1/12)	180	29	6	1	20	160	<1	2	2 strch, 1 fat
Quick Bread Mix, Carrot (1/12)	140	22	5	1	25	150	<1	2	1 1/2 strch, 1 fat
Quick Bread Mix, Cranberry (1/12)	160	30	4	1	20	160	<1	2	2 strch, 1 fat

Quick Bread Mix, Date (1/12)	180	32	4	1	20	160	1	3	2 strch, 1 fat
Quick Bread Mix, Nut (1/12)	170	27	6	1	20	190	1	3	2 strch, 1 fat
Quick Bread Mix, Pumpkin (1/12)	170	27	5	1	35	200	<1	3	2 strch, 1 fat
Roll/Bread Dough, Bread Sticks Garlic & Herb (1)	180	25	7	2	0	580	<1	4	1 1/2 strch, 1 fat
Roll/Bread Dough, Corn Bread Twist (1)	140	18	6	2	0	310	0	3	1 strch, 1 fat
Roll/Bread Dough, Crescent (1)	110	11	6	2	0	220	0	2	1 strch, 1 fat
Roll/Bread Dough, Pizza Crust (1/5)	150	9	2	0	0	380	4	5	1/2 strch
Roll/Bread Dough, Reduced Fat Crescents (1)	100	12	5	1	0	230	0	2	1 strch, 1 fat
Sweet Roll Dough & Icing, Cinnamon (1)	150	23	6	2	0	340	4	2	1 1/2 carb., 1 fat
Sweet Roll w/Icing, Apple Cinnamon (1)	150	23	6	2	0	320	<1	2	1 1/2 strch, 1 fat
Sweet Rolls, Caramel (1)	170	24	7	2	0	330	<1	2	1 1/2 carb., 1 fat
Sweet Rolls, Reduced Fat, Cinnamon w/Icing (1)	140	24	4	1	0	340	<1	2	1 1/2 carb., 1 fat
Toaster Strudel Pastries, Apple (1)	180	27	7	2	5	190	1	3	2 carb., 1 fat
Toaster Strudel Pastries, Blueberry (1)	180	26	7	2	5	200	1	3	2 carb., 1 fat
Toaster Strudel Pastries, Cherry (1)	180	27	7	2	5	200	1	3	2 carb., 1 fat
Toaster Strudel Pastries, Cinnamon (1)	190	26	8	2	5	200	1	3	2 carb., 2 fat

BREAD PRODUCTS & BAKED GOODS

Products	Cal.	Carb. (g)	Fat (g)	Sat. Fat (g)	Chol. (mg)	Sod. (mg)	Fib. (g)	Prot. (g)	Servings/Exchanges
Toaster Strudel Pastries, Cream Cheese (1)	190	23	10	4	15	230	0	3	1 1/2 carb., 2 fat
Toaster Strudel Pastries, Cream Cheese & Blueberry (1)	190	24	9	3	10	220	1	3	1 1/2 carb., 2 fat
Toaster Strudel Pastries, Cream Cheese & Strawberry (1)	190	24	9	3	10	220	1	3	1 1/2 carb., 2 fat
Toaster Strudel Pastries, French Toast-Style (1)	190	28	7	2	5	200	1	3	2 carb., 1 fat
Toaster Strudel Pastries, Raspberry (1)	180	26	7	2	5	200	1	3	2 carb., 1 fat
Toaster Strudel Pastries, Strawberry (1)	180	26	7	2	5	200	1	3	2 carb., 1 fat
Turnovers, Apple (1)	170	23	8	2	0	310	<1	2	1 1/2 carb., 2 fat
Turnovers, Cherry (1)	180	24	8	2	0	310	0	2	1 1/2 carb., 2 fat
PROGRESSO									
Bread Crumbs, Italian-Style (1/4 cup)	110	20	2	0	0	430	1	4	1 strch
Bread Crumbs, Parmesan (1/4 cup)	100	17	2	0	0	870	1	4	1 strch
Bread Crumbs, Plain (1/4 cup)	100	19	2	0	0	210	1	4	1 strch

SHAKE 'N BAKE

Coating Mix, BBQ Chicken or Pork (1/8 pkt)	45	9	1	0	0	410	0	0	1/2 strch
Coating Mix, Classic Italian (1/8 pkt)	40	7	<1	0	0	270	0	1	1/2 strch
Coating Mix, Honey Mustard (1/8 pkt)	45	9	1	0	0	300	0	0	1/2 strch
Coating Mix, Hot Spicy Chicken or Pork (1/8 pkt)	40	7	1	0	0	170	0	1	1/2 strch
Coating Mix, Mild Country (1/8 pkt)	35	5	2	1	0	240	0	0	1/2 strch
Coating Mix, Original Chicken (1/8 pkt)	40	7	1	0	0	220	0	1	1/2 strch
Coating Mix, Original Fish (1/4 pkt)	80	14	2	0	0	350	<1	2	1 strch
Coating Mix, Original Pork (1/8 pkt)	45	8	<1	0	0	230	0	1	1/2 strch
Coating Mix, Tangy Honey (1/8 pkt)	45	9	1	0	9	300	0	0	1/2 strch
Potato Mix, Crispy Cheddar (1/6 pkt)	30	2	2	2	5	380	0	2	1 fat
Potato Mix, Herb & Garlic (1/6 pkt)	20	5	0	0	0	380	0	0	free

STOVE TOP

Microwave Stuffing, Chicken (1/2 cup)	160	20	7	2	0	480	<1	4	1 strch, 1 fat
Microwave Stuffing, Corn Bread (1/2 cup)	160	20	7	2	0	480	<1	3	1 strch, 1 fat
Stuffing Mix for Beef (1/2 cup)	180	22	9	2	0	540	1	4	1 1/2 strch, 2 fat

BREAD PRODUCTS & BAKED GOODS

Products	Cal.	Carb. (g)	Fat (g)	Sat. Fat (g)	Chol. (mg)	Sod. (mg)	Fib. (g)	Prot. (g)	Servings/Exchanges
Stuffing Mix for Pork (1/2 cup)	170	20	9	2	0	530	1	4	1 strch, 2 fat
Stuffing Mix for Turkey (1/2 cup)	170	20	9	2	0	530	<1	4	1 strch, 2 fat
Stuffing Mix, Chicken Flavor (1/2 cup)	170	20	9	2	0	510	<1	4	1 strch, 2 fat
Stuffing Mix, Corn Bread (1/2 cup)	170	21	8	2	0	580	1	3	1 1/2 strch, 2 fat
Stuffing Mix, Low-Sodium Chicken (1/2 cup)	180	21	9	2	0	340	<1	4	1 1/2 strch, 2 fat
Stuffing Mix, San Francisco (1/2 cup)	170	20	9	2	0	530	1	4	1 strch, 2 fat
Stuffing Mix, Savory Herbs (1/2 cup)	170	20	9	2	0	530	1	4	1 strch, 2 fat
WEIGHT WATCHERS									
Coffee Cake, Cinnamon Streusel (1)	190	28	7	1	5	250	NA	3	2 carb., 1 fat
Muffins, Apple Spice (1)	160	29	5	1	NA	260	NA	3	2 strch, 1 fat
Muffins, Banana Nut (1)	170	32	5	1	10	250	NA	3	2 strch, 1 fat
Muffins, Blueberry (1)	170	32	5	1	10	220	NA	3	2 strch, 1 fat
Muffins, Honey Bran (1)	160	32	4	1	5	150	NA	3	2 strch, 1 fat
Rolls, Glazed Cinnamon (1)	180	31	5	1	5	170	NA	4	2 carb., 1 fat

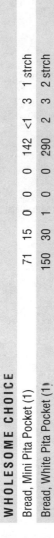

WHOLESOME CHOICE

Bread, Mini Pita Pocket (1)	71	15	0	0	142	<1	3	1 strch
Bread, White Pita Pocket (1)	150	30	1	0	290	2	3	2 strch

CANDY

Products	Cal.	Carb. (g)	Fat (g)	Sat. Fat (g)	Chol. (mg)	Sod. (mg)	Fib. (g)	Prot. (g)	Servings/Exchanges
Almond Roca (1 oz)	124	19	5	3	3	51	<1	2	1 carb., 1 fat
Almonds, Chocolate-Coated (1/4 cup)	234	16	18	3	<1	24	4	5	1 carb., 4 fat
Almonds, Sugar-Coated (7)	129	20	5	<1	0	6	1	2	1 carb., 1 fat
Butterscotch (5 pieces)	119	29	1	<1	3	13	0	<1	2 carb.
Candy Corn (26 pieces)	140	36	0	0	0	80	0	0	2 1/2 carb.
Caramel Apple (1 medium)	255	56	4	3	3	111	4	2	1 fruit, 4 carb., 1 fat
Caramels (3)	116	23	3	2	2	74	<1	1	1 1/2 carb., 1 fat
Chewing Gum (1 piece)	10	3	<1	0	0	<1	0	0	free
Chewing Gum, Sugar-Free (1 piece)	11	4	<1	0	0	<1	0	0	free
Cherries, Chocolate-Covered (2)	110	18	4	3	0	15	2	<1	1 carb., 1 fat
Divinity, Homemade (1 oz)	98	25	3	<1	0	13	0	<1	1 1/2 carb., 1 fat
Fruit Leather (0.5 oz)	49	12	<1	<1	0	9	<1	<1	1 carb.
Fudge, Chocolate, Homemade (1 oz)	108	23	3	1	4	18	4	4	1 1/2 carb., 1 fat

Food									Exchanges
Fudge, Chocolate Marshmallow, Homemade (1 oz)	118	20	5	3	7	29	0	<1	1 carb., 1 fat
Fudge, Chocolate w/Nuts, Homemade (1 oz)	124	20	6	3	6	27	<1	<1	1 carb., 1 fat
Fudge, Vanilla, Homemade (1 oz)	105	23	2	<1	5	19	0	<1	1 1/2 carb.
Fudge, Vanilla w/Nuts, Homemade (1 oz)	118	21	4	1	4	17	<1	<1	1 1/2 carb., 1 fat
Gumdrops (10 small)	139	36	0	0	0	16	0	0	2 1/2 carb.
Gummy Bears (10 small)	85	22	0	0	0	15	0	0	1 1/2 carb.
Hard Candy, All Flavors (1 oz)	106	28	0	0	0	11	0	0	2 carb.
Jellybeans (10)	40	10	<1	0	0	3	0	0	1/2 carb.
Lollipops (1)	22	6	0	0	0	2	0	0	1/2 carb.
Milk Chocolate Bar w/Almonds (1.5 oz)	216	22	14	7	8	30	3	4	1 1/2 carb., 3 fat
Milk Chocolate Bar w/Peanuts (1.5 oz)	235	16	18	5	4	17	2	7	1 carb., 4 fat
Mint Patty, Chocolate-Covered (1 small)	28	5	<1	<1	0	<1	<1	<1	1/2 carb.
Peanut Brittle, Homemade (1 oz)	129	20	5	1	4	128	<1	2	1 carb., 1 fat
Peanuts, Milk Chocolate-Coated (1/4 cup)	193	18	13	5	3	15	2	5	1 carb., 3 fat
Peanuts, Yogurt-Covered (1/4 cup)	194	16	13	3	1	15	2	4	1 carb., 3 fat

CANDY

Products	Cal.	Carb. (g)	Fat (g)	Sat. Fat (g)	Chol. (mg)	Sod. (mg)	Fib. (g)	Prot. (g)	Servings/Exchanges
Penuche Brown Sugar Fudge w/Nuts, Homemade (1 oz)	112	22	3	<1	2	28	<1	<1	1 1/2 carb.
Praline, Homemade (1 oz)	129	18	7	<1	0	18	<1	<1	1 carb., 1 fat
Raisins, Milk Chocolate-Covered (1/4 cup)	185	33	7	4	1	17	2	2	2 carb., 1 fat
Raisins, Yogurt-Covered (1/4 cup)	190	34	6	4	4	21	2	2	2 carb., 1 fat
Taffy, Homemade (1 oz)	107	26	<1	<1	3	25	0	0	2 carb.
Toffee, Homemade (1 oz)	154	18	9	6	30	53	0	0	1 carb., 2 fat
Truffles, Homemade (1 oz)	138	13	10	5	15	20	<1	2	1 carb., 2 fat
BREATHSAVERS									
Breath Mints (4)	60	16	0	0	0	0	0	0	1 carb
CADBURY'S									
Caramello Bar (1.6 oz)	220	29	10	6	10	60	<1	3	2 carb., 2 fat
CONCORDE									
Bit-O-Honey Chews (6 = 1.7 oz)	186	39	4	NA	<1	124	NA	1	2 1/2 carb., 1 fat

ESTEE

Item									
Caramels, Vanilla/Chocolate (5)	115	26	5	1	0	65	0	1	2 carb., 1 fat
Chocolately Covered Pretzels (7)	130	19	6	4	0	270	<1	2	1 carb., 1 fat
Gourmet Jelly Beans (26)	70	24	0	0	0	30	0	0	1 1/2 carb.
Fruit Gumdrops (23)	80	36	0	0	0	0	0	0	2 1/2 carb.
Gummy Bears (17)	100	30	0	0	0	5	0	3	2 carb.
Hard Candy, Butterscotch (2)	25	12	0	0	0	50	0	0	1 carb.
Hard Candy, Peppermint Swirls (3)	30	14	0	0	0	0	0	0	1 carb.
Licorice Gum Drops (11)	90	36	0	0	0	65	0	1	2 1/2 carb.
Milk Chocolate Bar, No Sucrose Added (7 squares)	230	17	17	10	20	65	0	4	1 carb., 3 fat
Milk Chocolate w/Almond Bar, No Sucrose Added (7 squares)	230	16	17	9	20	65	0	4	1 carb., 3 fat
Milk Chocolate w/Fruit & Nut Bar, No Sucrose Added (7 squares)	220	18	16	9	20	65	0	4	1 carb., 3 fat
Milk Chocolate w/Crisp Rice Bar, No Sucrose Added (7 squares)	370	29	26	15	30	110	0	7	2 carb., 3 fat

CANDY

Products	Cal.	Carb. (g)	Fat (g)	Sat. Fat (g)	Chol. (mg)	Sod. (mg)	Fib. (g)	Prot. (g)	Servings/Exchanges
Mint Candies (5)	30	16	0	0	0	0	0	0	1 carb.
Mint Chocolate Bar, No Sucrose Added (7 squares)	200	23	14	8	10	10	0	2	1 1/2 carb., 3 fat
Peanut Brittle (1.3 oz)	160	28	9	2	10	115	1	3	2 carb., 2 fat
Peanut Butter Cups (5)	200	19	12	7	<5	70	1	5	1 carb., 2 fat
Peanuts, Candy-Coated (1/4 cup)	200	23	9	4	<5	45	1	5	1 1/2 carb., 2 fat
Raisins, Chocolate-Coated (1/4 cup)	180	27	6	5	<5	45	1	3	2 carb., 1 fat
Toffee Candies (5)	30	16	0	0	0	0	0	0	1 carb.
HERSHEY'S									
5th Avenue Bar (2 oz)	280	38	12	5	<5	95	1	5	2 1/2 carb., 2 fat
Chocolate Kisses (9)	230	24	13	8	10	35	1	3	1 1/2 carb., 3 fat
Cookies & Cream Bar (1.55 oz)	220	25	12	7	5	95	0	4	1 1/2 carb., 2 fat
Golden Almond Chocolate Bar (2.8 oz)	448	35	30	13	12	52	4	10	2 carb., 6 fat
Golden Almond Solitaires (2.8-oz pkg)	443	37	29	12	10	44	3	9	2 1/2 carb., 6 fat
Good & Plenty Licorice (1.8 oz)	160	40	0	0	0	120	0	<1	2 1/2 carb.

Kit Kat Bar (1.5 oz)	220	27	11	7	<5	30	<1	3	2 carb., 2 fat
Krackel Bar (1.5 oz)	218	25	12	7	8	57	<1	3	1 1/2 carb., 2 fat
Milk Chocolate Bar (1.55 oz)	230	25	13	9	10	40	1	3	1 1/2 carb., 3 fat
Milk Chocolate Bar, Symphony (1.5 oz)	230	24	14	9	10	40	<1	3	1 1/2 carb., 3 fat
Mr. Goodbar (1.75 oz)	270	25	17	7	<5	20	2	5	1 1/2 carb., 3 fat
Reese's Peanut Butter Cups (2 = 1.6 oz)	250	25	14	5	<5	140	1	5	1 1/2 carb., 3 fat
Reese's Pieces (1.63-oz pkg)	230	26	11	7	0	90	1	6	2 carb., 2 fat
Reese's sticks (1.5 oz)	230	23	13	6	<5	110	1	4	1 1/2 carb., 3 fat
Rolos Caramel (1.91 oz)	260	36	11	6	10	110	0	3	2 1/2 carb., 2 fat
Skor Bar (1.4 oz)	210	23	12	7	20	110	0	2	1 1/2 carb., 2 fat
Special Dark Sweet Chocolate Bar (1.45 oz)	220	24	13	8	<5	0	3	2	1 1/2 carb., 3 fat
Sweet Escapes, Caramel & Peanut Butter (1.4 oz)	140	24	5	2	0	150	0	2	1 1/2 carb., 1 fat
Sweet Escapes, Chocolate Toffee Crisp (1.7 oz)	160	24	7	4	NA	80	NA	2	1 1/2 carb., 1 fat
Sweet Escapes, Triple Chocolate Wafer (1.4 oz)	160	28	5	3	0	60	NA	1	2 carb., 1 fat
Tootsie Rolls (6 bite-size)	160	33	3	4	0	40	<1	<1	2 carb.
Whatchamacallit Bar (1.7 oz)	220	29	10	7	5	100	<1	4	2 carb., 2 fat

CANDY

Products	Cal.	Carb. (g)	Fat (g)	Sat. Fat (g)	Chol. (mg)	Sod. (mg)	Fib. (g)	Prot. (g)	Servings/Exchanges
Whoppers Chocolate Malted Milk Balls (18)	180	29	7	6	0	95	<1	1	1 carb., 2 fat
KRAFT									
Butter Mints (7 = 0.5 oz)	60	14	0	0	0	25	0	0	1 carb.
Caramels (5 = 1.5 oz)	170	32	3	1	3	110	0	2	2 carb., 1 fat
Fudgies (5 = 1.5 oz)	180	32	5	3	0	90	0	1	2 carb., 1 fat
M & M MARS									
3 Musketeers Bar (2.13 oz)	260	46	8	5	5	110	1	2	3 carb., 2 fat
Almond Bar (1.76 oz)	240	31	13	5	5	70	1	3	2 carb., 2 fat
Kudos Nutty Fudge Snack Bar (1.3 oz)	200	20	12	NA	5	55			1 carb., 2 fat
M&M's, Chocolate (1.7-oz pkg)	240	34	10	6	5	30	1	2	2 carb., 2 fat
M&M's, Peanut (1.74-oz pkg)	250	30	13	5	5	25	2	5	2 carb., 3 fat
Milky Way Bar (2.05 oz)	270	41	10	5	5	95	1	2	3 carb., 2 fat
Snickers Bar (2.07 oz)	280	35	14	5	5	140	1	4	3 carb., 3 fat
Starburst Fruit Chews (2.07 oz)	240	48	5	1	0	0	0	0	3 carb., 1 fat

Twix Caramel Cookie Bar (2 oz)	280	37	14	5	5	115	1	3	2 1/2 carb., 3 fat

NESTLE

100 Grand Bar (1.5 oz)	200	30	8	5	10	75	1	2	2 carb., 2 fat
Baby Ruth Bar (2.1 oz)	270	36	13	7	0	130	2	4	2 1/2 carb., 3 fat
Buncha Crunch Bar (1.4 oz)	200	26	10	6	10	60	<1	2	2 carb., 2 fat
Bittyfinger (1.36 oz, 2 bars)	170	27	7	4	0	85	<1	2	2 carb., 1 fat
Butterfinger Bar (2.1 oz)	270	42	11	5	0	130	1	3	3 carb., 2 fat
Butterfinger BB's (1.7-oz bag)	230	33	9	6	0	95	1	2	2 carb., 2 fat
Chunky Bar (1.4 oz)	210	24	11	6	5	20	1	3	1 1/2 carb., 2 fat
Crunch Bar (1.4 oz)	230	29	12	7	10	65	<1	2	2 carb., 2 fat
Demet's Turtles (1)	83	10	5	<5	<5	16	<1	1	1/2 carb., 1 fat
Flipz-Milk Chocolate (1 oz, 1 bar)	130	20	6	4	<5	130	<1	2	1 carb., 1 fat
Flipz-Peanut Butter (1 oz, 1 bar)	140	19	6	4	0	140	<1	3	1 carb., 1 fat
Flipz-White Fudge (1 oz, 1 bar)	130	19	6	5	0	130	0	2	1 carb., 1 fat
Goobers Chocolate-Covered Peanuts (1.38-oz bag)	210	20	13	5	5	15	1	4	1 carb., 3 fat
Milk Chocolate Bar (1.45 oz)	220	26	13	8	10	25	<1	2	1 carb., 2 fat

CANDY

Products	Cal.	Carb. (g)	Fat (g)	Sat. Fat (g)	Chol. (mg)	Sod. (mg)	Fib. (g)	Prot. (g)	Servings/Exchanges
Mocha Crunch (1.3 oz)	200	21	12	7	10	65	0	2	1 1/2 carb., 2 fat
Oh Henry! Bar (0.9 oz—1 bar)	120	16	5	3	<5	60	0	2	1 carb., 1 fat
Pearson Nips, Caramel (2)	60	11	2	1	0	40	0	0	1 carb.
Pearson Nips, Chocolate (2)	60	11	2	1	0	40	0	0	1 carb.
Pearson Nips, Chocolate Parfait (2)	60	10	2	1	0	30	0	0	1 carb.
Pearson Nips, Coffee (2)	50	10	2	2	0	40	0	0	1 carb.
Pearson Nips, Peanut Butter Parfait (2)	60	10	2	2	0	45	0	<1	1 carb.
Raisinets (1.58 oz)	190	31	8	5	<5	15	1	2	2 carb., 2 fat
Sno Caps (2.3-oz box)	300	48	13	8	0	0	3	2	3 carb., 3 fat
Treasures w/Butterfinger (3 pieces)	180	24	9	5	5	40	<1	2	1 1/2 carb., 2 fat
Treasures, Caramel (3 pieces)	180	22	9	6	5	55	<1	1	1 1/2 carb., 2 fat
Treasures, Peanut Butter (4 pieces)	250	23	17	7	5	90	1	4	1 1/2 carb., 3 fat
Turtles Caramel Chocolate (2 = 1.2 oz)	160	20	9	3	<5	30	<1	2	1 carb., 2 fat
White Crunch (1.4 oz)	220	23	13	8	10	70	0	3	1 1/2 carb., 3 fat

PETER PAUL

Almond Joy Bar (1.76 oz)	240	29	13	8	0	70	2	2	2 carb., 3 fat
Mounds Bar (1.9 oz)	250	31	13	11	0	80	3	2	2 carb., 2 fat

PLANTER'S

Peanut Bar (1.6 oz)	230	22	14	2	0	70	2	6	1 1/2 carb., 3 fat

Y & S

Nibs Cherry (2.25 oz)	220	49	2	0	0	135	0	2	3 carb.
Twizzlers Strawberry (3 pieces)	120	27	<1	0	0	85	0	1	2 carb.

YORK

Peppermint Patty (large, 1.5 oz)	170	34	3	2	0	10	<1	<1	2 carb., 1 fat

CEREALS

Products	Cal.	Carb. (g)	Fat (g)	Sat. Fat (g)	Chol. (mg)	Sod. (mg)	Fib. (g)	Prot. (g)	Servings/Exchanges
Bulgur (1/2 cup)	76	17	<1	0	0	5	4	3	1 strch
Corn Grits, White or Yellow, Cooked (1/2 cup)	73	16	<1	<1	0	0	<1	2	1 strch
Cream of Rice, Cooked (1/2 cup)	64	14	<1	<1	0	1	<1	1	1 strch
Cream of Rye, Cooked (1/2 cup)	54	12	<1	<1	0	175	2	1	1 strch
Cream of Wheat, Cooked (1/2 cup)	66	14	<1	<1	0	71	<1	2	1 strch
Farina, Cooked (1/2 cup)	59	12	<1	<1	0	0	2	2	1 strch
Granola, Homemade (1/2 cup)	285	32	15	3	0	15	6	9	2 strch, 3 fat
Honey Bran Cereal (1 cup)	60	14	<1	<1	0	101	2	2	1 strch
Kasha or Buckwheat Groats, Cooked (1/2 cup)	91	20	<1	<1	0	4	2	3	1 strch
Millet, Cooked (1/4 cup)	72	14	<1	<1	0	1	<1	2	1 strch
Multi-Grain Cereal, Cooked (1/2 cup)	100	20	1	<1	0	380	2	3	1 strch
Oatmeal Cereal, Cooked (1/2 cup)	73	13	1	<1	0	1	2	3	1 strch
Wheatena, Cooked (1/2 cup)	68	15	<1	<1	0	3	3	2	1 strch

GENERAL MILLS

Basic 4 (1 cup)	200	43	3	0	0	320	3	4	3 strch
Body Buddies Natural Fruit (1 cup)	120	26	1	0	0	290	0	2	2 starch
Boo Berry (1 cup)	120	27	1	0	0	210	0	1	2 starch
Cheerios (1 cup)	110	22	2	0	0	280	3	3	1 1/2 strch
Cheerios, Apple Cinnamon (3/4 cup)	120	25	2	0	0	160	1	2	1 1/2 strch
Cheerios, Honey Nut (1 cup)	120	24	2	0	0	270	2	3	1 1/2 strch
Cheerios Plus, Multi-Grain (1 cup)	110	24	1	0	0	200	3	3	1 1/2 strch
Chex, Corn (1 cup)	110	26	0	0	0	280	0	2	2 strch
Chex, Honey Nut (3/4 cup)	110	26	1	0	0	220	0	1	2 starch
Chex, Multi-Bran (1 cup)	200	49	2	0	0	390	7	4	3 strch
Chex, Rice (1 1/4 cup)	120	27	0	0	0	290	0	2	2 starch
Chex, Wheat (1 cup)	180	40	1	0	0	420	5	5	2 1/2 strch
Cinnamon Grahams (3/4 cup)	120	26	1	0	0	230	1	1	2 starch
Cinnamon Toast Crunch (3/4 cup)	130	24	4	<1	0	210	1	1	1 1/2 strch
Cocoa Puffs (1 cup)	120	26	1	0	0	170	0	1	2 starch

CEREALS

Products	Cal.	Carb. (g)	Fat (g)	Sat. Fat (g)	Chol. (mg)	Sod. (mg)	Fib. (g)	Prot. (g)	Servings/Exchanges
Cookie Crisp (1 cup)	120	27	1	0	0	180	0	1	2 strch
Count Chocula (1 cup)	120	26	1	0	0	180	0	1	2 starch
Country Corn Flakes (1 cup)	110	26	0	0	0	260	0	2	2 starch
Crispy Wheat 'N Raisins (1 cup)	190	45	1	0	0	270	4	4	3 strch
Fiber One (1/2 cup)	60	24	1	0	0	130	13	2	1 1/2 strch
Frankenberry (1 cup)	120	27	1	0	0	210	0	1	2 starch
French Toast Crunch (3/4 cup)	120	26	2	0	0	180	0	1	2 strch
Frosted Cheerios (1 cup)	120	26	1	0	0	210	1	2	2 starch
Golden Grahams (3/4 cup)	120	25	1	0	0	270	1	1	1 1/2 strch
Honey Nut Clusters (3/4 cup)	210	47	2	0	0	230	3	4	3 strch
Kaboom (1 1/4 cup)	120	24	1	0	0	290	1	2	1 1/2 starch
Kix (1 1/3 cup)	120	26	<1	0	0	270	1	2	1 1/2 strch
Kix, Berry Berry (3/4 cup)	120	26	2	0	0	170	0	1	2 strch
Lucky Charms (1 cup)	120	25	1	0	0	210	1	2	1 1/2 strch

Millenios (1 cup)	120	25	1	0	0	180	1	2	1 1/2 starch
Nature Valley Low Fat Fruit Granola (2/3 cup)	210	44	3	0	0	210	3	4	3 starch, 1 fat
Nesquik Chocolate (3/4 cup)	120	25	2	0	0	190	0	1	1 1/2 starch
Oatmeal Crisp, Almond (1 cup)	220	42	5	<1	0	240	4	5	3 starch, 1 fat
Oatmeal Crisp, Apple Cinnamon (1 cup)	210	45	2	0	0	250	4	5	3 starch
Oatmeal Crisp, Raisin (1 cup)	210	44	2	0	0	210	4	5	3 strch
Raisin Nut Bran (3/4 cup)	200	41	4	<1	0	250	5	4	3 strch
Reese's Peanut Butter Puffs (3/4 cup)	130	24	3	<1	0	200	0	2	1 1/2 starch, 1 fat
Sunrise (3/4 cup)	110	26	<1	0	0	190	1	1	2 starch
Team Cheerios (1 cup)	120	25	1	0	0	210	1	2	1 1/2 starch
Total Brown Sugar & Oat (3/4 cup)	110	25	1	0	0	170	1	2	1 1/2 starch
Total Corn Flakes (1 1/3 cup)	110	26	0	0	0	200	0	2	2 strch
Total Raisin Bran (1cup)	180	43	1	0	0	240	5	4	3 starch
Total Whole-Grain (3/4 cup)	110	24	1	<1	0	200	3	3	2 strch
Trix (1 cup)	120	27	1	0	0	200	1	1	2 strch
Wheat Hearts (1/4 cup dry)	130	26	1	0	0	0	2	5	2 starch

CEREALS

Products	Cal.	Carb. (g)	Fat (g)	Sat. Fat (g)	Chol. (mg)	Sod. (mg)	Fib. (g)	Prot. (g)	Servings/Exchanges
Wheaties (1 cup)	110	24	1	0	0	220	3	3	1 1/2 strch
Wheaties, Frosted (3/4 cup)	110	27	0	0	0	200	0	1	2 strch
Wheaties Raisin Bran (1 cup)	180	45	1	0	0	250	5	4	3 starch
HEALTH VALLEY									
100% Blue Corn (1 oz)	90	19	1	NA	0	10	3	3	1 strch
Fat-Free Granola O's, Almond (1 oz)	90	19	0	0	0	5	5	3	1 strch
Fat-Free Granola O's, Apple Cinnamon (1 oz)	90	19	0	0	0	5	5	3	1 strch
Fat-Free High Fiber O's (1 oz)	90	19	0	0	0	5	5	3	1 strch
Organic Amaranth Flakes (1 oz)	90	20	0	0	0	10	3	3	1 strch
KASHI									
Kashi (1/2 cup)	170	30	3	0	0	15	6	6	2 strch
Kashi Medley (1/2 cup)	100	20	1	0	0	50	2	4	1 strch
Puffed Kashi (1 cup)	70	13	<1	0	0	0	2	3	1 strch

KELLOGG'S

All-Bran (1/2 cup)	80	24	1	0	0	65	10	4	1 1/2 strch
All-Bran w/Extra Fiber (1/2 cup)	50	20	1	0	0	120	13	3	1 strch
Apple Jacks (1 cup)	120	30	0	0	0	150	1	1	2 strch
Bran Buds (1/3 cup)	80	24	1	0	0	200	13	2	1 1/2 strch
Cocoa Frosted Flakes (3/4 cup)	120	28	0	0	0	170	0	1	2 starch
Cocoa Krispies (3/4 cup)	120	27	1	<1	0	190	1	1	2 strch
Complete Oat Bran Flakes (3/4 cup)	110	23	1	0	0	210	4	3	1 1/2 starch
Complete Wheat Bran Flakes (3/4 cup)	90	23	<1	0	0	210	5	3	1 1/2 strch
Corn Flakes (1 cup)	100	24	0	0	0	200	1	2	1 1/2 strch
Corn Pops (1 cup)	120	28	0	0	0	120	0	1	2 strch
Country Inn Specialties, Green Gables Inn Blend (1/2 cup)	210	37	6	4	0	160	4	4	2 1/2 starch, 1 fat
Country Inn Specialties, Greyfield Inn Blend (3/4 cup)	210	38	6	1	0	220	3	3	2 1/2 starch, 1 fat

CEREALS

Products	Cal.	Carb. (g)	Fat (g)	Sat. Fat (g)	Chol. (mg)	Sod. (mg)	Fib. (g)	Prot. (g)	Servings/Exchanges
Country Inn Specialties, Inn at Ormsby Hill Blend (1 cup)	220	49	2	1	0	300	3	4	3 starch
Cracklin' Oat Bran (3/4 cup)	190	35	7	2	0	170	6	4	2 strch, 2 fat
Crispix (1 cup)	110	25	0	0	0	210	1	2	2 strch
Froot Loops (1 cup)	120	28	1	<1	0	150	1	1	2 strch
Froot Loops, Marshmallow Blasted (1 cup)	120	27	<1	0	0	105	0	1	2 starch
Frosted Flakes (3/4 cup)	120	28	0	0	0	150	1	1	2 strch
Healthy Choice Almond Crunch w/Raisins (1 cup)	210	45	3	0	0	230	5	5	3 starch, 1 fat
Healthy Choice Low Fat Granola (1/2 cup)	190	39	3	<1	0	120	3	4	2 1/2 starch, 1 fat
Healthy Choice Low Fat Granola w/Raisins (2/3 cup)	220	48	3	1	0	150	3	5	3 starch, 1 fat
Healthy Choice Mueslix Raisin & Almond Crunch (2/3 cup)	200	41	3	0	0	160	4	5	2 starch, 1 fat

Healthy Choice Toasted Brown Sugar Squares (1 cup)	190	44	1	0	0	5	5	5	3 starch
Honey Crunch Flakes (3/4 cup)	120	26	1	0	210	1	2	2 starch
Just Right w/Fruit & Nut (1 cup)	220	49	2	0	280	3	4	3 strch
Mini-Wheats, Apple Cinnamon (3/4 cup)	180	44	1	0	20	5	4	3 starch
Mini-Wheats-Blueberry (3/4 cup)	180	43	1	0	20	5	4	3 starch
Mini-Wheats, Frosted Original (5 biscuits)	180	41	1	0	5	5	5	3 strch
Mini-Wheats, Frosted Bite Size (24 biscuits)	200	48	1	0	5	6	6	3 strch
Nut & Honey Crunch (1 1/4 cup)	223	45	3	<1	370	<1	4	3 strch
Product 19 (1 cup)	100	25	0	0	210	1	2	1 1/2 strch
Raisin Bran (1 cup)	190	45	2	0	350	8	5	3 strch
Raisin Bran Crunch (1 cup)	190	44	1	0	200	4	3	3 starch
Rice Krispies (1 1/4 cup)	120	29	0	0	320	<1	2	2 strch
Rice Krispies, Apple Cinnamon (3/4 cup)	112	27	0	0	223	<1	2	2 strch
Rice Krispies, Razzle Dazzle (3/4 cup)	110	25	0	0	170	0	1	1 1/2 starch
Rice Krispies Treats (3/4 cup)	120	26	2	0	190	0	1	2 strch

CEREALS

Products	Cal.	Carb. (g)	Fat (g)	Sat. Fat (g)	Chol. (mg)	Sod. (mg)	Fib. (g)	Prot. (g)	Servings/Exchanges
Smacks (3/4 cup)	100	24	<1	0	0	50	1	2	2 strch
Smart Start (1 cup)	180	43	<1	0	0	330	2	3	3 starch
Special K (1 cup)	110	23	0	0	0	220	1	6	1 1/2 strch
Special K Plus (1 cup)	210	47	2	0	0	250	3	4	3 starch
MALT-O-MEAL									
Berry Colossal Crunch (3/4 cup)	120	26	2	0	0	220	1	1	2 starch
Cocoa Comets (3/4 cup)	120	27	1	0	0	190	<1	1	2 strch
Colossal Crunch (3/4 cup)	120	25	2	0	0	230	1	1	1 1/2 starch
Corn Bursts (1 cup)	120	29	0	0	0	120	0	1	2 strch
Crispy Rice (1 cup)	110	26	0	0	0	320	0	2	2 strch
Frosted Flakes (3/4 cup)	110	27	0	0	0	200	<1	2	2 strch
Frosted Mini Spooners (1 cup)	190	45	1	0	0	0	6	5	3 strch
Golden Puffs (3/4 cup)	100	26	0	0	0	40	<1	2	2 strch
Hot Wheat Cereal, Chocolate (3 Tbsp dry)	120	28	0	0	0	0	1	3	2 strch

Food	Cal	Carb	Fat			Sod			Exchanges
Hot Wheat Cereal, Maple & Brown Sugar (3 Tbsp dry)	120	28	0	0	0	0	0	1	3	2 strch
Hot Wheat Cereal, Quick Original (3 Tbsp dry)	120	27	0	0	0	0	1	4	2 strch
Puffed Rice (1 cup)	60	13	0	0	0	0	0	1	1 strch
Puffed Wheat (1 cup)	50	11	0	0	0	0	1	2	1 strch
Toasty O's (1 cup)	110	22	2	0	0	260	3	3	1 1/2 strch
Toasty O's, Apple & Cinnamon (3/4 cup)	120	25	2	0	0	160	1	2	1 1/2 strch
Toasty O's, Frosted (1 cup)	120	25	1	0	0	210	1	7	1 1/2 strch
Toasty O's, Honey & Nut (1 cup)	110	24	1	0	0	270	2	3	1 1/2 strch
Tootie Fruities (1 cup)	120	26	1	0	0	140	<1	1	2 strch

NABISCO

Food	Cal	Carb	Fat			Sod			Exchanges
100% Bran Cereal (1/3 cup)	80	23	<1	0	0	120	8	4	1 1/2 strch
Shredded Wheat (2 biscuits)	160	38	<1	0	0	0	5	5	2 1/2 strch
Shredded Wheat Bites, Frosted (1 cup)	190	44	1	0	0	10	5	4	3 strch
Shredded Wheat Bites, Honey Nut (1 cup)	200	43	2	0	0	40	4	5	3 strch
Shredded Wheat, Spoon-Size (1 cup)	170	41	<1	0	0	0	5	5	3 strch

CEREALS

Products	Cal.	Carb. (g)	Fat (g)	Sat. Fat (g)	Chol. (mg)	Sod. (mg)	Fib. (g)	Prot. (g)	Servings/Exchanges
Shredded Wheat & Bran (1 1/4 cup)	200	47	1	0	0	0	8	7	3 strch
NATURE VALLEY									
Granola, Fruit & Nut (1 oz)	130	19	5	1	0	45	1	2	1 strch, 1 fat
Granola, Cinnamon Raisin (1/3 cup)	120	20	4	<1	0	50	1	2	1 strch, 1 fat
Granola, Toasted Oat (1/3 cup)	130	20	5	<1	0	50	1	2	1 strch, 1 fat
POST									
Alpha-Bits (1 cup)	130	27	2	0	0	210	1	3	2 strch
Alpha-Bits, Marshmallow (1 cup)	120	25	1	0	0	160	0	2	1 1/2 strch
Banana Nut Crunch (1 cup)	250	43	6	1	0	240	4	5	3 strch, 1 fat
Blueberry Morning (1 1/4 cup)	220	43	3	<1	0	250	2	4	3 strch, 1 fat
Bran Flakes (3/4 cup)	100	24	<1	0	0	220	5	3	1 1/2 strch
Cocoa Pebbles (3/4 cup)	120	26	1	1	0	160	0	1	1 1/2 strch
Cranberry Almond Crunch (1 cup)	220	44	3	0	0	200	3	4	3 strch, 1 fat
Fruit & Fiber, Date/Raisin/Walnut (1 cup)	210	42	3	<1	0	250	5	4	3 strch, 1 fat

Cereal	Cal								Exchanges
Fruit & Fiber, Peach/Raisin/Almond (1 cup)	210	42	3	<1	0	260	5	4	3 strch, 1 fat
Fruity Pebbles (3/4 cup)	110	24	1	<1	0	160	0	<1	1 1/2 strch
Grape Nuts (1/2 cup)	200	47	1	0	0	350	5	6	3 strch
Grape Nuts Flakes (3/4 cup)	100	24	1	0	0	140	5	6	1 1/2 strch
Golden Crisp (3/4 cup)	110	25	0	0	0	40	0	1	1 1/2 strch
Great Grains Crunchy Pecan (2/3 cup)	220	38	6	1	0	190	4	5	2 1/2 strch, 1 fat
Great Grains, Raisin/Date/Pecan (2/3 cup)	210	39	5	<1	0	160	4	4	2 1/2 strch, 1 fat
Honey Bunches of Oats (3/4 cup)	120	25	2	<1	0	190	1	2	1 1/2 strch, 1 fat
Honey Bunches of Oats & Almonds (3/4 cup)	130	24	3	<1	0	180	1	3	1 1/2 strch, 1 fat
Honeycombs (1 1/3 cup)	110	26	<1	0	0	220	<1	2	2 strch
Raisin Bran (1 cup)	190	47	1	0	0	300	8	4	3 strch
Toasties Corn Flakes (1 cup)	100	24	0	0	0	270	1	2	1 1/2 strch
Waffle Crisp (1 cup)	130	24	3	0	0	120	0	2	1 1/2 strch, 1 fat
QUAKER									
100% Natural Granola, Low Fat (2/3 cup)	210	44	3	NA	0	140	3	5	3 strch, 1 fat

CEREALS

Products	Cal.	Carb. (g)	Fat (g)	Sat. Fat (g)	Chol. (mg)	Sod. (mg)	Fib. (g)	Prot. (g)	Servings/Exchanges
100% Natural Granola, Raisin (1/2 cup)	230	34	9	4	0	20	3	5	2 strch, 2 fat
100% Natural Granola, Regular (1/2 cup)	220	31	9	NA	0	20	3	5	2 strch, 2 fat
Apple Zaps (1 cup)	120	27	1	NA	0	135	1	1	2 strch
Cap'n Crunch (3/4 cup)	110	23	2	0	0	200	1	1	1 1/2 strch
Cap'n Crunch Oops! All Berries (1 cup)	130	27	2	NA	0	180	1	2	2 strch
Cap'n Crunch Peanut Butter (3/4 cup)	110	22	3	<1	0	200	1	2	1 1/2 strch, 1 fat
Cap'n Crunch w/Crunchberries (3/4 cup)	100	22	2	0	0	180	1	1	1 1/2 strch
Cinnamon Crunch (1 cup)	120	25	2	NA	0	230	1	2	1 1/2 strch
Cocoa Blasts (1 cup)	130	29	1	<1	0	140	1	1	2 strch
Crunchy Corn Bran (1 cup)	90	23	1	<1	0	250	5	5	2 strch
Frosted Flakers (3/4 cup)	120	28	0	NA	0	200	0	1	2 strch
Frosted Oats (1 cup)	110	23	2	NA	0	230	1	2	1 1/2 strch
Frosted Shedded Wheat (1 cup)	200	45	1	NA	0	0	4	5	3 strch
Fruitangy Oh's (1 cup)	120	27	1	NA	0	150	1	2	2 strch

Honey Crisp Corn Flakes (3/4 cup)	110	27	0	NA	0	260	1	2	2 strch
Honey Grahams (3/4 cup)	110	23	2	NA	0	230	1	2	1 1/2 strch
Honey Nut Oats (3/4 cup)	110	24	1	NA	0	220	1	2	1 1/2 strch
Hot Oat Bran (1/2 cup)	150	25	3	<1	0	230	6	7	1 1/2 strch, 1 fat
Instant Hot Oatmeal (1 pkt)	100	19	2	0	0	80	3	4	1 1/2 strch, 1 fat
Instant Hot Oatmeal, Apple & Cinnamon (1 pkt)	130	27	2	<1	0	170	3	3	2 strch
Instant Hot Oatmeal, Bananas & Cream (1 pkt)	140	26	3	<1	0	160	2	3	2 strch, 1 fat
Instant Hot Oatmeal, Blueberry & Cream (1 pkt)	140	26	3	<1	0	180	2	3	2 strch, 1 fat
Instant Hot Oatmeal, Chocolate Chip Cookie (1 pkt)	160	32	3	<1	0	200	3	4	2 strch, 1 fat
Instant Hot Oatmeal, Cinnamon Spice (1 pkt)	170	36	2	0	0	240	3	4	2 1/2 strch
Instant Hot Oatmeal, Cookies 'n Cream (1 pkt)	160	31	3	<1	0	200	2	4	2 strch, 1 fat
Instant Hot Oatmeal, Dinosaur Eggs (1 pkt)	200	38	4	2	0	240	3	4	2 1/2 strch, 1 fat
Instant Hot Oatmeal, Maple/Brown Sugar (1 pkt)	160	33	2	0	0	240	3	4	2 strch
Instant Hot Oatmeal, Peaches & Cream (1 pkt)	140	27	3	<1	0	180	2	3	2 strch
Instant Hot Oatmeal, Raisin/Date/Walnut (1 pkt)	140	27	3	<1	0	240	3	3	2 strch, 1 fat

CEREALS

Products	Cal.	Carb. (g)	Fat (g)	Sat. Fat (g)	Chol. (mg)	Sod. (mg)	Fib. (g)	Prot. (g)	Servings/Exchanges
Instant Hot Oatmeal, S'mores (1 pkt)	160	32	3	<1	0	220	2	4	2 strch, 1 fat
Instant Hot Oatmeal, Strawberries & Cream (1 pkt)	140	27	3	<1	0	180	2	3	2 strch
King Vitamin (1 1/2 cup)	120	26	1	0	0	260	1	2	2 strch
Kretschmer Honey Crunch Wheat Germ (1 2/3 Tbsp)	50	8	1	0	0	0	1	4	1/2 strch
Kretschmer Wheat Bran (1/4 cup)	30	10	1	0	0	0	7	3	1/2 strch
Kretschmer Wheat Germ (2 Tbsp)	50	6	1	0	0	0	2	4	1/2 strch
Life (3/4 cup)	120	25	2	0	0	160	2	3	1 1/2 strch
Life, Cinnamon (3/4 cup)	120	26	1	0	0	150	2	3	2 strch
Marshmallow Safari (3/4 cup)	140	29	2	NA	0	210	1	2	2 strch
Mother's Butter Bumpers (1.2 oz)	130	26	3	<1	0	270	1	3	2 strch, 1 fat
Mother's Cinnamon Oat Crunch (2 oz)	230	48	3	<1	0	250	5	6	3 strch, 1 fat
Mother's Groovy Grahams (1 oz)	100	24	<1	0	0	240	1	2	1 1/2 strch
Mother's Harvest Oat Flakes w/Apples & Almonds (1 oz)	120	24	2	0	0	170	2	3	1 1/2 strch

Mother's Harvest Oat Flakes (1 oz)	110	23	1	0	0	200	2	3	1 1/2 strch
Mother's Honey Roundups (1 oz)	110	24	<1	0	0	170	1	2	1 1/2 strch
Mother's Toasted Oat Bran (1.1 oz)	120	24	2	0	0	200	3	4	1 1/2 strch
Multi-Grain Hot Cereal (1/2 cup)	130	29	2	0	0	10	5	5	2 strch
Oat Bran (1 1/4 cup)	210	43	3	<1	0	210	6	7	3 strch
Oh's, Honey Graham (3/4 cup)	110	23	2	<1	0	180	1	1	1 1/2 strch
Old-Fashioned Hot Oats (1/2 cup)	150	27	3	<1	0	0	4	5	2 strch, 1 fat
Popeye Puffed Rice (1 cup)	50	12	0	0	0	0	0	1	1 strch
Popeye Puffed Wheat (1 1/4 cup)	50	11	0	0	0	0	1	2	1 strch
Quick Hot Oats (1/2 cup)	150	27	3	<1	0	0	4	5	2 strch, 1 fat
Quick 'N Hearty Microwave Oatmeal, Apple Spice (1 pkt)	170	35	2	<1	0	310	3	4	2 strch
Quick 'N Hearty Microwave Oatmeal, Brown Sugar Cinnamon (1 pkt)	150	31	2	<1	0	260	3	4	2 strch
Quick 'N Hearty Microwave Oatmeal, Cinnamon Raisin (1 pkt)	170	35	2	<1	0	270	3	4	2 strch

CEREALS

Products	Cal.	Carb. (g)	Fat (g)	Sat. Fat (g)	Chol. (mg)	Sod. (mg)	Fib. (g)	Prot. (g)	Servings/Exchanges
Quick 'N Hearty Microwave Oatmeal, Honey Bran (1 pkt)	150	31	2	<1	0	250	3	4	2 strch
Quick 'N Hearty Microwave Oatmeal, Regular (1 pkt)	110	19	2	<1	0	150	2	4	1 strch
Quisp (1 cup)	110	23	2	NA	0	190	1	1	1 1/2 strch
Rice Crisps (1 cup)	110	26	0	NA	0	290	0	2	2 strch
Shredded Wheat (3 biscuits)	220	50	2	<1	0	0	7	7	3 strch
Sweet Crunch (1 cup)	110	23	2	<1	0	190	1	1	1 1/2 strch
Sweet Puffs (1 cup)	130	30	1	0	0	80	2	2	2 strch
Toasted Oatmeal, Honey Nut (1 cup)	190	40	3	NA	0	180	3	4	2 1/2 strch, 1 fat
Toasted Oatmeat, Original (1 cup)	190	40	2	NA	0	220	4	5	2 1/2 strch
Toasted Oatmeal Squares, Cinnamon (1 cup)	230	47	3	NA	0	270	5	8	3 strch, 1 fat
Toasted Oatmeal Squares, Regular (1 cup)	220	43	3	NA	0	260	4	7	3 strch, 1 fat

Toasted Oats (1 cup)	110	23	2	N/A	0	280	2	3	1 1/2 strch
Unprocessed Bran (1/3 cup)	35	11	21	0	0	0	0	8	3	1 strch
Whole-Wheat Natural Hot Cereal (1/2 cup)	130	30	1	0	0	0	4	5	2 strch

RALSTON

Sun Flakes (3/4 cup)	110	23	1	0	0	210	<1	2	1 1/2 strch

CHEESE AND CHEESE PRODUCTS

Products	Cal.	Carb. (g)	Fat (g)	Sat. Fat (g)	Chol. (mg)	Sod. (mg)	Fib. (g)	Prot. (g)	Servings/Exchanges
American Processed (1 oz)	106	<1	9	6	27	406	0	6	1 high-fat meat
Cheddar (1 oz)	114	<1	9	6	<1	176	0	7	1 high-fat meat
Cheddar/Colby, Low-Fat (1 oz)	49	<1	2	2	6	174	0	7	1 lean meat
Cheese, Fat-Free (1 oz)	37	3	0	0	0	384	0	6	1 very lean meat
Colby & Monterey Jack (1 oz)	111	0	9	6	30	192	0	7	1 high-fat meat
Cottage Cheese, 2%, Reduced-Fat (1/4 cup)	50	2	1	<1	5	227	0	8	1 very lean meat
Cottage Cheese, 4.5% (1/4 cup)	54	1	2	2	8	213	0	7	1 lean meat
Cottage Cheese, Dry (1/4 cup)	31	<1	<1	<1	2	5	0	6	1 very lean meat
Cottage Cheese, Nonfat (1/4 cup)	35	3	0	0	5	210	0	7	1 very lean meat
Feta (1 oz)	74	1	6	4	25	313	0	4	1 med-fat meat
Goat Cheese, Semi-Soft (1 oz)	103	<1	9	6	22	146	0	6	1 high-fat meat
Monterey Jack (1 oz)	106	0	9	5	27	152	0	7	1 high-fat meat
Mozzarella, Light (1 oz)	65	0	3	2	15	180	0	8	1 lean meat

Mozzarella, Part-Skim (1 oz)	72	<1	5	3	16	132	0	7	1 med-fat meat
Parmesan, Grated (2 Tbsp)	46	<1	3	2	8	186	0	4	1 lean meat
Ricotta, Part-Skim (1/4 cup)	86	3	5	3	19	78	0	7	1 med-fat meat
String Cheese Stick (1)	72	<1	5	3	16	132	0	7	1 med-fat meat
Swiss (1 oz)	107	1	8	5	26	74	0	8	1 high-fat meat
Yogurt Cheese (1 oz)	22	3	<1	<1	<1	22	0	2	free

ALPINE LACE

American (1 oz)	90	2	7	4	20	200	0	6	1 high-fat meat
Cheddar, Reduced-Fat (1 oz)	80	1	5	3	20	95	0	7	1 med-fat meat
Colby, Reduced-Fat (1 oz)	80	1	5	4	20	85	0	7	1 med-fat meat
Fat-Free Free N' Lean Singles (1 oz)	40	1	0	0	5	260	0	8	1 very lean meat
Monterey Jack, Reduced-Fat (1 oz)	80	1	5	4	15	75	0	7	1 med-fat meat
Mozzarella, Part Skim (1 oz)	70	1	5	3	15	75	0	7	1 med-fat meat
Muenster, Reduced-Sodium (1 oz)	100	1	9	6	25	85	0	7	1 high-fat meat
Provolone (1 oz)	70	1	5	5	15	85	0	7	1 med-fat meat
Swiss, Light (1 oz)	100	1	7	4	20	35	0	8	1 high-fat meat

CHEESE AND CHEESE PRODUCTS

Products	Cal.	Carb. (g)	Fat (g)	Sat. Fat (g)	Chol. (mg)	Sod. (mg)	Fib. (g)	Prot. (g)	Servings/Exchanges
Swiss, Natural (1 oz)	90	1	6	4	1	35	0	8	1 med-fat meat
BREAKSTONE									
Cottage Cheese, 1/2% Dry Curd (1/4 cup)	45	3	0	0	<5	90	0	7	1 very lean meat
Cottage Cheese, Fat Free (1/2 cup)	80	6	0	0	5	440	0	13	2 very lean meat
Cottage Cheese, 2% Low-Fat, Small Curd (1/2 cup)	90	4	3	2	15	390	0	13	2 lean meat
Cottage Cheese, 4% Milkfat, Large Curd (1/2 cup)	120	5	5	3	25	400	0	13	2 lean meat
Cottage Cheese, 4% Milkfat, Small Curd (1/2 cup)	120	5	5	3	25	400	0	13	2 lean meat
Cream Cheese, Temp-Tee Whipped (2 Tbsp)	80	<1	8	5	25	70	0	2	2 fat
Ricotta (1/4 cup)	110	3	8	5	25	90	0	7	1 high-fat meat
DI GIORNO									
100% Romano, Grated (2 tsp)	20	0	2	1	5	75	0	2	free
100% Romano, Shredded (2 Tbsp)	20	0	2	1	5	70	0	2	free
100% Parmesan, Shredded (2 Tbsp)	20	0	2	1	5	75	0	2	free

HEALTHY CHOICE

Cheese Food, Fat-Free Singles (1 oz)	40	3	0	0	5	390	0	6	1 very lean meat
Cream Cheese, Fat-Free (1 oz)	30	2	0	0	5	200	0	6	1 very lean meat
Cream Cheese, Fat-Free, Herb & Garlic (1 oz)	30	2	0	0	5	200	0	6	1 very lean meat
Mozzarella, Fat-Free Shredded (1 oz)	40	1	0	0	5	200	0	9	1 very lean meat
Mozzarella Stick, Natural Fat-Free (1 oz)	40	1	0	0	5	200	0	9	1 very lean meat
Natural Cheddar, Fat-Free, Shredded (1 oz)	40	1	0	0	5	200	0	9	1 very lean meat
Pizza Cheese, Fat-Free Shredded (1 oz)	40	1	0	0	5	200	0	9	1 very lean meat

KNUDSEN

Cottage Cheese, 2% Lowfat (1/2 cup)	100	5	3	2	15	400	0	14	2 very lean meat
Cottage Cheese, 1 1/2% Lowfat w/Pineapple (1/2 cup)	120	14	2	1	10	330	0	11	1 fruit, 2 very lean meat
Cottage Cheese, Fat-Free (1/2 cup)	80	4	0	0	5	380	0	14	2 very lean meat
Cottage Cheese On The Go! 2% Lowfat (4 oz)	90	5	2	2	15	370	0	13	2 very lean meat
Cottage Cheese On The Go!, 2% Lowfat w/ Pineapple (4 oz)	110	13	2	1	10	300	0	10	1 fruit, 1 lean meat

CHEESE AND CHEESE PRODUCTS

Products	Cal.	Carb. (g)	Fat (g)	Sat. Fat (g)	Chol. (mg)	Sod. (mg)	Fib. (g)	Prot. (g)	Servings/Exchanges
Creamed Cottage Cheese, 4%, Large Curd (1/2 cup)	130	4	5	4	30	330	0	16	2 lean meat
Creamed Cottage Cheese, 4%, Small Curd (1/2 cup)	120	4	5	4	25	400	0	14	2 lean meat
KRAFT									
American Pasteurized Processed Cheese, Light 'N' Lively (3/4 oz)	45	2	3	2	10	280	0	5	1 lean meat
Baby Swiss (1 oz)	110	0	9	6	25	110	0	7	1 high-fat meat
Cheddar (1 oz)	110	<1	9	6	30	180	0	7	1 high-fat meat
Cheddar, Fat Free, Shredded (1/4 cup)	40	1	0	0	<5	270	0	9	1 very lean meat
Cheddar, Natural 2% Reduced Fat (1 oz)	90	<1	6	4	20	240	0	7	1 med-fat meat
Cheddar, Shredded (1/4 cup)	100	<1	8	6	30	170	0	6	1 high-fat meat
Cheddar, 2% Reduced Fat Mild, Shredded (1/4 cup)	80	<1	6	4	20	220	0	7	1 med-fat meat

Food									
Cheddar, Natural 2% Reduced Fat Sharp (1 oz)	90	<1	6	4	20	240	0	7	1 med-fat meat
Cheese Spread, Bacon (2 Tbsp)	90	<1	8	5	25	570	0	5	1 high fat meat
Cheese Spread, Roka Brand Blue (2 Tbsp)	80	2	7	5	20	340	0	3	1 high fat meat
Cheese Spread, Pimento (2 Tbsp)	80	3	6	4	20	170	0	2	1 med-fat meat
Cheese Spread, Pineapple (2 Tbsp)	70	4	5	4	15	115	0	2	1 med-fat meat
Cheez Whiz Cheese Sauce (2 Tbsp)	90	3	7	5	20	540	0	4	1 med-fat meat
Cheez Whiz Light Cheese Sauce (2 Tbsp)	80	6	3	2	15	540	0	6	1/2 carb., 1 lean meat
Cheez Whiz Jalapeno Pepper Cheese Spread (2 Tbsp)	90	3	7	5	25	510	0	4	1 high-fat meat
Cheez Whiz Mild Salsa Cheese Sauce (2 Tbsp)	100	3	7	5	25	530	0	4	1 high-fat meat
Cheez Whiz Squeezable Cheese Sauce (2 Tbsp)	100	4	8	4	15	470	0	2	2 fat
Colby (1 oz)	110	<1	9	6	30	180	0	7	1 high-fat meat
Colby, Natural 2% Reduced Fat (1 oz)	80	0	6	4	20	220	0	7	1 med-fat meat
Colby & Monterey Jack, Shredded (1/4 cup)	100	<1	8	6	25	170	0	6	1 high-fat meat
Cracker Barrel, Spreadable Sharp Cheddar (2 Tbsp)	80	<1	8	5	20	180	0	3	1 high-fat meat
Cream Cheese, Neufchatel, Philadelphia (1 oz)	70	<1	6	4	20	120	0	3	1 med-fat meat
Cream Cheese, Philadelphia Brick (1 oz)	100	<1	10	6	30	90	0	2	2 fat

CHEESE AND CHEESE PRODUCTS

Products	Cal.	Carb. (g)	Fat (g)	Sat. Fat (g)	Chol. (mg)	Sod. (mg)	Fib. (g)	Prot. (g)	Servings/Exchanges
Cream Cheese, Philadelphia Brick, Fat Free (1 oz)	30	2	0	0	<5	140	0	4	1 very lean meat
Cream Cheese, Philadelphia Brick w/Chives (1 oz)	90	<1	9	6	25	135	0	2	2 fat
Cream Cheese, Philadelphia Soft (2 Tbsp)	100	1	10	7	30	100	0	2	2 fat
Cream Cheese, Philadelphia Soft, Cheesecake (2 Tbsp)	110	4	9	6	25	95	0	2	2 fat
Cream Cheese, Philadelphia Soft, Chive & Onion (2 Tbsp)	110	2	10	7	30	135	0	1	2 fat
Cream Cheese, Philadelphia Soft, Fat-Free (2 Tbsp)	30	2	0	0	<5	200	0	5	1 very lean meat
Cream Cheese, Philadelphia Soft, Light (2 Tbsp)	70	2	5	4	15	150	0	3	1 fat
Cream Cheese, Philadelphia Soft, Honey Nut (2 Tbsp)	110	4	10	6	30	150	0	2	2 fat
Cream Cheese, Philadelphia Soft, Pineapple (2 Tbsp)	100	4	9	6	25	100	0	1	2 fat
Cream Cheese, Philadelphia Soft, Smoked Salmon (2 Tbsp)	100	1	9	6	30	200	0	2	2 fat

Food									
Cream Cheese, Philadelphia Soft, Strawberry (2 Tbsp)	110	5	9	6	25	100	0	1	2 fat
Cream Cheese, Philadelphia Whipped (2 Tbsp)	70	<1	7	5	25	85	0	1	1 fat
Grated Nonfat Topping (2 tsp)	15	3	0	0	0	75	0	<1	free
Grated Parm Plus!, Garlic Herb (2 tsp)	15	2	0	0	0	75	0	<1	free
Grated Parm Plus!, Zesty Red Pepper (2 tsp)	15	2	0	0	0	110	0	<1	free
Loaf Old English Sharp Pasteurized Processed American (1 oz)	100	<1	9	5	25	370	0	6	1 high-fat meat
Monterey Jack (1 oz)	110	0	9	6	30	190	0	6	1 high-fat meat
Monterey Jack, Natural 2% Reduced Fat (1 oz)	80	<1	6	4	20	240	0	7	1 med-fat meat
Monterey Jack, Shredded (1/4 cup)	100	<1	8	6	<1	170	0	6	1 high-fat meat
Monterey Jack & Jalapeño Pepper (1 oz)	110	<1	9	6	30	190	0	7	1 high-fat meat
Mozzarella, Fat-Free Natural, Shredded (1/4 cup)	45	2	0	0	<5	340	<1	9	1 very lean meat
Mozzarella, Whole-Milk, Shredded (1/3 cup)	100	1	8	5	25	220	0	7	1 high-fat meat
Mozzarella, Part-Skim (1 oz)	80	<1	5	4	15	200	0	8	1 med-fat meat
Mozzarella, Part-Skim, String Cheese (1 piece)	80	0	6	4	20	240	0	7	1 med-fat meat

CHEESE AND CHEESE PRODUCTS

Products	Cal.	Carb. (g)	Fat (g)	Sat. Fat (g)	Chol. (mg)	Sod. (mg)	Fib. (g)	Prot. (g)	Servings/Exchanges
Parmesan, Grated (2 tsp)	20	0	2	1	2	75	0	2	free
Pizza Cheese, Smoke-Flavored Mozzarella & Provolone (1/4 cup)	90	<1	7	5	20	200	0	6	1 high-fat meat
Pizza Style Four-Cheese, Shredded (1/4 cup)	90	<1	7	5	20	220	0	6	1 high-fat meat
Provolone Cheese Slices w/Smoke Flavor (1 slice)	150	<1	11	8	35	370	0	11	1 1/2 high-fat meat
Romano, Grated (2 tsp)	20	0	2	1	<5	70	0	2	free
Singles American 2% Reduced Fat (3/4-oz slice)	50	2	3	2	10	320	0	5	1 lean meat
Singles American Pasteurized Processed Cheese (3/4 oz)	70	2	5	4	15	280	0	4	1 med-fat meat
Singles Fat-Free Pasteurized Processed American Cheese Slice (3/4 oz slice)	30	2	0	0	<5	290	0	5	1 very lean meat
Singles Fat-Free Pasteurized Processed Sharp Cheddar Cheese (2/3 oz slice)	35	3	0	0	3	300	0	5	1 very lean meat

Singles Fat-Free Pasteurized Processed Swiss Cheese (3/4 oz slice)	30	3	0	0	0	270	0	5	1 very lean meat
Singles Fat-Free Pasteurized Processed White Cheese (3/4 oz slice)	30	3	0	0	<5	300	0	5	1 very lean meat
Singles Pasteurized Processed Cheese Food w/Pimento (3/4 oz slice)	70	2	5	4	15	290	0	4	1 med-fat meat
Singles Pasteurized Processed Monterey Cheese (3/4 oz slice)	70	2	5	4	15	290	0	4	1 med-fat meat
Singles Pasteurized Processed Sharp Cheddar Cheese (3/4 oz)	70	2	5	4	15	290	0	4	1 med-fat meat
Singles Pasteurized Processed Sharp Cheddar Cheese (3/4 oz slice)	70	<1	6	4	20	300	0	4	1 med-fat meat
Singles Pasteurized Processed Swiss Cheese Food (3/4 oz slice)	70	1	5	4	15	320	0	4	1 med-fat meat
Singles Pasteurized Processed White American Cheese (3/4 oz slice)	70	2	5	4	2	280	0	4	1 med-fat meat

CHEESE AND CHEESE PRODUCTS

Products	Cal.	Carb. (g)	Fat (g)	Sat. Fat (g)	Chol. (mg)	Sod. (mg)	Fib. (g)	Prot. (g)	Servings/Exchanges
Swiss Cheese, Shredded (1/3 cup)	100	<1	8	5	25	45	0	7	1 high-fat meat
Swiss Cheese Slices, 2% Reduced Fat (1 slice)	130	<1	9	6	25	90	0	11	1 1/2 med-fat meat
Taco Cheese, Shredded (1/3 cup)	120	1	10	7	30	240	0	7	1 high-fat meat
Velveeta Cheese Spread (1 oz)	90	3	6	4	25	420	0	5	1 med-fat meat
Velveeta Cheese Spread, Mexican, Mild or Hot (1 oz)	90	3	6	4	20	420	0	5	1 med-fat meat
Velveeta Reduced Fat Processed Cheese (1 oz)	60	3	3	2	10	440	0	5	1 lean meat
Velveeta Shredded Pasteurized Processed Cheese Food (1/4 cup)	130	3	9	6	30	500	0	8	1 high-fat meat
LIFETIME									
Cheddar, Fat-Free (1 oz)	40	1	0	0	5	225	0	8	1 very lean meat
Cheddar, Fat-Free (1/4 cup)	45	1	0	0	5	244	0	9	1 very lean meat
Mexican Cheese, Fat-Free, Mild (1 oz)	40	1	0	0	5	225	0	8	1 very lean meat
Monterey Jack, Fat-Free (1 oz)	40	1	0	0	5	225	0	8	1 very lean meat
Mozzarella, Fat-Free (1/4 cup)	44	1	0	0	5	244	0	9	1 very lean meat

Food									
Swiss, Fat-Free (1 oz)	40	1	0	0	5	225	0	8	1 very lean meat
SARGENTO									
Edam Cheese (1 oz)	100	<1	8	NA	25	270	0	7	1 high-fat meat
Feta Cheese	80	1	6	NA	25	320	0	4	1 high-fat meat
Italian Style Cheese, Grated (1 oz)	110	1	8	NA	26	105	0	8	1 high-fat meat
Limburger Cheese (1 oz)	90	<1	8	NA	25	230	0	4	1 high-fat meat
Taco Cheese (1 oz)	110	<1	9	NA	27	160	0	7	1 high-fat meat
STELLA FOODS									
Aged Provolone (1 oz)	100	<1	8	5	20	290	0	7	1 high-fat meat
Blue Cheese (1 oz)	100	<1	8	5	20	390	0	6	1 high-fat meat
Feta (1 oz)	80	1	6	5	25	310	0	5	1 med-fat meat
Fontinella (1 oz)	100	<1	7	4	30	330	0	8	1 high-fat meat
Italian Cheese, Sharp (1 oz)	100	<1	7	5	30	330	0	8	1 high-fat meat
Lorraine Cheese, Smoked (1 oz)	110	<1	9	5	25	30	0	7	1 high-fat meat
Lorraine Cheese w/Chive & Onion (1 oz)	110	<1	9	5	25	30	0	7	1 high-fat meat
Mozzarella (1 oz)	80	<1	6	4	15	180	0	8	1 med-fat meat

CHEESE AND CHEESE PRODUCTS

Products	Cal.	Carb. (g)	Fat (g)	Sat. Fat (g)	Chol. (mg)	Sod. (mg)	Fib. (g)	Prot. (g)	Servings/Exchanges
Mozzarella, Whole-Milk (1 oz)	90	<1	7	5	20	180	0	6	1 high-fat meat
Parmesan, Dried Grated (1 Tbsp)	35	0	3	2	10	130	0	3	1 fat
Provolone, Lite (1 oz)	70	<1	4	2	20	120	0	8	1 med-fat meat
Provolone, Mello (1 oz)	100	<1	7	4	20	290	0	7	1 high-fat meat
Ricotta, Part-Skim (1/4 cup)	85	3	5	3	20	75	0	7	1 med-fat meat
Romano, Fresh Grated (1 Tbsp)	30	0	2	2	5	75	0	2	1 fat
WEIGHT WATCHERS									
Cheddar, Natural Mild Yellow (1 oz)	80	1	5	3	15	150	0	8	1 med-fat meat
Cheddar Cheese Slices, Fat-Free, Sharp (2 slices)	30	2	0	0	0	310	0	?	1 very lean meat
Cheddar Cheese Spread, Sharp (2 Tbsp)	70	7	3	2	10	190	0	4	1/2 strch, 1 lean meat
Colby Cheese, Natural (1 oz)	80	1	5	2	15	130	0	8	1 med-fat meat
Cottage Cheese, 1% (1/2 cup)	90	4	1	<1	NA	460	0	14	2 very lean meat
Cottage Cheese, 2% (1/2 cup)	100	4	2	2	NA	460	0	14	2 very lean meat
Cream Cheese, Substitute (1 oz)	35	1	2	1	NA	40	0	3	1 fat

Barnes & Noble Booksellers
4140 W Jefferson Blvd. Bldg J
Ft. Wayne IN 46804
(219) 432-3343
08-10-03 S02036 R002

Courtship   7.50
0515127213
Diabetes Carbohydrate an   14.95
1580400507

SUB TOTAL   22.45
SALES TAX   1.35
TOTAL   23.80

AMOUNT TENDERED
CASH   25.00

TOTAL PAYMENT   25.00
CHANGE   1.20
        Thank you for Shopping at
        Barnes & Noble Booksellers
#93891 08-10-03 12:39P jr

days with a receipt from any Barnes & Noble store.

Store Credit issued for new and unread books and unopened music after 30 days or without a sales receipt. Credit issued at <u>lowest sale price</u>.
We gladly accept returns of new and unread books and unopened music from bn.com with a bn.com receipt for store credit at the bn.com price.

Full refund issued for new and unread books and unopened music within 30 days with a receipt from any Barnes & Noble store.
Store Credit issued for new and unread books and unopened music after 30 days or without a sales receipt. Credit issued at <u>lowest sale price</u>.
We gladly accept returns of new and unread books and unopened music from bn.com with a bn.com receipt for store credit at the bn.com price.

Full refund issued for new and unread books and unopened music within 30 days with a receipt from any Barnes & Noble store.
Store Credit issued for new and unread books and unopened music after 30 days or without a sales receipt. Credit issued at <u>lowest sale price</u>.
We gladly accept returns of new and unread books and unopened music from bn.com with a bn.com receipt for store credit at the bn.com price.

Full refund issued for new and unread books and unopened music within 30 days with a receipt from any Barnes & Noble store.

Monterey Jack, Natural (1 oz)	80	1	5	2	15	120	0	8	1 med-fat meat
Mozarella Cheese, Natural Shredded (1 oz)	80	1	4	2	15	150	0	8	1 med-fat meat
Parmesan Italian Topping, Fat-Free, Grated (1 tsp)	15	2	0	0	0	45	0	?	free
Swiss Cheese Slices, Natural (1 oz)	90	1	5	3	15	50	0	9	1 med-fat meat

COMBINATION FOODS AND FROZEN ENTREES

Products	Cal.	Carb. (g)	Fat (g)	Sat. Fat (g)	Chol. (mg)	Sod. (mg)	Fib. (g)	Prot. (g)	Servings/Exchanges
Beef Burgundy (1 cup)	285	10	11	3	91	110	2	34	1/2 carb., 5 lean meat
Beef Stroganoff & Noodles (1 cup)	342	21	20	8	73	454	2	20	1 1/2 carb., 2 med-fat meat, 2 fat
Beef w/Macaroni & Tomato Sauce, Homemade (1 cup)	254	26	10	4	39	862	3	16	2 carb., 2 med-fat meat
Burrito, Bean (1)	224	36	7	4	2	493	4	7	2 1/2 carb., 1 fat
Burrito, Beef (1)	262	30	11	6	32	746	<1	13	2 carb., 1 med-fat meat, 1 fat
Cabbage Rolls, Stuffed (8 oz)	179	23	6	1	11	551	4	8	1 1/2 carb., 1 med-fat meat, 1 fat
Chicken & Noodles, Homemade (1 cup)	367	26	19	6	96	600	2	22	2 carb., 2 med-fat meat, 2 fat
Chicken a la King, Homemade (1 cup)	468	12	34	13	186	760	1	27	1 carb., 3 med-fat meat, 4 fat
Chicken Tetrazzini (1 cup)	372	28	20	7	50	813	2	19	2 carb., 2 med-fat meat, 2 fat
Chiles Rellenos (1)	425	7	35	17	165	620	1	23	1/2 carb., 3 med-fat meat, 4 fat

Food									Exchanges
Chili Con Carne w/Beans & Rice (1 cup)	297	46	8	4	25	1162	6	11	3 carb, 2 fat
Chili Con Carne, w/o Beans (1 cup)	350	21	19	7	81	1407	4	25	1 1/2 carb, 3 med-fat meat, 1 fat
Chimichanga, Beef & Bean (1)	249	26	12	3	24	242	3	11	2 carb, 1 med-fat meat, 1 fat
Chop Suey, Shrimp, w/Noodles (1 cup)	277	22	12	2	122	937	2	21	1 1/2 carb, 2 med-fat meat
Chop Suey & Noodles, Beef (1 cup)	425	31	25	5	46	818	3	22	2 carb, 2 med-fat meat, 3 fat
Chow Mein, Beef, No Noodles (1 cup)	275	12	16	4	54	774	2	22	1 carb, 3 med-fat meat
Chow Mein, Shrimp, w/Noodles (1 cup)	277	22	12	2	122	937	2	21	1 1/2 carb, 2 med-fat meat
Corndog (1)	460	56	19	5	79	973	NA	17	4 carb, 1 med-fat meat, 3 fat
Corned Beef Hash, Canned (1 cup)	398	24	25	12	73	1188	1	19	1 1/2 carb, 2 med-fat meat, 3 fat
Curry, Beef (1 cup)	437	13	32	7	70	1323	3	27	1 carb, 3 med-fat meat, 3 fat
Eggplant Parmesan (1 cup)	320	17	22	10	57	683	3	15	1 carb, 2 med-fat meat, 2 fat
Enchilada, Beef & Cheese (1)	323	31	18	9	40	1319	NA	12	2 carb, 1 med-fat meat, 3 fat
Enchilada, Chicken (1)	195	16	9	4	36	312	2	13	1 carb, 2 med-fat meat
Fajita, Chicken (1)	405	50	13	3	41	439	4	22	3 carb, 2 med-fat meat, 1 fat

COMBINATION FOODS & FROZEN ENTREES

Products	Cal.	Carb. (g)	Fat (g)	Sat. Fat (g)	Chol. (mg)	Sod. (mg)	Fib. (g)	Prot. (g)	Servings/Exchanges
Goulash, Beef, w/Noodles (1 cup)	341	23	14	4	88	457	2	30	1 1/2 carb., 3 med-fat meat
Lasagna (8 oz)	302	27	12	NA	34	885	NA	22	2 carb., 2 med-fat meat
Macaroni & Cheese (1 cup)	228	26	10	4	NA	730	NA	9	2 carb., 2 med-fat meat
Meat Loaf, Beef & 1/3 Pork (1 slice)	205	5	14	5	84	381	<1	15	2 med-fat meat, 1 fat
Meat Tamale (1)	183	16	10	4	24	229	3	7	1 carb., 1 med-fat meat, 1 fat
Meat Tortellini (1 cup)	372	33	15	5	238	797	1	25	2 carb., 3 med-fat meat
Moo Goo Gai Pan (1 cup)	281	12	20	5	39	327	3	15	2 vegetable, 2 med-fat meat, 2 fat
Pepper, Stuffed Green Bell (1)	229	20	12	5	34	201	2	11	1 carb., 1 vegetable, 2 med-fat meat, 2 fat
Pizza, Cheese, Thin Crust (1/4 of 10-inch)	317	28	17	7	20	770	NA	14	2 carb., 2 med-fat meat, 1 fat
Pizza, Meat, Thin Crust (1/4 of 10-inch)	368	29	21	7	29	1000	NA	15	2 carb., 2 med-fat meat, 2 fat
Pot Pie (7 oz)	450	35	28	NA	34	778	NA	13	2 carb., 2 med-fat meat, 4 fat
Quesadilla (1)	199	21	10	4	14	255	1	6	1 1/2 carb., 2 fat

Food									Exchanges/Choices
Quiche Lorraine (1/8 pie)	508	20	39	18	205	549	<1	20	1 carb, 3 med-fat meat, 5 fat
Ravioli, Cheese w/Tomato Sauce (1)	336	38	14	6	160	1541	2	14	2 1/2 carb., 1 med-fat meat, 2 fat
Salad, Carrot Raisin (1/2 cup)	202	21	14	2	10	117	2	1	1/2 fruit, 2 vegetable, 3 fat
Salad, Chef-Style (1 1/2 cup)	267	5	16	8	140	743	NA	26	1 vegetable, 3 med-fat meat
Salad, Egg (1/2 cup)	293	2	28	6	287	333	0	8	1 med-fat meat, 5 fat
Salad, Potato, No Egg (1/2 cup)	134	16	7	1	5	345	2	2	1 carb., 1 fat
Salad, Seafood (1/2 cup)	166	3	12	2	64	274	<1	13	2 med-fat meat
Salad, Shrimp (1/2 cup)	141	3	9	2	103	196	<1	13	2 med-fat meat
Salad, Three-Bean (1/2 cup)	70	7	4	<1	0	257	2	2	1/2 carb., 1 fat
Salad, Tuna (1/2 cup)	192	10	10	2	13	412	0	16	1/2 carb., 2 med-fat meat
Salad, Waldorf (1/2 cup)	201	6	20	2	10	118	1	2	1/2 fruit, 4 fat
Salmon Patty/Cake (4.5 oz)	261	14	16	4	57	657	1	16	1 carb., 2 med-fat meat, 1 fat
Shepherd's Pie, Beef (1 cup)	287	31	10	3	41	702	3	18	2 carb., 2 med-fat meat
Sloppy Joe Gravy/Sauce, Beef (1 cup)	380	24	23	9	81	1246	3	21	1 1/2 carb., 2 med-fat meat, 3 fat

COMBINATION FOODS & FROZEN ENTREES

Products	Cal.	Carb. (g)	Fat (g)	Sat. Fat (g)	Chol. (mg)	Sod. (mg)	Fib. (g)	Prot. (g)	Servings/Exchanges
Spaghetti w/Meatballs (1 cup)	258	29	10	2	NA	1220	NA	12	2 carb., 2 med-fat meat
Shrimp, Stuffed (1 cup)	276	9	14	3	221	694	<1	28	1/2 carb., 4 lean meat
Shrimp w/Noodles & Cheese Sauce (1 cup)	350	24	15	6	220	698	2	28	1 1/2 carb., 3 med-fat meat
Souffle, Cheese, Homemade (1 cup)	197	6	14	6	194	299	<1	12	2 med-fat meat, 1 fat
Souffle, Spinach (1 cup)	219	3	18	7	184	763	3	12	2 med-fat meat, 2 fat
Sukiyaki (1 cup)	175	6	8	3	154	762	1	19	1/2 carb., 3 lean meat
Swedish Meatballs w/Cream Sauce (1 cup)	404	17	23	10	162	1157	<1	31	1 carb., 4 med-fat meat, 1 fat
Sweet & Sour Pork w/Rice (1 cup)	269	40	6	2	29	906	1	13	2 1/2 carb., 1 med-fat meat
Taco, Chicken (1)	173	9	8	3	45	106	1	15	1/2 carb., 2 med-fat meat
Tostada, Bean & Cheese (1)	223	27	10	5	30	543	7	10	2 carb., 1 med-fat meat, 1 fat
Tostada, Bean & Chicken (1)	248	18	11	5	53	434	3	20	1 carb., 2 med-fat meat
Tuna-Noodle Casserole (9 oz)	259	34	8	NA	NA	1043	NA	13	2 carb., 2 med-fat meat
Turkey-Noodle Casserole (1 cup)	326	29	13	4	84	732	2	23	2 carb., 2 med-fat meat, 2 fat
Veal Parmigiana (1 cup)	350	15	20	8	138	755	1	27	1 strch, 3 med-fat meat

ARMOUR CLASSICS

Chicken & Noodle Dinner (11 oz)	230	23	7	NA	50	160	NA	19	1 1/2 carb., 2 med-fat meat
Chicken Fettuccine Dinner (11 oz)	260	28	9	NA	50	660	NA	17	2 carb., 2 med-fat meat
Chicken Mesquite Dinner (9.5 oz)	370	42	16	NA	55	660	NA	15	3 carb., 2 med-fat meat, 1 fat
Chicken Parmigiana Dinner (11.5 oz)	370	27	19	NA	75	1060	NA	22	2 carb., 2 med-fat meat, 2 fat
Chicken, Wine & Mushroom Dinner (10.75 oz)	280	24	11	NA	50	900	NA	22	1 1/2 carb., 3 med-fat meat
Glazed Chicken Dinner (10.75 oz)	300	24	16	NA	60	960	NA	15	1 1/2 carb., 2 med-fat meat, 1 fat
Meat Loaf Dinner (1 oz)	300	33	10	5		600			2 carb., 2 med-fat meat
Salisbury Steak Dinner (11.25 oz)	350	26	17	NA	55	1430	NA	22	2 carb., 2 med-fat meat, 1 fat
Swedish Meatballs Dinner (11.25 oz)	330	23	18	NA	80	1140	NA	19	1 1/2 carb., 2 med-fat meat, 2 fat
Turkey & Dressing Dinner (11.5 oz)	320	34	12	NA	50	1280	NA	19	2 carb., 2 med-fat meat
Veal Parmigiana Dinner (11.25 oz)	400	34	22	NA	55	1220	NA	18	2 carb., 1 med-fat meat, 3 fat

ARMOUR LITE

Beef Steak Dinner (10 oz)	290	25	9	NA	30	440	NA	27	1 1/2 carb., 3 lean meat

COMBINATION FOODS & FROZEN ENTREES

Products	Cal.	Carb. (g)	Fat (g)	Sat. Fat (g)	Chol. (mg)	Sod. (mg)	Fib. (g)	Prot. (g)	Servings/Exchanges
Chicken Burgundy Dinner (10 oz)	210	25	2	NA	45	780	NA	23	1 1/2 carb., 3 very lean meat
Shrimp Creole Dinner (11.25 oz)	260	53	2	NA	45	900	NA	6	3 1/2 carb.
Sweet & Sour Chicken (11 oz)	240	39	2	NA	35	870	NA	18	2 1/2 carb., 2 very lean meat
BANQUET									
Beef Enchilada Meal (11 oz)	370	54	12	5	20	1330	8	10	3 1/2 carb., 1 med-fat meat, 1 fat
Beef Patty w/Country Style Vegetables (9.5 oz)	310	22	20	8	40	1090	3	11	1 1/2 carb., 1 med-fat meat, 3 fat
Cheese Enchilada Meal (11 oz)	380	56	10	4	20	1500	9	12	4 carb., 1 med-fat meat, 1 fat
Chicken & Dumplings w/Gravy Meal (10 oz)	270	35	9	3	40	780	3	13	2 carb., 1 med-fat meat, 1 fat
Chicken Chow Mein Meal (9 oz)	210	28	7	2	30	850	3	9	2 carb., 1 med-fat meat
Chicken Fried Beef Steak Meal (10 oz)	420	39	23	12	35	1200	4	15	2 1/2 carb., 1 med-fat meat, 4 fat
Chicken Parmigiana Meal (9.5 oz)	320	29	15	5	50	900	3	10	2 carb., 2 med-fat meat, 1 fat

									Exchanges
Chicken Enchilada Meal (11 oz)	350	54	10	3	25	1580	9	12	3 1/2 carb., 1 med-fat meat, 1 fat
Extra Helping Chicken Fried Beef Steak Dinner (16 oz)	820	63	50	23	70	2260	8	29	4 carb., 2 med-fat meat, 8 fat
Extra Helping Meat Loaf Dinner (16 oz)	610	24	40	15	110	1940	6	29	3 carb., 3 med-fat meat, 5 fat
Extra Helping Salisbury Steak Dinner (16.5 oz)	740	37	54	21	130	2200	7	27	2 1/2 carb., 3 med-fat meat, 8 fat
Extra Helping Turkey & Gravy w/Dressing Dinner (17 oz)	630	57	32	5	80	2250	10	28	4 carb., 3 med-fat meat, 1 fat
Chicken Lo Mein (10.5 oz)	270	43	6	1		1060			3 carb., 1 fat
Chicken Pasta Primavera (9.5 oz)	320	40	12	5	25	840	5	11	3 carb., 1 med-fat meat, 1 fat
Fettuccine Alfredo (9.5 oz)	350	40	15	7	25	850	4	11	2 1/2 carb., 1 med-fat meat, 2 fat
Grilled Chicken (9.9 oz)	330	37	13	3	50	1210	3	16	2 1/2 strch, 1 med-fat meat, 2 fat

COMBINATION FOODS & FROZEN ENTREES

Products	Cal.	Carb. (g)	Fat (g)	Sat. Fat (g)	Chol. (mg)	Sod. (mg)	Fib. (g)	Prot. (g)	Servings/Exchanges
Lasagna w/Meat Sauce (9.5 oz)	260	38	8	2	10	820	5	10	2 1/2 carb., 1 med-fat meat, 1 fat
Macaroni & Cheese (9.5 oz)	320	44	11	4	20	970	4	11	3 carb., 1 med-fat meat, 1 fat
Mexican-Style Enchilada Combination Meal (11 oz)	360	55	11	5	20	1390	9	10	3 1/2 carb., 1 med-fat meat, 1 fat
Oriental-Style Chicken w/Egg Rolls (9 oz)	260	36	9	3	40	790	3	10	2 carb., 1 med-fat meat, 1 fat
Pasta w/White Cheddar Broccoli (9.5 oz)	320	48	11	6	15	810	4	11	3 carb., 1 med-fat meat, 1 fat
Pork Cutlet Meal (10.25 oz)	420	38	25	7	38	1060	4	11	2 1/2 carb., 1 med-fat meat, 4 fat
Pot Pie, Beef (7 oz)	400	38	23	11	30	1000	1	9	2 1/2 carb., 5 fat
Pot Pie, Chicken (7 oz)	380	36	22	9	40	950	1	10	2 1/2 carb., 4 fat
Pot Pie, Vegetable Cheese (7 oz)	340	39	17	7	10	920	1	6	2 1/2 carb., 3 fat
Salisbury Steak Meal (9.5 oz)	380	28	24	12	60	1140	4	12	2 carb., 2 med-fat meat, 1 fat
Southern Fried Chicken Meal (8.75 oz)	560	40	33	8	100	1540	3	26	2 1/2 carb., 3 med-fat meat, 4 fat

Food	Cal	Carb	Fat	Sat Fat	Chol	Sod	Fiber	Prot	Exchanges
Turkey & Gravy w/Dressing Meal (9.25 oz)	270	30	11	4	55	1060	3	14	2 carb., 2 med-fat meat
Veal Parmigiana Meal (9 oz)	360	35	19	6	25	960	7	13	2 carb., 1 med-fat meat, 2 fat
Vegetable Lasagna (10.5 oz)	260	41	6	2		850		3	3 carb., 1 fat
White Meat Fried Chicken Meal (8.75 oz)	480	40	28	11	100	1100	3	18	2 1/2 carb., 2 med-fat meat, 4 fat

BETTY CROCKER

Food	Cal	Carb	Fat	Sat Fat	Chol	Sod	Fiber	Prot	Exchanges
Chicken Helper, Cheddar & Broccoli (1 cup)	310	30	9	3	65	780	1	28	2 carb., 3 lean meat
Chicken Helper, Chicken & Herb Rice (1 cup)	260	26	7	2	60	490	<1	24	2 carb., 2 lean meat
Chicken Helper, Chicken & Stuffing (1 cup)	290	28	9	2	60	830	1	25	2 carb., 3 lean meat
Chicken Helper, Chicken Fried Rice (1 cup)	260	23	8	2	120	730	1	24	1 1/2 carb., 3 lean meat
Chicken Helper, Fettuccine Alfredo (1 cup)	290	28	8	3	65	830	1	26	2 carb., 3 lean meat
Chicken Helper, Roasted Garlic (1 cup)	290	29	8	3	65	730	1	27	2 carb., 3 lean meat
Hamburger Helper, Beef Taco (1 cup)	280	31	10	4	50	960	2	19	2 carb., 2 med-fat meat
Hamburger Helper, Beef Teriyaki (1 cup)	290	34	10	4	50	990	2	18	2 carb., 2 med-fat meat
Hamburger Helper, Cheeseburger Macaroni (1 cup)	360	33	16	6	65	940	1	23	2 carb., 2 med-fat meat, 1 fat

COMBINATION FOODS & FROZEN ENTREES

Products	Cal.	Carb. (g)	Fat (g)	Sat. Fat (g)	Chol. (mg)	Sod. (mg)	Fib. (g)	Prot. (g)	Servings/Exchanges
Hamburger Helper, Cheesy Hashbrowns (1 cup)	400	39	19	6	60	530	2	21	2 1/2 carb., 2 med-fat meat, 2 fat
Hamburger Helper, Fettuccine Alfredo (1 cup)	300	26	13	6	55	860	0	20	2 carb., 2 med-fat meat, 1 fat
Hamburger Helper Lasagna (1 cup)	270	29	10	4	50	1000	2	19	2 carb., 2 med-fat meat
Hamburger Helper, Mushroom & Wild Rice (1 cup)	310	30	12	5	55	880	2	20	2 carb., 2 med-fat meat
Hamburger Helper, Pizzabake (1 cup)	270	28	10	4	45	720	<1	17	2 carb., 2 med-fat meat
Hamburger Helper, Potato Stroganoff (1 cup)	260	24	11	5	50	880	2	18	1 1/2 carb., 2 med-fat meat
Hamburger Helper, Potatoes AuGratin (1 cup)	280	25	13	5	55	730	2	18	1 1/2 carb., 2 med-fat meat, 1 fat
Hamburger Helper, Rice Oriental (1 cup)	280	32	10	4	50	990	0	18	2 carb., 2 med-fat meat
Hamburger Helper, Stroganoff (1 cup)	320	30	13	5	55	830	0	21	2 carb., 2 med-fat meat, 1 fat
Skillet Chicken Helper, Stir-Fried Chicken (1 cup)	270	30	9	2	105	760	1	18	2 carb., 2 med-fat meat
Suddenly Salad, Caesar (3/4 cup)	220	30	9	2	0	580	1	5	2 carb., 2 fat
Suddenly Salad, Classic Pasta (3/4 cup)	250	38	8	1	0	910	2	7	2 1/2 carb., 2 fat

Food									
Suddenly Salad, Ranch & Bacon (3/4 cup)	330	30	20	3	15	480	1	7	2 carb., 4 fat
Suddenly Salad, Roasted Garlic Parmesan (3/4 cup)	260	33	11	2	10	770	1	7	2 carb., 2 fat
Tuna Helper, Cheesy Broccoli (1 cup)	290	38	9	3	20	860	1	15	2 1/2 carb., 2 med-fat meat
Tuna Helper, Creamy Pasta (1 cup)	300	31	13	4	20	910	1	14	2 carb., 1 med-fat meat, 1 fat
Tuna Helper, Fettuccine Alfredo (1 cup)	310	32	14	4	15	950	1	14	2 carb., 2 med-fat meat, 1 fat
Tuna Helper, Pasta Salad (2/3 cup)	380	26	27	3	10	730	1	10	2 carb., 1 med-fat meat, 4 fat
Tuna Helper, Tetrazzini (1 cup)	300	34	12	4	20	1040	1	14	2 carb., 2 med-fat meat
Tuna Helper, Tuna Melt (1 cup)	300	34	13	4	20	900	1	12	2 carb., 1 med-fat meat, 1 fat
Tuna Helper, Tuna Pot Pie (1 cup)	440	40	24	7	10	1080	1	18	2 1/2 carb., 2 med-fat meat, 3 fat
BIRD'S EYE CLASSIC									
Broccoli w/Cauliflower Carrot Butter (1/2 cup)	55	8	2	1	5	240	3	2	2 vegetable
Broccoli w/Cheese Sauce (1/2 cup)	70	7	3	2	0	425	2	4	1 vegetable, 1 fat
Cauliflower w/Cheese Sauce (1/2 cup)	65	7	3	2	7	380	2	4	1 vegetable, 1 fat
Peas & Potatoes w/Cream Sauce (1/2 cup)	75	12	2	<1	4	380	3	4	1 strch
Small Onions w/Cream Sauce (1/2 cup)	60	10	2	<1	4	325	2	2	2 vegetable

COMBINATION FOODS & FROZEN ENTREES

Products	Cal.	Carb. (g)	Fat (g)	Sat. Fat (g)	Chol. (mg)	Sod. (mg)	Fib. (g)	Prot. (g)	Servings/Exchanges
Sweet Corn w/Butter Sauce (1/2 cup)	115	23	3	1	5	215	2	3	1 1/2 strch, 1 fat
BUDGET GOURMET									
Beef SirloinTips w/Country Gravy (10 oz)	310	21	18	NA	40	570	NA	16	1 1/2 carb., 2 med-fat meat, 2 fat
Beef Stroganoff (8.6 oz)	250	30	7	4	35	580	4	16	2 carb., 2 lean meat
Chicken & Fettuccine (10 oz)	380	33	19	10	85	810	3	20	2 carb., 2 med-fat meat, 2 fat
Chinese Style Vegetables w/Chicken (10 oz)	280	47	7	1	10	590	NA	11	3 carb., 1 fat
Fettuccine w/Meat Sauce (10 oz)	290	34	10	NA	25	980	NA	16	2 carb., 1 med-fat meat, 1 fat
Lasagna, Three-Cheese (10 oz)	370	38	16	10	60	870	5	20	2 1/2 carb., 2 med-fat meat, 1 fat
Light & Healthy Oriental Chicken (9 oz)	280	44	6	1	20	690	NA	19	3 carb., 1 med-fat meat
Linguine w/Shrimp (10 oz)	330	33	15	NA	75	1250	NA	15	2 carb., 1 med-fat meat, 2 fat
Pepper Steak & Rice (10 oz)	290	38	8	3	40	1060	4	18	2 1/2 carb., 2 med-fat meat

Item									Exchanges
Potato & Broccoli w/Cheese Sauce (10.5 oz)	300	40	10	4	30	740	NA	13	2 1/2 carb., 1 med-fat meat, 1 fat
Rigatoni in Cream Sauce (10.8 oz)	290	44	7	3	30	710	NA	19	3 carb., 1 med-fat meat
Roasted Chicken (11.2 oz)	280	34	7	NA	40	1110	NA	19	2 carb., 2 med-fat meat, 2 fat
Seafood Marinara (11.5 oz)	320	43	9	NA	70	690	NA	16	3 carb., 1 med-fat meat, 3 fat
Seafood Newburg (10 oz)	350	43	12	NA	70	660	NA	17	3 carb., 1 med-fat meat, 1 fat
Side Dish, Macaroni & Cheese (5.3 oz)	210	23	8	NA	25	370	NA	9	1 1/2 carb., 1 med-fat meat, 1 fat
Side Dish, Spinach Au Gratin (5.5 oz)	221	12	17	8	40	410	2	7	1 carb., 1 med-fat meat, 2 fat
Shrimp & Fettuccine (9.5 oz)	375	38	20	NA	145	660	NA	10	2 1/2 carb., 1 med-fat meat, 3 fat
Sirloin Salisbury Steak (8.6 oz)	240	27	8	3	40	550	2	16	2 carb., 2 med-fat meat
Special Selections Beef Stroganoff (9 oz)	260	28	8	4	35	500	3	18	2 carb., 2 med-fat meat
Special Selections French Recipe Chicken (9 oz)	200	19	8	3	30	950	4	13	1 1/2 carb., 1 med-fat meat, 1 fat
Special Selections Lasagna w/Meat Sauce (10 oz)	250	31	7	3	30	690	3	15	2 carb., 1 med-fat meat

COMBINATION FOODS & FROZEN ENTREES

Products	Cal.	Carb. (g)	Fat (g)	Sat. Fat (g)	Chol. (mg)	Sod. (mg)	Fib. (g)	Prot. (g)	Servings/Exchanges
Special Selections Mandarin Chicken (10 oz)	250	37	5	1	45	850	4	16	2 1/2 carb., 1 med-fat meat
Special Selections, Turkey w/Scalloped Noodles (9 oz)	440	44	20	10	115	840	2	19	3 carb., 1 med-fat meat, 3 fat
Swedish Meatballs (11.2 oz)	450	40	22	NA	70	1110	NA	23	2 1/2 carb., 2 med-fat meat, 2 fat
Sweet & Sour Chicken & Rice (10 oz)	350	53	7	NA	40	640	NA	18	3 1/2 carb., 1 med-fat meat
Teriyaki Chicken (12 oz)	360	44	12	NA	55	610	NA	20	3 carb., 2 med-fat meat
Turkey a la King w/Rice (10 oz)	390	36	18	NA	75	740	NA	20	2 1/2 carb., 2 med-fat meat, 2 fat
Turkey Breast, Dijon (11.2 oz)	340	37	12	NA	65	860	NA	20	2 1/2 carb., 2 med-fat meat
CELESTE									
Pizza, Cheese (1/4)	315	28	17	7	20	690	2	14	2 carb., 1 med-fat meat, 2 fat
Pizza, Deluxe (1/4)	380	29	22	7	20	870	3	16	2 carb., 1 med-fat meat, 3 fat
Pizza, Pepperoni (1/4)	370	29	21	7	15	940	2	15	2 carb., 1 med-fat meat, 3 fat
Pizza, Sausage (1/4)	375	30	22	7	15	900	3	16	2 carb., 1 med-fat meat, 3 fat

Pizza, Supreme (1/4)	380	29	24	7	15	970	3	17	2 carb., 2 med-fat meat, 3 fat
Pizza-For-One, Cheese (1)	500	48	25	11	40	1070	4	21	3 carb., 2 med-fat meat, 3 fat
Pizza-For-One, Vegetable (1)	490	44	26	NA	NA	1200	NA	20	3 carb., 2 med-fat meat, 3 fat

CHEF AMERICA

Croissant Pockets, Egg, Sausage & Cheese (1)	340	39	15	6	95	740	2	12	2 1/2 strch, 1 med-fat meat, 2 fat
Croissant Pockets, Philly Steak & Cheese (1)	350	37	16	8	50	790	2	15	2 1/2 strch, 1 med-fat meat, 2 fat
Hot Pockets, Ham/Cheese (1)	320	39	12	6	40	620	3	14	2 1/2 carb., 1 med-fat meat, 1 fat
Hot Pockets, Pepperoni Pizza (1)	350	41	15	7	40	640	4	13	3 carb., 1 med-fat meat, 2 fat
Hot Pockets, Pizza Mini's, Double Cheese (1)	240	32	9	4	15	430	3	7	2 strch, 2 fat
Hot Pockets, Pizza Mini's (1)	250	31	11	4	15	500	3	7	2 strch, 2 fat
Lean Pockets, Chicken Fajita (1)	270	41	7	3	30	580	5	11	3 carb., 1 med-fat meat
Lean Pockets, Turkey/Broccoli/Cheese (1)	250	35	7	3	35	540	4	12	2 carb., 1 med-fat meat

COMBINATION FOODS & FROZEN ENTREES

Products	Cal.	Carb. (g)	Fat (g)	Sat. Fat (g)	Chol. (mg)	Sod. (mg)	Fib. (g)	Prot. (g)	Servings/Exchanges
CHEF BOYARDEE									
Beef Ravioli (8.7 oz)	230	37	5	2	15	1180	4	8	2 1/2 carb., 1 fat
Macaroni w/Cheese (7.5 oz)	170	33	2	1	25	970	2	7	2 carb.
Spaghetti w/Meatballs (8.5 oz)	250	34	9	4	20	940	2	9	2 carb., 2 fat
CHEF MATE									
Corned Beef Hash (1 cup)	485	29	30	13	90	1595	6	24	2 carb., 3 med-fat meat, 3 fat
Italian Rotini & Meatballs (1 cup)	270	28	11	4	20	1390	2	12	2 carb., 1 med-fat meat, 1 fat
Macaroni and Cheese (1 cup)	280	35	11	6	30	1345	3	11	2 carb., 1 med-fat meat, 1 fat
Oriental Beef & Vegetables (1 cup)	190	25	6	<1	15	1150	1	9	1 1/2 carb., 1 med-fat meat
Oriental Chicken & Vegetables (1 cup)	210	24	8	2	40	1170	1	11	1 1/2 carb., 1 med-fat meat, 1 fat
Oriental Vegetables (1 cup)	180	27	7	1	0	1410	3	3	2 carb., 1 fat
Sausage n' Shells (1 cup)	382	19	28	9	55	990	1	15	1 carb., 2 med-fat meat, 4 fat

CHUN KING

	Cal.	Carb.	Fat	Sat. Fat	Chol.	Sod.	Fiber	Prot.	Exchanges
Chicken Imperial (13 oz)	300	54	1	NA	NA	1540	NA	17	3 1/2 carb., 1 lean meat
Chow Mein, Chicken (13 oz)	370	53	6	NA	NA	1560	NA	25	3 1/2 carb., 2 lean meat
Crunchy Walnut Chicken (13 oz)	310	49	5	NA	NA	1700	NA	16	3 carb., 1 med-fat meat
Pepper Beef (13 oz)	310	53	3	NA	NA	1300	NA	17	3 carb., 1 fat
Sweet & Sour Pork (13 oz)	400	78	5	NA	NA	1460	NA	11	3 carb., 1 med-fat meat
Szechwan Beef (13 oz)	340	57	3	NA	NA	1810	NA	20	3 1/2 carb., 1 lean meat

DI GIORNO

	Cal.	Carb.	Fat	Sat. Fat	Chol.	Sod.	Fiber	Prot.	Exchanges
Stuffed Ravioli, Light Cheese (1 cup)	280	40	7	4	40	400	2	15	3 carb., 1 lean meat
Stuffed Ravioli, Sun Dried Tomato (1 1/3 cups)	380	48	14	8	55	600	3	17	3 carb., 1 med-fat meat, 2 fat
Stuffed Ravioli w/Italian Sausage (1 1/4 cups)	350	45	12	6	55	570	3	14	3 carb., 1 med-fat meat, 1 fat
Stuffed Tortellini, Pesto (1 cup)	320	46	8	5	45	430	3	16	3 carb., 1 med-fat meat, 1 fat
Stuffed Tortellini, Three Cheese (3/4 cup)	250	37	7	4	35	300	2	11	2 1/2 carb., 1 med-fat meat

DINING LITE

	Cal.	Carb.	Fat	Sat. Fat	Chol.	Sod.	Fiber	Prot.	Exchanges
Cheese Cannelloni (9 oz)	310	38	9	NA	70	650	NA	19	2 1/2 carb., 2 med-fat meat
Chicken a la King (9 oz)	240	30	7	NA	40	780	NA	14	2 carb., 1 med-fat meat

COMBINATION FOODS & FROZEN ENTREES

Products	Cal.	Carb. (g)	Fat (g)	Sat. Fat (g)	Chol. (mg)	Sod. (mg)	Fib. (g)	Prot. (g)	Servings/Exchanges
Fettuccine (9 oz)	290	33	12	NA	35	1020	NA	12	2 carb., 1 med-fat meat, 1 fat
Lasagna (9 oz)	260	36	6	NA	30	800	NA	14	2 1/2 carb., 1 med-fat meat
Oriental Pepper Steak (9 oz)	260	33	6	NA	40	1050	NA	18	2 carb., 2 lean meat
Salisbury Steak (9 oz)	200	14	8	NA	55	1000	NA	18	1 carb., 2 med-fat meat
Spaghetti w/Beef (9 oz)	220	25	8	NA	20	440	NA	12	1 1/2 carb., 1 med-fat meat, 1 fat
Teriyaki Beef (9 oz)	270	36	5	NA	45	850		20	2 1/2 carb., 2 lean meat
FRANCO-AMERICAN									
Beef Ravioli w/Meat Sauce (7.5 oz)	250	35	8	NA	NA	920	NA	10	2 1/2 carb., 1 fat
Macaroni & Cheese (7.4 oz)	170	24	6	NA	NA	1059	NA	6	1 1/2 carb., 1 fat
Spaghetti w/Meatballs (7.4 oz)	220	25	9	NA	NA	950	NA	9	1 1/2 carb., 1 med-fat meat, 1 fat
Spaghetti w/Tomato & Cheese Sauce (7.4 oz)	180	36	2	1	NA	840	NA	5	3 carb.
SpaghettiOs w/Franks (7.5 oz)	220	26	9	NA	NA	1000	NA	8	2 carb., 2 fat

									Exchanges
SpaghettiOs w/Meatballs (1 cup)	260	31	11	5	20	1150	5	11	2 carb, 1 med-fat meat, 1 fat
SpaghettiOs, Tomato & Cheese Sauce (7 oz)	160	31	2	<1	5	840	2	5	2 carb.

GREAT STARTS

Burrito, Sausage (3.5 oz)	240	24	12	4	60	500	1	9	1 1/2 carb., 1 med-fat meat, 1 fat
Burrito w/Scrambled Eggs (3.5 oz)	200	25	8	3	60	510	2	8	1 1/2 carb., 1 med-fat meat, 1 fat
Burrito w/Scrambled Eggs, Bacon (3.5 oz)	250	27	11	4	90	540	2	10	2 carb., 1 med-fat meat, 1 fat
Eggs & Silver Dollar Pancake (4.3 oz)	250	22	14	6	290	540	1	9	1 1/2 carb., 1 med-fat meat, 2 fat
French Toast, Cinnamon (5.6 oz)	440	34	28	12	150	580	2	14	2 carb., 1 med-fat meat, 5 fat
Muffin, Egg Bacon Cheese (4 oz)	290	25	15	6	95	750	2	14	1 1/2 carb., 1 med-fat meat, 2 fat
Pancakes w/Bacon (4.6 oz)	400	42	20	7	100	1030	1	12	3 carb., 4 fat
Pancakes w/Sausage (6 oz)	490	52	25	11	90	950	3	14	3 1/2 carb., 1 med-fat meat, 4 fat

COMBINATION FOODS & FROZEN ENTREES

Products	Cal.	Carb. (g)	Fat (g)	Sat. Fat (g)	Chol. (mg)	Sod. (mg)	Fib. (g)	Prot. (g)	Servings/Exchanges
Sandwich, Egg & Cheese (4.3 oz)	350	30	20	8	110	890	1	12	2 carb., 1 med-fat meat, 3 fat
Scrambled Eggs & Bacon (5.3 oz)	290	17	19	9	240	700	1	11	1 carb., 1 med-fat meat, 3 fat
Scrambled Eggs & Sausage (6.3 oz)	360	21	26	10	280	800	3	12	1 1/2 carb., 1 med-fat meat, 5 fat
GREEN GIANT									
Create A Meal Fajita Style (10 oz)	430	40	16	6	70	1300	4	32	2 strch, 2 vegetable, 3 med-fat meat
Create A Meal Hearty Vegetable Stew (1 1/4 cups)	280	25	9	2	55	1000	16	23	1 strch, 2 vegetable, 2 med-fat meat
Create A Meal Oven Roasted Homestyle Pot Roast (2 cups)	370	33	13	3	70	860	5	29	2 strch, 1 vegetable, 3 med-fat meat
Create A Meal Oven Roasted, Garlic Herb (1 3/4 cups)	360	37	9	2	70	760	6	32	2 strch, 1 vegetable, 3 lean meat
Create A Meal Oven Roasted, Parmesan Herb (1 3/4 cups)	330	27	11	3	75	1080	5	31	1 1/2 strch, 1 vegetable, 3 lean meat

Food									Exchanges
Create A Meal/Ground Beef, Beefy Noodle (1 1/4 cups)	350	31	14	5	70	1130	3	26	1 1/2 strch, 1 vegetable, 3 med-fat meat
Create A Meal/Ground Beef, Homestyle Stew (1 cup)	340	25	16	6	70	1310	4	24	1 strch, 1 vegetable, 3 med-fat meat
Create A Meal/Ground Beef, Skillet Lasagna (1 1/4 cups)	350	33	13	5	70	830	3	26	2 strch, 1 vegetable, 3 med-fat meat
Create A Meal Stir-Fry, Broccoli (1 1/3 cups)	290	16	13	3	60	1160	4	27	3 vegetables, 3 med-fat meat
Create A Meal Stir-Fry, Vegetable Almond (1 1/3 cups)	320	20	12	2	65	1070	5	32	1 strch, 1 vegetable, 4 lean meat
Create A Meal Stir-Fry Vegetables, LoMein (2 1/3 cups)	320	35	7	2	60	980	4	30	1 strch, 4 vegetable
Create A Meal Stir-Fry Vegetables, Sweet & Sour (1 1/4 cups)	290	29	7	1	60	460	5	27	1 strch, 3 vegetable, 3 lean meat
Create A Meal Stir-Fry Vegetables, Szechuan (1 3/4 cups)	310	20	14	3	60	1390	4	26	1/2 strch, 2 vegetable, 3 med-fat meat
Create A Meal Stir-Fry Vegetables, Teriyaki (1 3/4 cups)	230	18	6	1	55	920	4	27	4 vegetable, 3 lean meat

COMBINATION FOODS & FROZEN ENTREES

Products	Cal.	Carb. (g)	Fat (g)	Sat. Fat (g)	Chol. (mg)	Sod. (mg)	Fib. (g)	Prot. (g)	Servings/Exchanges
Rice & Broccoli, Frozen (1 pkg)	320	44	12	4	15	1000	2	8	3 strch, 2 fat
Rice Medley, Frozen (1 pkg)	240	46	3	2	5	880	3	6	3 strch, 1 fat
Rice Pilaf, Frozen (1 pkg)	230	44	3	2	5	1020	3	6	3 strch, 1 fat
HEALTHY CHOICE									
Beef & Peppers Cantonese (11.5 oz)	280	32	7	3	55	480	5	22	2 carb., 2 lean meat
Beef Broccoli Bejing (12 oz)	300	45	5	2	25	420	6	21	3 carb., 2 lean meat
Beef Macaroni (8.5 oz)	220	34	4	2	20	450	5	12	2 strch, 1 med-fat meat
Beef Pepper Steak Oriental (9.5 oz)	260	34	5	3	35	520	2	19	2 carb., 2 lean meat
Beef Stroganoff (11 oz)	310	44	7	3	60	440	3	19	3 carb., 2 lean meat
Bowl Creations, Chili & Cornbread (9.5 oz)	340	49	7	3	30	600	11	21	3 strch., 2 lean meat
Bowl Creations, Turkey Divan (9.5 oz)	250	31	6	2	25	600	5	18	2 strch., 2 lean meat
Bowl Creations, Roasted Potatoes w/Ham (8.5 oz)	200	26	3	2	30	600	6	17	2 strch, 2 very lean meat
Cheddar Broccoli Potatoes (10.5 oz)	330	53	7	3	25	550	6	13	3 1/2 carb., 1 fat
Chicken & Vegetables Marsala (11.5 oz)	240	32	4	2	30	440	3	20	2 carb., 2 very lean meat

Chicken Broccoli Alfredo (11.5 oz)	300	34	7	3	50	530	2	25	2 carb., 3 lean meat
Chicken Cacciatore (10.75 oz)	340	52	5	2	20	590	6	21	3 1/2 carb., 1 med-fat meat
Chicken Dijon (11 oz)	270	33	5	2	40	470	6	23	2 carb., 2 lean meat
Chicken Fettuccine Alfredo (8.5 oz)	280	35	7	3	40	410	3	22	2 carb., 2 lean meat
Chicken Francesca (12.5 oz)	330	46	6	3	30	600	4	23	3 carb., 2 lean meat
Chicken Parmigiana (11.5 oz)	330	46	8	3	40	490	3	19	3 carb., 2 med-fat meat
Chicken Teriyaki (11 oz)	270	37	6	3	37	600	3	17	2 1/2 carb., 2 lean meat
Country Glazed Chicken (8.5 oz)	230	30	4	2	45	480	3	17	2 carb., 2 lean meat
Country Herb Chicken (12.15 oz)	320	44	8	3	45	540	3	18	3 carb., 1 med-fat meat
Country Inn Roast Turkey (10 oz)	250	28	6	2	28	530	4	20	2 carb., 3 lean meat
Fiesta Chicken Fajitas (7 oz)	260	36	4	1	30	410	4	21	2 1/2 carb., 2 lean meat
French Bread Pizza, Cheese (6 oz)	340	51	5	8	15	480	5	22	3 1/2 carb., 2 lean meat
French Bread Pizza, Pepperoni (6 oz)	340	49	5	2	20	580	6	24	3 carb., 2 lean meat
French Bread Pizza, Vegetable (6 oz)	280	44	4	2	10	480	5	17	3 strch. 1 med-fat meat
Hearty Handfuls, Chicken & Broccoli (6.1 oz)	320	51	5	2	20	580	5	17	3 1/2 strch, 1 med-fat meat
Hearty Handfuls, Ham & Cheese (6.1 oz)	320	50	5	2	25	590	4	19	3 strch., 1 med-fat meat

COMBINATION FOODS & FROZEN ENTREES

Products	Cal.	Carb. (g)	Fat (g)	Sat. Fat (g)	Chol. (mg)	Sod. (mg)	Fib. (g)	Prot. (g)	Servings/Exchanges
Hearty Handfuls, Philly Beef Steak (6.1 oz)	290	47	5	2	25	550	5	16	3 strch., 1 med-fat meat
Herb Baked Fish (10.9 oz)	340	54	7	2	35	480	5	16	3 1/2 strch., 1 med-fat meat
Honey Mustard Chicken (9.5 oz)	290	38	6	3	40	520	1	21	2 1/2 carb., 2 lean meat
Lasagna Roma (13.5 oz)	420	59	9	3	35	580	6	26	4 carb., 2 med-fat meat
Manicotti w/Three-Cheese (11 oz)	300	40	9	3	35	550	5	15	2 1/2 carb., 1 med-fat meat, 1 fat
Mesquite Beef Barbeque (11 oz)	320	38	9	3	55	490	5	21	2 1/2 carb., 2 med-fat meat
Mesquite Chicken Barbeque (10.5 oz)	310	48	5	2	55	480	6	18	3 1/2 carb., 2 lean meat
Sesame Chicken (9.75 oz)	250	38	4	1	35	600	2	16	2 1/2 carb., 1 med-fat meat
Sesame Chicken (10.8 oz)	360	54	7	2	20	600	4	19	2 1/2 carb., 2 lean meat
Shrimp & Vegetables (11.8 oz)	270	39	6	3	50	580	6	15	2 1/2 carb., 1 med-fat meat
Southwestern Glazed Chicken (10.2 oz)	260	30	6	3	40	450	4	21	2 carb., 2 lean meat
Stuffed Pasta Shells (10.35 oz)	370	60	6	3	20	570	5	18	4 carb., 1 med-fat meat
Swedish Meatballs (9.1 oz)	280	35	6	3	50	590	3	22	2 carb., 2 lean meat

Traditional Beef Tips (11.25 oz)	260	32	6	3	40	390	6	20	2 carb., 2 lean meat
Traditional Meat Loaf (12 oz)	330	52	7	4	35	460	6	15	3 carb., 2 med-fat meat
Traditional Salisbury Steak (11.5 oz)	330	48	7	3	50	470	6	18	3 carb., 1 med-fat meat
Vegetable Pasta Italiano (10 oz)	250	48	3	2	10	480	6	9	3 carb.
Yankee Pot Roast (11 oz)	290	38	7	3	55	460	4	19	2 1/2 carb., 2 lean meat

HORMEL

Kid's Kitchen Beans & Weiners (7.5 oz)	310	36	13	4	45	731	NA	13	2 1/2 carb., 1 med-fat meat, 2 fat
Kid's Kitchen Beefy Mac (7.5 oz)	200	25	6	2	25	780	NA	11	1 1/2 carb., 1 med-fat meat
Kid's Kitchen Cheezy Mac'n Cheese (7.5 oz)	260	28	11	6	45	650	NA	12	2 carb., 1 med-fat meat, 1 fat
Kid's Kitchen Spaghetti & Mini Meatballs (7.5 oz)	220	26	8	4	20	880	NA	11	2 carb., 1 med-fat meat, 1 fat

KIDS CUISINE

Big-League Hamburger Pizza (8.3 oz)	400	61	11	4	25	530	6	14	4 carb., 1 med-fat meat, 1 fat
Buckaroo Beef Patty Sandwich w/Cheese (8.5 oz)	410	58	15	7	30	500	4	12	4 carb., 1 med-fat meat, 2 fat
Circus Show Corn Dog (8.8 oz)	490	70	20	7	30	800	5	8	4 1/2 carb., 4 fat

COMBINATION FOODS & FROZEN ENTREES

Products	Cal.	Carb. (g)	Fat (g)	Sat. Fat (g)	Chol. (mg)	Sod. (mg)	Fib. (g)	Prot. (g)	Servings/Exchanges
Cosmic Chicken Nuggets (9.1 oz)	500	50	25	10	45	1070	5	18	3 carb., 1 med-fat meat, 4 fat
High-Flying Fried Chicken (10.1 oz)	440	48	20	9	70	940	5	18	3 carb., 2 med-fat meat, 2 fat
Magical Macaroni & Cheese (10.6 oz)	440	72	13	8	15	870	4	10	5 carb., 3 fat
Pirate Pizza w/Cheese (8 oz)	430	71	11	3	30	480	5	12	5 carb., 1 med-fat meat, 1 fat
Raptor Ravioli w/Cheese (9.8 oz)	320	60	5	2	15	780	5	7	4 carb., 1 fat
LA CHOY									
Almond Chicken w/Rice Entree (9.75 oz)	270	40	8	NA	42	1092	3	14	2 1/2 carb., 1 med-fat meat, 1 fat
Chicken Chow Mein Entree, Canned (3/4 cup)	240	47	2	<1	19	1420	1	8	3 carb.
Oriental Chicken w/Noodles Entree (9 oz)	160	23	4	1	13	1163	4	11	1 1/2 carb., 1 med-fat meat
Shrimp Chow Mein Entree, Canned (3/4 cup)	50	7	1	0	19	860	2	3	1/2 carb.
Sweet & Sour Noodles w/Pork Entree, Canned (3/4 cup)	250	48	4	1	18	1540	1	6	3 carb., 1 fat

LEAN CUISINE

American Favorites Baked Chicken (8 5/8 oz)	230	31	4	2	35	520	5	18	2 carb., 2 lean meat
American Favorites Baked Fish (9 oz)	270	36	6	2	45	540	3	17	2 1/2 carb., 2 lean meat
American Favorites Beef Pot Roast (9 oz)	210	25	6	2	30	570	6	13	1 1/2 carb., 2 lean meat
American Favorites, Chicken Medallions (9 3/8 oz)	260	27	9	3	25	520	3	17	2 strch., 2 med-fat meat
American Favorites Country Vegetables & Beef (9 oz)	210	33	4	1	25	590	3	11	2 carb., 1 med-fat meat
American Favorites, Honey Roasted Chicken (8 1/2 oz)	270	42	6	2	25	590	4	13	3 strch., 1 med-fat meat
American Favorites Meat Loaf & Whipped Potatoes (9 3/8 oz)	250	30	6	3	50	590	4	18	2 carb., 2 lean meat
American Favorites Roasted Turkey Breast (9 3/4 oz)	270	49	3	<1	20	590	5	13	3 carb., 2 lean meat
American Favorites Salisbury Steak (9 1/2 oz)	280	29	8	4	60	590	4	24	2 carb., 3 lean meat
Angel Hair Pasta (10 oz)	260	46	5	1	0	470	2	9	2 carb., 1 fat
Café Classics Beef Peppercorn (8 3/4 oz)	220	23	7	2	35	580	2	15	1 1/2 carb., 1 med-fat meat

COMBINATION FOODS & FROZEN ENTREES

Products	Cal.	Carb. (g)	Fat (g)	Sat. Fat (g)	Chol. (mg)	Sod. (mg)	Fib. (g)	Prot. (g)	Servings/Exchanges
Café Classics, Beef Portabello (9 oz)	220	24	7	4	35	590	2	14	1 1/2 strch, 1 med-fat meat
Café Classics Bow Tie Pasta & Chicken (9 1/2 oz)	250	34	5	1	45	530	3	16	2 carb., 2 lean meat
Café Classics Cheese Lasagna w/Chicken Scalopini (10 oz)	290	33	8	2	30	590	3	21	2 carb., 2 med-fat meat
Café Classics Chicken & Vegetables (10 1/2 oz)	270	33	6	2	25	590	4	20	2 carb., 2 lean meat
Café Classics Chicken a l'Orange (9 oz)	260	40	1	<1	40	320	2	22	2 1/2 carb., 2 very lean meat
Café Classics Chicken Breast in Wine Sauce (8 1/8 oz)	210	23	6	2	35	560	2	15	1 1/2 carb., 2 lean meat
Café Classics Chicken Carbonara (9 oz)	280	33	8	2	30	580	2	18	2 carb., 2 med-fat meat
Café Classics Chicken in Peanut Sauce (9 oz)	290	35	6	2	30	590	4	23	2 carb., 2 lean meat
Café Classics Chicken Mediterranean (10 oz)	260	38	4	1	25	590	2	17	2 1/2 carb., 2 lean meat
Café Classics Chicken Parmesan (10 7/8 oz)	260	31	7	3	30	590	4	19	2 carb., 2 lean meat
Café Classics Chicken Piccata (9 oz)	270	41	6	2	25	530	2	13	3 carb., 1 med-fat meat
Café Classics, Chicken w/Basil Cream Sauce (8 1/2 oz)	270	35	7	2	35	580	3	16	2 strch, 1 med-fat meat

Café Classics Fiesta Chicken (8 1/2 oz)	270	36	5	<1	30	590	4	19	2 1/2 carb., 2 lean meat
Café Classics Glazed Chicken (8 1/2 oz)	240	25	6	1	55	480	0	22	1 1/2 carb., 2 lean meat
Café Classics Grilled Chicken Salsa (8 7/8 oz)	270	36	7	3	45	570	4	15	2 1/2 carb., 1 med-fat meat
Café Classics Herb-Roasted Chicken (8 oz)	200	24	5	1	25	510	3	15	1 1/2 carb., 2 lean meat
Café Classics Honey Mustard Chicken (8 oz)	260	40	4	1	35	550	3	15	2 1/2 carb., 1 med-fat meat
Café Classics Honey Roasted Pork (9 1/2 oz)	250	32	6	3	45	590	3	17	2 strch., 2 lean meat
Café Classics Oriental Beef (9 1/4 oz)	240	35	4	2	30	590	2	17	2 carb., 2 lean meat
Cheese Cannelloni (9 1/8 oz)	230	28	4	2	15	570	3	20	2 carb., 1 med-fat meat
Cheese Ravioli (8 1/2 oz)	270	40	7	3	45	580	5	11	2 1/2 carb., 1 med-fat meat
Chicken Chow Mein w/Rice (9 oz)	220	33	5	1	35	560	3	12	2 carb., 1 med-fat meat
Chicken Enchilada Suiza w/Mexican-Style Rice (9 oz)	280	48	5	2	25	520	3	11	3 carb., 1 med-fat meat
Chicken Fettuccine (9 1/4 oz)	300	38	6	3	50	590	3	24	2 1/2 carb., 2 lean meat
Chicken Lasagna (10 oz)	270	30	8	3	35	590	5	19	2 strch., 2 med-fat meat
Chicken Pie (9 1/2 oz)	290	35	9	3	30	570	5	18	2 1/2 carb., 1 med-fat meat, 1 fat

COMBINATION FOODS & FROZEN ENTREES

Products	Cal.	Carb. (g)	Fat (g)	Sat. Fat (g)	Chol. (mg)	Sod. (mg)	Fib. (g)	Prot. (g)	Servings/Exchanges
Deluxe Cheddar Potato (10 3/8 oz)	270	40	7	4	20	590	6	12	2 1/2 carb., 1 med-fat meat
Fettuccine Alfredo (9 oz)	300	47	7	3	15	550	2	12	3 carb., 1 med-fat meat
Fettuccine Primavera (10 oz)	270	38	7	3	15	580	4	13	2 1/2 carb., 1 med-fat meat
French Bread Pizza, Cheese (6 oz)	320	48	7	4	15	580	4	15	3 carb., 2 lean meat
French Bread Pizza, Deluxe (6 1/8 oz)	300	46	6	3	25	590	4	16	3 carb., 3 lean meat
French Bread Pizza, Pepperoni (5 1/4 oz)	310	46	7	3	20	590	3	15	3 carb., 2 med-fat meat
French Bread Pizza, Sun Dried Tomatoes (5 1/4 oz)	340	48	8	5	20	580	3	19	3 strch, 2 med-fat meat
Hearty Portions, Chicken & BBQ Sauce (13 7/8 oz)	380	54	8	2	50	790	6	24	3 1/2 strch, 2 med-fat meat
Hearty Portions, Grilled Chicken & Penne Pasta (14 oz)	380	50	7	3	40	850	6	30	3 strch, 3 lean meat
Hearty Portions, Homestyle Beef Stroganoff (14 1/4 oz)	350	44	9	3	30	890	9	23	3 strch, 2 med-fat meat
Hearty Portions, Jumbo Rigatoni w/Meatballs (15 3/8 oz)	440	64	9	4	35	820	7	25	4 strch, 2 med-fat meat

Hearty Portions, Roasted Chicken w/Mushrooms (12 1/2 oz)	340	44	6	2	35	850	4	27	3 strch, 3 lean meat
Hearty Portions, Salisbury Steak (15 1/2 oz)	340	40	7	3	50	850	10	28	2 1/2 strch, 3 lean meat
Homestyle Turkey (9 3/8 oz)	230	30	5	1	40	590	3	17	2 carb., 2 lean meat
Lasagna, Classic Cheese (11 1/2 oz)	280	40	5	3	15	560	6	19	2 1/2 carb, 2 lean meat
Lasagna, Vegetable (10 1/2 oz)	260	35	7	3	20	590	5	15	2 carb., 1 med-fat meat
Lasagna w/Meat Sauce (10 1/2 oz)	290	37	6	4	25	560	4	21	2 1/2 carb., 2 lean meat
Macaroni & Beef (10 oz)	270	43	4	2	25	590	4	15	3 carb., 1 med-fat meat
Macaroni and Cheese (10 oz)	290	45	6	4	15	560	4	14	3 strch, 1 med-fat meat
Mandarin Chicken (9 oz)	250	38	4	<1	25	590	3	15	2 1/2 strch, 1 med-fat meat
Marinara Twist (10 oz)	240	42	3	1		440			3 carb.
Penne Pasta w/Tomato Basil Sauce (10 oz)	270	52	4	1	0	350	5	8	3 1/2 strch, 1 fat
Skillet Sensations, Beef Fajita (6 oz)	300	48	4	2	25	760	6	19	3 strch, 1 med-fat meat
Skillet Sensations, Beef Teriyaki & Rice (6 oz)	280	48	3	1	25	700	5	14	3 strch, 1 lean meat
Skillet Sensations, Chicken Oriental (6 oz)	280	46	3	<1	15	790	6	17	3 strch, 1 lean meat
Skillet Sensations, Roasted Beef & Potatoes (6 oz)	290	38	7	3	35	760	9	18	2 1/2 strch, 2 lean meat

COMBINATION FOODS & FROZEN ENTREES

Products	Cal.	Carb. (g)	Fat (g)	Sat. Fat (g)	Chol. (mg)	Sod. (mg)	Fib. (g)	Prot. (g)	Servings/Exchanges
Spaghetti w/Meat Sauce (11 1/2 oz)	290	50	5	2	20	570	7	11	3 carb., 1 med-fat meat
Spaghetti w/Meatballs (9 1/2 oz)	280	40	6	2	20	570	4	16	2 1/2 carb., 2 lean meat
Stuffed Cabbage w/Whipped Potatoes (9 1/2 oz)	170	24	5	2	15	380	5	8	1 1/2 carb., 1 med-fat meat
Swedish Meatballs w/Pasta (9 1/8 oz)	290	38	6	3	45	580	3	21	2 1/2 carb., 2 lean meat
Teriyaki Stir-Fry (10 oz)	290	48	4	<1	25	590	4	17	3 strch, 1 med-fat meat
Three-Bean Chili w/Rice (10 oz)	250	38	6	2	5	590	9	10	2 1/2 carb., 1 fat
MORTON									
Breaded Chicken Patty Meal (6.75 oz)	290	24	17	4	35	840	4	10	1 1/2 carb., 1 med-fat meat, 2 fat
Chicken Nuggets Meal (7 oz)	340	31	19	5	30	470	2	12	2 carb., 1 med-fat meat, 3 fat
Chili Gravy w/Beef Enchilada & Tamale (10 oz)	260	40	7	3	5	1000	4	8	2 1/2 carb., 1 fat
Fried Chicken Meal (9 oz)	470	30	30	10	90	1100	3	20	2 carb., 2 med-fat meat, 4 fat
Gravy & Charbroiled Beef Patty Meal (9 oz)	310	26	18	9	30	1210	5	10	2 carb., 1 med-fat meat, 2 fat

Food								Exchanges
Gravy & Salisbury Steak Meal (9 oz)	310	24	20	8	30	1100	3	7	1 1/2 carb., 1 med-fat meat, 1 fat
Gravy & Turkey w/Dressing Meal (9 oz)	240	27	10	4	40	1200	4	10	2 carb., 1 med-fat meat, 1 fat
Macaroni & Cheese (6.5 oz)	240	34	8	4	20	1190	3	9	2 carb., 2 fat
Spaghetti w/Meat Sauce (8.5 oz)	200	30	6	3	5	750	4	5	2 carb., 1 fat
Veal Parmigiana w/Tomato Sauce (8.75 oz)	280	30	15	5	25	950	4	8	2 carb., 3 fat
Vegetable Pot Pie w/Beef (7 oz)	340	35	21	9	20	1380	2	8	2 carb., 4 fat
Vegetable Pot Pie w/Chicken (7 oz)	320	32	18	7	25	1040	2	8	2 carb., 3 fat
Vegetable Pot Pie w/Turkey (7 oz)	310	29	18	9	25	1060	2	8	2 carb., 3 fat
OLD EL PASO									
Burrito, Bean & Cheese (1)	300	44	9	5	15	840	3	12	3 carb., 1 med-fat meat, 1 fat
Burrito, Beef/Bean, Medium (1)	320	46	10	4	5	800	3	12	3 carb., 1 med-fat meat, 1 fat
Chimichanga, Beef (1)	360	37	20	5	10	470	3	9	2 1/2 carb., 4 fat
Chimichanga, Chicken (1)	340	39	16	4	20	540	2	11	2 1/2 carb., 1 med-fat meat, 2 fat
Pizza Burrito, Cheese (1)	240	27	9	4	20	430	0	13	2 carb., 1 med-fat meat, 1 fat

COMBINATION FOODS & FROZEN ENTREES

Products	Cal.	Carb. (g)	Fat (g)	Sat. Fat (g)	Chol. (mg)	Sod. (mg)	Fib. (g)	Prot. (g)	Servings/Exchanges
Pizza Burrito, Pepperoni (1)	260	31	10	5	20	510	0	12	2 carb., 1 med-fat meat, 1 fat
Pizza Burrito, Sausage (1)	250	32	9	4	15	420	0	11	2 carb., 1 med-fat meat, 1 fat
Side Dishes, Chili w/Beans (1 cup)	240	19	11	3	30	770	6	17	1 strch, 2 med-fat meat
Side Dishes, Spanish Rice (1 cup)	130	28	1	0	0	1340	2	3	2 strch
Side Dishes, Tamales in Chili Gravy (3)	320	31	19	7	30	590	5	7	2 strch, 4 fat
ORE IDA									
Baked BBQ Sauce w/Beef Pocket (5 oz)	350	48	11	3	20	580	2	14	3 carb., 1 med-fat meat, 1 fat
Chicken Broccoli Cheese Pocket (5 oz)	330	43	11	3	30	590	3	14	3 carb., 1 med-fat meat, 1 fat
Chicken Fajita Pocket (4 oz)	250	35	8	2	10	390	3	11	2 carb., 1 med-fat meat, 1 fat
Fried Beef Cheddar Pocket (6 oz)	440	36	24	7	55	760	2	18	2 1/2 carb., 2 med-fat meat, 3 fat
Ham & Cheese Pocket (5 oz)	370	46	15	6	35	880	3	14	3 carb., 1 med-fat meat, 2 fat
Pepperoni Pizza Pocket (6 oz)	510	50	26	7	35	1040	4	19	3 carb., 1 med-fat meat, 4 fat
Pizza Deluxe Pocket (5 oz)	400	39	19	7	40	590	3	18	2 1/2 carb., 2 med-fat meat, 2 fat

Food	Cal	Carb	Fat	Sat Fat	Chol	Sod	Fiber	Prot	Exchanges
Turkey Swiss Broccoli Pocket (6 oz)	380	49	14	5	35	690	3	18	3 carb., 1 med-fat meat, 2 fat
OSCAR MAYER									
Lunchables Bologna/American (4.5-oz pkg)	480	20	38	17	80	1520	4	18	1 1/2 carb., 2 med-fat meat, 5 fat
Lunchables Deluxe Turkey/Ham (5.1-oz pkg)	370	23	20	10	60	1760	NA	23	1 1/2 carb., 2 med-fat meat, 2 fat
Lunchables Fun Pack Bologna w/Wild Cherry (1 pkg)	530	48	28	13	70	1140	2	12	3 1/2 carb., 1 med-fat meat, 5 fat
Lunchables Fun Pack Extra Cheesy Pizza w/Fruit Punch (1 pkg)	450	61	15	9	30	720	2	17	4 carb., 1 med-fat meat, 2 fat
Lunchables Fun Pack Ham w/Fruit Punch (1 pkg)	440	48	20	9	50	1270	1	15	3 1/2 carb., 2 med-fat meat, 2 fat
Lunchables Fun Pack Low-Fat Ham w/Fruit Punch (1 pkg)	330	54	9	5	35	1120	<1	17	3 1/2 carb., 2 med-fat meat
Lunchables Fun Pack Low-Fat Turkey/Cheddar (4.3 oz)	250	18	9	5	35	1600	2	18	1 carb., 2 med-fat meat

COMBINATION FOODS & FROZEN ENTREES

Products	Cal.	Carb. (g)	Fat (g)	Sat. Fat (g)	Chol. (mg)	Sod. (mg)	Fib. (g)	Prot. (g)	Servings/Exchanges
Lunchables Fun Pack Low-Fat Turkey w/Pacific Cooler Juice Drink (1 pkg)	360	61	9	5	30	1190	<1	15	4 carb., 1 med-fat meat, 1 fat
Lunchables Fun Pack Pepperoni Pizza w/Orange (1 pkg)	460	55	16	8	35	830	2	16	3 1/2 carb., 1 med-fat meat, 2 fat
Lunchables Fun Pack Taco Bell Tacos (1 pkg)	460	69	13	6	35	950	2	20	4 1/2 carb., 2 med-fat meat, 1 fat
Lunchables Fun Pack Turkey w/Pacific Cooler Juice Drink (1 pkg)	450	51	20	9	50	1340	1	15	3 1/2 carb., 1 med-fat meat, 3 fat
Lunchables, Grilled Burgers (1 pkg)	460	67	14	8	40	1060	1	15	4 1/2 carb., 1 med-fat meat, 2 fat
Lunchables Ham/Cheddar (4.5-oz pkg)	370	18	25	11	70	1680	2	21	1 carb., 3 med-fat meat, 2 fat
Lunchables Ham/Swiss (4.5-oz pkg)	340	18	21	10	65	1660	NA	22	1 carb., 3 med-fat meat, 1 fat
Lunchables, Pancakes & Bac'n Bites (1 pkg)	560	107	11	3	70	480	<1	8	7 carb., 2 fat
Lunchables Pizza, Extra Cheesy (4.5-oz pkg)	300	28	13	7	30	690	2	17	2 carb., 1 med-fat meat, 2 fat

Lunchables Pizza, Pepperoni/Mozzarella (4.5-oz pkg)	310	28	15	7	35	790	2	15	2 carb., 1 med-fat meat, 2 fat
Lunchables Taco Bell Nachos (4.5-oz pkg)	380	39	21	5	10	1060	3	19	2 1/2 carb., 2 med-fat meat, 2 fat
Lunchables Turkey/Monterey Jack (4.5-oz pkg)	360	18	22	11	75	1600	NA	21	1 1/2 carb., 2 med-fat meat, 2 fat
Lunchables, Waffles & Sausage (1 pkg)	550	100	14	3	55	520	<1	9	7 carb., 3 fat
PAPPALO'S									
Pizza, Cheese (1/4 of 12")	310	41	7	4	30	440	4	20	3 carb., 2 lean meat
Pizza-For-One, Pepperoni (7.1 oz)	525	65	20	7	38	985	3	23	4 carb., 2 med-fat meat, 2 fat
PATIO									
Enchilada Dinner, Beef (12 oz)	370	52	12	5	25	1700	8	12	3 1/2 carb., 1 med-fat meat, 1 fat
Enchilada Dinner, Cheese (12 oz)	370	54	12	5	25	1570	7	11	3 1/2 carb., 1 med-fat meat, 1 fat
Enchilada Dinner, Chicken (12 oz)	400	60	12	4	35	1470	8	13	4 carb., 1 med-fat meat, 1 fat

COMBINATION FOODS & FROZEN ENTREES

Products	Cal.	Carb. (g)	Fat (g)	Sat. Fat (g)	Chol. (mg)	Sod. (mg)	Fib. (g)	Prot. (g)	Servings/Exchanges
Fiesta Dinner (12 oz)	350	53	11	6	25	1760	7	11	3 1/2 carb., 1 med-fat meat, 1 fat
Mexican-Style Dinner (13.25 oz)	470	59	19	8	30	2210	10	15	4 carb., 1 med-fat meat, 2 fat
Ranchera Dinner (13 oz)	470	55	22	10	35	2670	9	13	3 1/2 carb., 1 med-fat meat, 3 fat
PROGRESSO									
Ravioli, Beef (1 cup)	260	45	5	2	5	940	4	9	3 carb., 1 fat
Ravioli, Cheese (1 cup)	220	43	2	1	<5	930	4	7	3 carb.
RED BARON									
Breakfast Sandwich, Sausage Scrapple (1)	380	34	21	8	65	730	2	15	2 carb., 1 med-fat meat, 3 fat
Pizza Deep Dish Singles, Pepperoni (1)	530	47	31	11	35	90	2	18	3 carb., 1 med-fat meat, 5 fat
Pizza Pouches, Ham & Cheese (1)	355	36	17	6	41	1052	NA	15	2 1/2 carb., 1 med-fat meat, 2 fat

Pizza, Sausage Combination (1/5 of 12")	340	31	18	7	25	690	2	14	2 carb., 1 med-fat meat, 3 fat
SPAGO									
Pizza, 5-Grain, Whole-Wheat, Artichoke Hearts (2.7 oz)	170	19	7	NA	NA	12	NA	8	1 carb., 1 med-fat meat
Pizza, 5-Grain, Whole-Wheat, Spicy Chicken (2.7 oz)	180	18	8	NA	23	320	NA	9	1 carb., 1 med-fat meat, 1 fat
STOUFFER'S									
Beef Pie (10 oz)	440	36	25	10	55	1140	4	18	2 1/2 carb., 2 med-fat meat, 3 fat
Beef Stroganoff (9.8 oz)	390	30	20	7	85	1100	2	23	2 carb., 2 med-fat meat, 2 fat
Cheese Manicotti (9 oz)	360	34	16	9	40	850	4	19	2 carb., 2 med-fat meat, 1 fat
Chicken a la King (9.5 oz)	350	41	13	4	40	800	2	17	3 strch, 1 med-fat meat, 2 fat
Chicken Pie (8 oz)	430	35	25	8	40	1150	5	17	2 strch, 2 med-fat meat, 3 fat
Chili w/Beans (8.75 oz)	270	29	10	4	35	1130	8	15	2 strch, 2 fat

COMBINATION FOODS & FROZEN ENTREES

Products	Cal.	Carb. (g)	Fat (g)	Sat. Fat (g)	Chol. (mg)	Sod. (mg)	Fib. (g)	Prot. (g)	Servings/Exchanges
Creamed Chipped Beef & Biscuit (4.4 oz)	160	8	10	5	35	620	0	10	1/2 carb., 1 med-fat meat, 1 med-fat meat, 1 fat
Enchilada, Chicken (4.8 oz)	220	22	11	5	30	570	2	8	1 1/2 carb., 1 med-fat meat, 1 fat
Fettuccine Alfredo (10 oz)	460	47	23	13	70	910	3	16	3 strch, 1 med-fat meat, 4 fat
Green Bean Mushroom Casserole (4 oz)	130	12	8	2	2	450	2	3	1 vegetable, 1/2 strch, 1 fat
Green Pepper Steak (10.5 oz)	330	45	9	3	35	650	3	17	3 carb., 1 med-fat meat, 1 fat
Green Peppers, Stuffed (10 oz)	200	27	5	2	20	820	3	11	2 carb., 1 med-fat meat
Ham w/Asparagus Bake (9.6 oz)	520	32	36	14		1040		23	2 carb., 2 med-fat meat, 5 fat
Hearty Portions, Beef Pot Roast (16 oz)	370	44	11	5	45	1410	8	23	3 strch, 2 med-fat meat
Hearty Portions, Chicken Pot Pie (8 oz)	590	49	37	12	40	1240	4	15	3 strch, 1 med-fat meat, 6 fat
Hearty Portions, Meatloaf w/Mashed Potatoes (17 oz)	480	46	23	10	90	1580	8	23	3 strch, 2 med-fat meat, 3 fat

Food									Exchanges
Hearty Portions, Roast Turkey Breast (16 oz)	490	52	20	6	35	1880	6	25	3 1/2 strch, 2 med-fat meat, 2 fat
Homestyle Baked Chicken Breast (8.9 oz)	260	18	11	6	65	680	3	22	1 carb., 3 lean meat
Homestyle Beef Pot Roast (8.9 oz)	250	29	8	3	35	780	4	16	2 carb., 2 med-fat meat
Homestyle Chicken and Dumplings (10 oz)	280	33	8	4	55	1000	0	19	2 strch, 2 med-fat meat
Homestyle Chicken Fettuccine (10.5 oz)	350	28	14	4	50	1040	2	28	2 carb., 4 lean meat
Homestyle Chicken Parmigiana (12 oz)	460	54	16	4	45	1060	5	24	3 1/2 carb., 2 med-fat meat, 1 fat
Homestyle Fish & Macaroni & Cheese (9 oz)	430	37	21	5	70	930	2	24	2 1/2 carb., 1 med-fat meat, 2 fat
Homestyle Fried Chicken (8.9 oz)	400	38	17	6	55	950	2	23	2 1/2 carb., 2 med-fat meat, 1 fat
Homestyle Meat Loaf (9.9 oz)	390	28	21	11	90	840	3	22	2 carb., 2 med-fat meat, 2 fat
Homestyle Roast Turkey (9.6 oz)	310	27	13	6	50	930	3	22	2 carb., 2 med-fat meat, 1 fat
Homestyle Salisbury Steak (9.6 oz)	380	28	18	8	60	1170	1	26	2 carb., 3 med-fat meat, 1 fat
Homestyle Veal Parmigana (11.6 oz)	430	49	17	5	80	1120	6	21	3 carb., 2 med-fat meat, 1 fat

COMBINATION FOODS & FROZEN ENTREES

Products	Cal.	Carb. (g)	Fat (g)	Sat. Fat (g)	Chol. (mg)	Sod. (mg)	Fib. (g)	Prot. (g)	Servings/Exchanges
Lasagna, Vegetable (10.5 oz)	440	43	20	8	35	1110	5	21	3 carb., 2 med-fat meat, 2 fat
Lasagna, Five-Cheese (10.8 oz)	360	40	13	7	35	960	6	21	2 1/2 carb., 2 med-fat meat, 1 fat
Lasagna w/Meat Sauce (10.5 oz)	370	39	14	7	45	1050	4	23	2 1/2 carb., 2 med-fat meat, 1 fat
Pizza, French Bread Sausage (6 oz)	420	48	18	7	20	1260	3	17	3 carb., 2 med-fat meat, 2 fat
Pizza, French Bread Double Cheese (6 oz)	430	44	21	7	20	990	3	17	3 carb., 2 med-fat meat, 2 fat
Pizza, French Bread Grilled Vegetable (5.8 oz)	350	48	12	5	10	500	3	12	3 carb., 2 fat
Pizza, Pepperoni (5.6 oz)	430	46	20	8	15	990	3	16	3 carb., 1 med-fat meat, 3 fat
Macaroni & Cheese (6 oz)	320	31	16	7	30	990	3	13	2 carb., 1 med-fat meat, 2 fat
Macaroni w/Beef (11.5 oz)	420	40	20	8	50	1530	5	20	2 1/2 carb., 2 med-fat meat, 2 fat
Noodles Romanoff (6 oz)	240	27	11	3	25	610	2	8	2 carb., 2 fat
Side Dish, Corn Soufflé (4 oz)	170	21	7	2	55	540	1	5	1 1/2 strch, 1 fat

Side Dish, Creamed Spinach (4.5 oz)	160	8	12	4	15	380	2	4	1 vegetable, 2 fat
Side Dish, Potatoes Au Gratin (4.6 oz)	150	20	5	4	15	510	3	6	1 carb., 1 fat
Side Dish, Scalloped Potatoes (4.6 oz)	140	17	6	1	<5	450	2	4	1 carb., 1 fat
Skillet Sensations, Broccoli and Beef (12.5 oz)	310	52	3	2	25	1350	3	18	2 vegetable, 2 1/2 strch, 1 med-fat meat
Skillet Sensations, Chicken Alfredo (12.5 oz)	490	63	16	6	30	1240	9	23	4 strch, 2 med-fat meat, 1 fat
Skillet Sensations, Chicken and Grilled Vegetables (12.5 oz)	440	62	9	4	30	1330	6	27	4 strch, 2 med-fat meat
Skillet Sensations, Teriyaki Chicken (12.5 oz)	340	59	3	1	30	1350	3	20	4 strch, 1 med-fat meat
Spaghetti & Meatballs (12.6 oz)	440	56	15	5	50	830	5	19	3 1/2 carb., 1 med-fat meat, 2 fat
Swedish Meatballs (10.3 oz)	470	45	22	8	65	970	2	23	3 carb., 2 med-fat meat, 2 fat
Tuna-Noodle Casserole (10 oz)	320	37	10	4	40	1130	0	20	2 1/2 carb., 2 med-fat meat
Turkey Pie (10 oz)	530	36	33	9	65	1040	3	21	2 1/2 carb., 2 med-fat meat, 5 fat
Turkey Tetrazzini (10 oz)	360	33	17	7	55	1060	1	19	2 carb., 2 med-fat meat, 1 fat

COMBINATION FOODS & FROZEN ENTREES

Products	Cal.	Carb. (g)	Fat (g)	Sat. Fat (g)	Chol. (mg)	Sod. (mg)	Fib. (g)	Prot. (g)	Servings/Exchanges
SWANSON									
Bean and Frankfurter (10.5 oz)	440	53	19	NA	NA	900	NA	14	3 1/2 carb., 1 med-fat meat, 3 fat
BBQ Beef Entrée (11 oz)	460	51	17	NA	NA	860	NA	30	3 1/2 carb., 3 med-fat meat
Beef Enchilada Dinner (13.75 oz)	480	55	21	NA	NA	1350	NA	17	4 carb., 1 med-fat meat, 3 fat
Beef Entrée (11.25 oz)	310	38	6	NA	NA	770	NA	26	2 1/2 carb., 3 lean meat
Beef Pie (7 oz)	370	36	19	5	NA	730		12	2 1/2 carb., 1 med-fat meat, 3 fat
Budget Chicken Parmigiana Meal (10.5 oz)	300	35	15	NA	NA	780	NA	7	2 carb., 1 med-fat meat, 2 fat
Chicken A La King, Canned (5 1/4 oz)	190	9	12	NA	NA	690	NA	10	1/2 carb., 1 med-fat meat, 1 fat
Chicken Cacciatore (10.95 oz)	260	33	8	NA	NA	1030	NA	15	2 carb., 1 med-fat meat, 1 fat
Chicken Grilled w/Garlic Sauce (10 oz)	310	39	9	NA	30	630	NA	17	2 1/2 carb., 1 med-fat meat, 1 fat

Food	Cal								Exchanges
Chicken Nibbles (3.25 oz)	300	19	19	NA	NA	690	NA	12	1 carb., 1 med-fat meat, 3 fat
Chicken Nibbles (4.3 oz)	340	29	20	NA	NA	730	NA	10	2 carb., 1 med-fat meat, 3 fat
Chicken Nuggets (3 oz)	230	14	14	NA	NA	360	NA	13	1 carb., 1 med-fat meat, 2 fat
Chicken Pot Pie (7 oz)	380	35	22	NA	NA	810	NA	11	2 carb., 1 med-fat meat, 3 fat
Chicken w/Dumplings, Canned (7.5 oz)	220	19	11	NA	NA	980	NA	11	1 carb., 1 med-fat meat, 1 fat
Fish'n Chips (6.5 oz)	340	37	16	NA	NA	670	NA	11	2 1/2 carb., 1 med-fat meat, 2 fat
Fried Chicken Dinner, Dark Meat (9.75 oz)	560	55	28	NA	NA	1130	NA	22	4 carb., 1 med-fat meat, 5 fat
Fried Chicken Dinner, White Meat (10.25 oz)	550	60	25	NA	NA	1460	NA	22	4 carb., 2 med-fat meat, 3 fat
Ham Entrée (9 oz)	300	26	13	NA	NA	1080	NA	19	2 carb., 2 med-fat meat, 1 fat
Hungry Man Beef Pie (16 oz)	610	58	31	NA	NA	1370	NA	24	4 carb., 4 med-fat meat, 4 fat
Hungry Man Beef Steak Dinner (16.75 oz)	640	41	37	NA	NA	1600	NA	35	3 carb., 4 med-fat meat, 3 fat
Hungry Man Boneless Chicken Dinner (17.75 oz)	700	65	28	NA	NA	1530	NA	48	4 carb., 5 med-fat meat, 1 fat
Hungry Man Chicken Pie (16 oz)	630	57	35	NA	NA	1600	NA	22	4 carb., 1 med-fat meat, 6 fat
Hungry Man Fried Chicken Dinner, Dark Meat (14.4 oz)	860	77	45	NA	NA	1660	NA	36	5 carb. 3 med-fat meat, 6 fat

COMBINATION FOODS & FROZEN ENTREES

Products	Cal.	Carb. (g)	Fat (g)	Sat. Fat (g)	Chol. (mg)	Sod. (mg)	Fib. (g)	Prot. (g)	Servings/Exchanges
Hungry Man Fried Chicken, Mostly White Meat (16.7 oz)	870	80	46	NA	NA	2150	NA	35	5 carb., 3 med-fat meat, 6 fat
Hungry Man Mexican-Style Dinner (20.25 oz)	820	88	41	NA	NA	2080	NA	25	6 carb., 1 med-fat meat, 7 fat
Hungry Man Turkey Dinner, Mostly White Meat (17 oz)	550	61	18	NA	NA	1810	NA	36	4 carb., 3 med-fat meat, 1 fat
Hungry Man Turkey Pie (16 oz)	650	57	36	NA	NA	1470	NA	24	4 carb., 1 med-fat meat, 6 fat
Lasagna Entrée (10.5 oz)	400	39	15	NA	NA	1070	NA	26	2 1/2 carb., 3 med-fat meat
Macaroni & Cheese Entrée (12.25 oz)	370	43	15	NA	NA	1070	NA	13	3 carb., 1 med-fat meat, 2 fat
Mexican-Style Meal (14.25 oz)	490	62	18	NA	NA	1760	NA	19	4 carb., 1 med-fat meat, 3 fat
Noodles & Chicken (10.5 oz)	280	45	8	NA	NA	740	NA	7	3 carb., 2 fat
Plump & Juicy Fried Chicken (3.25 oz)	290	17	18	NA	NA	610	NA	15	1 carb., 2 med-fat meat, 2 fat
Pork Loin Dinner (10.75 oz)	280	27	12	NA	NA	790	NA	20	2 carb., 2 med-fat meat
Rib Sandwich Dinner (10.25 oz)	340	50	10	NA	25	690	NA	13	3 carb., 1 med-fat meat, 1 fat

Food									Exchanges
Salisbury Steak Dinner (10 oz)	320	22	16	NA	NA	980	NA	21	1 1/2 carb, 2 med-fat meat, 1 fat
Seafood Creole (9 oz)	240	40	6	NA	NA	810	NA	7	2 1/2 carb, 1 fat
Sirloin Beef Tips & Noodles (7 oz)	160	16	5	NA	NA	550	NA	12	1 carb, 1 med-fat meat
Spaghetti & Meatballs (12.5 oz)	390	46	17	NA	NA	1100	NA	14	3 carb, 1 med-fat meat, 2 fat
Swedish Meatballs Entrée (10 oz)	350	37	11	NA	NA	700	NA	26	2 1/2 carb, 3 lean meat
Turkey Breast Meat w/Pasta (11.25 oz)	310	36	9	NA	NA	670	NA	22	2 1/2 carb, 2 med-fat meat
Turkey Dinner, Mostly White Meat (11.5 oz)	350	42	11	NA	NA	1090	NA	21	3 carb, 2 med-fat meat
Turkey Pot Pie (7 oz)	380	36	21	NA	NA	720	NA	11	2 1/2 carb, 1 med-fat meat, 3 fat
Turkey w/Gravy & Dressing (9 oz)	290	30	11	NA	NA	1010	NA	18	2 carb, 2 med-fat meat
Veal Parmigiana (12.25 oz)	430	42	20	NA	NA	1010	NA	20	3 carb, 2 med-fat meat, 2 fat
TOMBSTONE									
Pizza-For-One, Extra Cheese (7 oz)	520	41	28	13	50	940	3	26	3 carb., 2 med-fat meat, 4 fat
Pizza-For-One, Pepperoni (7 oz)	550	41	32	14	55	1160	3	25	2 1/2 carb, 3 med-fat meat, 3 fat

COMBINATION FOODS & FROZEN ENTREES

Products	Cal.	Carb. (g)	Fat (g)	Sat. Fat (g)	Chol. (mg)	Sod. (mg)	Fib. (g)	Prot. (g)	Servings/Exchanges
Pizza-For-One, Supreme (7.7 oz)	550	42	32	14	55	1090	3	24	3 carb., 2 med-fat meat, 4 fat
TOTINO'S									
Party Pizza, Combination, Family (1/3)	400	47	18	4	20	990	3	17	3 carb., 1 med-fat meat, 3 fat
Party Pizza, Canadian Bacon (1/2)	330	42	13	2	10	860	3	15	3 carb., 1 med-fat meat, 2 fat
Party Pizza, Cheese (1/2)	290	40	10	3	15	530	2	13	2 1/2 carb., 1 med-fat meat, 1 fat
Party Pizza, Pepperoni (1/2)	380	41	19	4	15	980	3	14	3 carb., 1 med-fat meat, 3 fat
Party Pizza, Sausage, Family (1/3)	410	48	18	4	15	870	4	16	3 carb., 1 med-fat meat, 3 fat
Pan Pizza, Sausage & Pepperoni (1/6)	330	35	15	7	25	560	NA	16	2 carb., 1 med-fat meat, 2 fat
Pizza-For-One, Combination (4.2 oz)	290	26	16	4	15	730	1	10	2 carb., 1 med-fat meat, 2 fat
Pizza-For-One, Pepperoni (4 oz)	290	26	16	4	15	700	1	10	2 carb., 1 med-fat meat, 2 fat
Pizza Rolls, Hamburger (10)	230	26	10	NA	NA	417	NA	9	2 carb., 1 med-fat meat, 1 fat
Pizza Rolls, Pepperoni (10)	384	39	19	5	31	865	2	14	2 1/2 carb., 1 med-fat meat, 3 fat

Item	Cal								Exchanges/Choices
Pizza Rolls, Sausage (10)	350	40	15	3	25	630	3	14	2 1/2 carb., 1 med-fat meat, 2 fat
Select Pizza, Supreme (1/3)	347	29	18	7		772			2 carb., 2 med-fat meat, 2 fat
Select Pizza, Two-Cheese & Pepperoni (1/3)	363	30	20	8		823			2 carb., 2 med-fat meat, 2 fat

WEIGHT WATCHERS

Item	Cal								Exchanges/Choices
Barbecue-Glazed Chicken (7.5 oz)	220	26	4	1	48	405	NA	19	2 carb., 2 lean meat
BBQ Glazed Chicken (7.5 oz)	217	26	4	<1	48	405	NA	19	2 carb., 2 lean meat
Beef Romanoff (9 oz)	230	29	7	3	20	540	NA	12	2 carb., 1 med-fat meat
Beef Stir Fry, Jade Garden (9 oz)	150	17	3	2	20	490	NA	13	1 carb., 1 lean meat
Broccoli & Cheese Baked Potato Entree (10.5 oz)	270	43	6	6	5	570	NA	10	3 carb., 1 fat
Cantonese Beef Stir Fry (9 oz)	200	27	4	1	15	530	NA	14	2 carb., 1 med-fat meat
Cheese Tortellini (9 oz)	310	50	6	1	15	570	NA	14	3 carb., 1 med-fat meat
Chicken Enchiladas Suiza Entree (9 oz)	283	33	10	4	64	517	4	16	2 carb., 1 med-fat meat, 1 fat
Chicken Fettuccine Entree (8.25 oz)	280	25	9	3	40	590	NA	22	1 1/2 carb., 3 lean meat
Chicken Oriental Entree (9 oz)	160	21	2	1	15	430	NA	15	1 1/2 carb., 1 lean meat
English Muffin Sandwich (4 oz)	240	29	8	2	15	540	NA	14	2 carb., 1 med-fat meat, 1 fat

COMBINATION FOODS & FROZEN ENTREES

Products	Cal.	Carb. (g)	Fat (g)	Sat. Fat (g)	Chol. (mg)	Sod. (mg)	Fib. (g)	Prot. (g)	Servings/Exchanges
Fettuccine Alfredo w/Broccoli (8 oz)	230	28	7	2	25	550	NA	15	2 carb., 1 med-fat meat
Grilled Salisbury Beef Steak (8.6 oz)	260	24	10	5	40	620	3	19	1 1/2 carb., 2 med-fat meat
Ham & Cheese Omelet (4 oz)	180	18	5	3	10	420	NA	14	1 carb., 1 med-fat meat
Hunan Rice & Vegetables (10.5 oz)	250	39	7	2	5	630	8	7	2 1/2 carb., 1 fat
Lasagna Entree, Italian Cheese (11 oz)	290	29	7	2	20	510	NA	28	2 carb., 3 lean meat
Lasagna, Garden (11 oz)	260	30	7	2	15	430	NA	19	2 carb., 2 lean meat
Lasagna w/Meat Sauce Entree (10.25 oz)	270	29	6	2	5	510		24	2 carb., 3 lean meat
London Broil (7.4 oz)	140	9	3	1	40	510	NA	18	1/2 carb., 2 very lean meat
Macaroni & Beef (9 1/2 oz)	220	31	4	2	10	510	NA	14	2 carb., 1 med-fat meat
Macaroni & Cheese (9 oz)	280	43	6	2	20	550	NA	15	3 carb., 1 med-fat meat
Manicotti and Ricotta (9.25 oz)	260	31	8	3	25	510	NA	17	3 carb., 1 med-fat meat, 1 fat
Penne Pasta and Ricotta (10 oz)	280	45	6	2	5	370	5	12	3 carb., 1 med-fat meat
Pizza, Cheese (6.03 oz)	300	36	7	2	10	310	NA	24	2 1/2 carb., 2 lean meat
Pizza, Pepperoni (6.08 oz)	320	36	8	2	15	550	NA	25	2 1/2 carb., 2 med-fat meat

Food									Exchanges/Choices
Risotto w/Cheese & Mushrooms (9 oz)	290	44	8	4	20	540	4	11	3 carb., 1 med-fat meat, 1 fat
Roast Orange Glazed Chicken (9 oz)	170	25	2	1	10	360	NA	14	1 1/2 carb., 2 very lean meat
Roast Turkey Meal (8.6 oz)	213	35	2	<1	24	504	3	15	2 carb., 1 lean meat
Sausage Biscuit (3 oz)	220	19	11	2	70	560	NA	11	1 carb., 1 med-fat meat, 1 fat
Sesame Chicken (9 oz)	200	23	4	2	10	420	NA	19	1 1/2 carb., 2 lean meat
Spaghetti w/Meat Sauce Entree (10 oz)	240	28	7	1	5	490	NA	16	2 carb., 1 med-fat meat
Stuffed Turkey Breast (8.5 oz)	270	31	8	3	60	520	NA	18	2 carb., 2 med-fat meat
Teriyaki Chicken (9 oz)	140	16	3	2	20	470	NA	13	1 carb., 1 fat
Tex-Mex Chicken (8.3 oz)	250	33	5	2	35	590	NA	18	2 carb., 2 lean meat
Three Cheese Rotini w/Vegetables (9 oz)	270	34	8	3	5	550	NA	14	2 carb., 1 med-fat meat, 1 fat
Tuna-Noodle Casserole (9 oz)	230	27	7	2	20	550	NA	15	2 carb., 1 med-fat meat

DESSERTS

Products	Cal.	Carb. (g)	Fat (g)	Sat. Fat (g)	Chol. (mg)	Sod. (mg)	Fib. (g)	Prot. (g)	Servings/Exchanges
Angel Food Cake (1 piece)	129	29	<1	<1	0	255	<1	3	2 carb.
Apple Brown Betty (3/4 cup)	264	46	8	4	17	295	4	4	3 carb., 2 fat
Apple Turnover (1)	289	36	15	4	0	262	1	3	2 1/2 carb., 3 fat
Bread Pudding w/Raisins (1/2 cup)	212	31	7	3	83	291	1	7	2 carb., 1 fat
Brownie (1 small)	115	18	5	1	15	88	<1	1	1 carb., 1 fat
Brownie w/Nuts (2-inch square)	140	20	7	1	9	83	<1	1	1 carb., 1 fat
Cake, Chocolate w/Chocolate Icing (1 piece)	234	35	11	3	29	214	2	3	2 carb., 2 fat
Cake, Frosted (2-inch square)	175	29	6	2	18	194	NA	2	2 carb., 1 fat
Cake, German Chocolate w/Icing (1 slice)	404	55	21	5	53	369	2	4	3 1/2 carb., 4 fat
Cake, Pound w/Butter (1 piece)	110	14	6	3	63	113	<1	2	1 carb., 1 fat
Cake, Unfrosted (2-inch square)	97	16	3	<1	18	168	NA	2	1 carb., 1 fat
Cake, White w/White Icing (1 piece)	266	45	10	4	6	166	<1	2	3 carb., 2 fat
Cake, Yellow w/Chocolate Icing (1 piece)	243	36	11	3	35	216	1	2	2 1/2 carb., 2 fat

Food								
Cake/Wafer Ice Cream Cone (1)	17	3	<1	<1	0	6	<1	<1	free
Cheesecake (1/12 cake)	257	20	18	9	44	166	<1	4	1 carb., 4 fat
Chocolate Chips, Semisweet (1/4 cup)	201	27	13	8	0	5	3	2	2 carb., 3 fat
Cobbler, Apple (3 x 3-inch piece)	199	35	6	1	1	304	2	2	2 carb., 1 fat
Cobbler, Cherry (3 x 3-inch piece)	198	34	6	1	1	311	1	2	2 carb., 1 fat
Cobbler, Peach (3 x 3-inch piece)	204	37	6	1	1	308	2	2	2 1/2 carb., 1 fat
Coconut Macaroons (1-2-inch)	97	17	3	3	0	59	<1	<1	1 carb., 1 fat
Coffee Cake, Cinnamon w/Crumb Topping (1 piece)	263	29	15	3	20	221	1	4	2 carb., 3 fat
Cookies (1-3-inch)	142	19	7	2	10	103	<1	2	1 carb., 1 fat
Cookies, Chocolate Chip (1)	78	9	5	1	5	55	<1	<1	1/2 carb., 1 fat
Cookies, Fat-Free (2)	68	16	<1	0	0	51	2	2	1 carb.
Cookies, Fortune (2)	61	13	<1	<1	2	44	<1	<1	1 carb.
Cookies, Lady Fingers (4)	161	26	4	1	161	65	<1	5	2 carb., 1 fat
Cookies, Oatmeal (1)	81	12	3	<1	0	69	<1	1	1 carb., 1 fat
Cookies, Peanut Butter (1)	73	8	4	<1	4	64	<1	1	1/2 carb., 1 fat
Cookies, Sandwich w/Creme Filling (2)	94	14	4	<1	NA	120	NA	1	1 carb., 1 fat

DESSERTS

Products	Cal.	Carb. (g)	Fat (g)	Sat. Fat (g)	Chol. (mg)	Sod. (mg)	Fib. (g)	Prot. (g)	Servings/Exchanges
Cookies, Shortbread (4)	161	21	8	2	6	146	<1	2	1 1/2 carb., 2 fat
Cookies, Snickerdoodle (1)	81	12	4	2	9	68	<1	<1	1 carb., 1 fat
Cookies, Soft Raisin (1)	60	10	2	<1	<1	51	<1	<1	1/2 carb.
Cookies, Sugar (1)	72	10	3	2	8	54	<1	<1	1/2 carb., 1 fat
Crepe, Chocolate-Filled (1)	119	15	5	2	58	148	<1	4	1 carb., 1 fat
Crepe, Fruit-Filled (1)	131	21	4	1	63	124	<1	4	1 1/2 carb., 1 fat
Crisp, Apple, Homemade (1/2 cup)	230	46	5	1	0	257	2	3	3 carb., 1 fat
Crisp, Cherry (3 x 3-inch piece)	146	24	6	<1	0	74	1	2	1 1/2 carb., 1 fat
Crisp, Peach (3 x 3-inch piece)	155	27	5	<1	0	70	2	2	2 carb., 1 fat
Cupcake, Chocolate w/Chocolate Icing (1)	154	23	7	2	19	140	1	2	1 1/2 carb., 1 fat
Cupcake, Frosted (1 small)	172	28	6	NA	NA	161	NA	2	2 carb., 1 fat
Custard, Homemade (1/2 cup)	148	15	7	3	123	109	0	7	1 carb., 1 fat
Fruit Juice Bar, Frozen, w/Cream (1)	87	19	1	<1	5	20	<1	1	1 carb.
Fruit Juice Bar, Frozen, 100% Juice (1, 3 oz)	75	19	<1	0	0	3	0	1	1 carb.

Frozen Yogurt, Fat-Free (1/3 cup)	60	12	0	0	0	58	NA	3	1 carb.
Frozen Yogurt, Low-Fat (1/3 cup)	66	14	1	<1	3	26	<1	2	1 carb.
Gelatin, Dessert (1/2 cup)	80	19	0	0	0	57	0	2	1 carb.
Gelatin Snacks, Grape (1)	80	18	0	0	0	45	0	1	1 carb.
Gelatin Snacks, Orange (1)	80	18	0	0	0	45	0	1	1 carb.
Gingersnaps (3)	87	16	2	<1	0	137	<1	1	1 carb.
Ice Cream (1/2 cup)	133	16	7	7	29	53	0	2	1 carb., 1 fat
Ice Cream, Fat-Free (1/2 cup)	90	20	0	0	0	65	NA	4	1 carb.
Ice Cream, Light (1/2 cup)	100	14	4	3	25	35	1	3	1 carb., 1 fat
Ice Cream, No Sugar Added (1/2 cup)	100	13	4	3	15	45	NA	3	1 carb., 1 fat
Ice Cream Bar, Creamsicle/Dreamsicle (1)	92	18	2	1	7	43	0	2	1 carb.
Ice Cream Bar, Drumstick (1)	157	18	9	4	21	48	<1	3	1 carb., 2 fat
Ice Cream Bar, Fudgesicle (1)	91	19	<1	<1	<1	55	<1	4	1 carb.
Ice Cream Sandwich (1)	144	22	6	3	20	36	<1	3	1 1/2 carb., 1 fat
Ice Pops/Popsicles, Double Stick (1)	92	24	0	0	0	15	0	0	1 1/2 carb.
Marshmallows (4 large)	90	23	<1	0	0	13	<1	<1	1 1/2 carb.

DESSERTS

Products	Cal.	Carb. (g)	Fat (g)	Sat. Fat (g)	Chol. (mg)	Sod. (mg)	Fib. (g)	Prot. (g)	Servings/Exchanges
Parfait, Lime (1/2 cup)	120	21	3	3	0	105	0	3	1 1/2 carb., 1 fat
Pie, Fruit, 2-Crust (1/6)	290	43	13	2	0	300	NA	2	3 carb., 3 fat
Pie, Pumpkin or Custard (1/8)	168	19	4	1	21	209	NA	4	1 carb., 2 fat
Pudding, Chocolate w/Whole Milk, Homemade (1/2 cup)	221	40	6	3	17	137	1	5	2 1/2 carb., 1 fat
Pudding, Regular (1/2 cup)	144	27	3	2	9	201	NA	4	2 carb., 1 fat
Pudding, Rice w/Raisins, Homemade (1/2 cup)	217	40	4	3	17	85	<1	6	2 1/2 carb., 1 fat
Pudding, Sugar-Free (1/2 cup)	90	13	2	2	9	420	<1	4	1 carb.
Pudding, Tapioca w/2% Milk (1/2 cup)	147	28	2	2	9	172	0	4	2 carb.
Pudding, Tapioca w/Whole Milk, Homemade (1/2 cup)	103	14	4	2	125	157	0	7	1 carb., 1 fat
Pudding, Vanilla w/Whole Milk, Homemade (1/2 cup)	130	20	4	3	16	113	0	4	1 carb., 1 fat
Pudding Pop, Chocolate (1)	72	12	2	2	<1	78	<1	2	1 carb.

Pudding Pop, Vanilla (1)	75	13	2	2	<1	50	0	2	1 carb.
Sherbet, Orange (1/2 cup)	132	29	2	1	5	44	0	1	2 carb.
Sorbet, Citrus Fruit (1/2 cup)	92	23	0	0	0	8	<1	<1	1 1/2 carb.
Sorbet, Non-Citrus Fruit (1/2 cup)	70	17	<1	<1	0	46	0	1	1 carb.
Sugar/Rolled Ice Cream Cone (1)	40	8	<1	<1	0	32	<1	<1	1/2 carb.
Topping, Butterscotch (2 Tbsp)	103	27	<1	<1	<1	143	<1	<1	2 carb.
Topping, Hot Fudge (2 Tbsp)	147	25	6	2	5	28	<1	2	1 1/2 carb., 1 fat
Topping, Marshmallow Creme (2 Tbsp)	118	30	<1	0	0	18	<1	<1	2 carb.
Topping, Whipped (2 Tbsp)	24	2	2	1	0	0	0	0	free
Topping, Whipped, Light (2 Tbsp)	19	2	1	<1	0	0	0	0	free

ARCHWAY

Coconut Macaroons (5)	106	12	6	5	0	38	<1	<1	1 carb., 1 fat
Cookie Jar Hermits (1)	95	17	3	<1	5	147	<1	1	1 carb., 1 fat
Cookies, Apple-Filled (1)	100	16	3	<1	<5	103	<1	1	1 carb., 1 fat
Cookies, Apple N' Raisin (1)	120	20	3	NA	10	170	1	2	1 carb., 1 fat
Cookies, Mud Pie (1)	110	15	5	2	5	105	1	<1	1 carb., 1 fat

DESSERTS

Products	Cal.	Carb. (g)	Fat (g)	Sat. Fat (g)	Chol. (mg)	Sod. (mg)	Fib. (g)	Prot. (g)	Servings/Exchanges
Cookies, Chocolate Chip (1)	50	7	3	NA	5	40	NA	1	1/2 carb., 1 fat
Cookies, Chocolate Chip & Toffee (1)	130	18	6	2	6	125	<1	1	1 carb., 1 fat
Cookies, Chocolate Chip, Sugar Free (1)	105	16	5	1	<1	65	<1	1	1 carb., 1 fat
Cookies, Cinnamon Honey Heart, Fat-Free (3)	105	25	0	0	0	125	1	1	1 1/2 carb.
Cookies, Cinnamon Apple (1)	105	17	4	<1	0	130	<1	1	1 carb., 1 fat
Cookies, Dark Molasses (1)	115	20	3	<1	0	150	<1	1	1 carb., 1 fat
Cookies, Date-Filled Oatmeal (1)	100	17	3	<1	<5	100	<1	1	1 carb., 1 fat
Cookies, Devil's Food, Fat-Free (1)	70	16	<1	<1	0	80	<1	1	1 carb.
Cookies, Dutch Cocoa (1)	100	17	3	<1	<5	87	<1	1	1 carb., 1 fat
Cookies, Frosty Lemon (1)	112	17	5	2	0	110	<1	1	1 carb., 1 fat
Cookies, Frosty Orange (1)	113	17	5	1	0	95	<1	1	1 carb., 1 fat
Cookies, Fruit & Honey Bar (1)	105	18	3	<1	6	107	<1	1	1 carb., 1 fat
Cookies, Gingersnaps, Reduced Fat (3)	140	24	4	<1	0	140	<1	1	1 1/2 carb., 1 fat
Cookies, Iced Gingersnaps (3)	170	26	7	2	0	130	<1	1	2 carb., 1 fat

Cookies, Iced Molasses (1)	114	20	4	1	0	130	<1	1	1 carb., 1 fat
Cookies, Iced Oatmeal (1)	125	18	5	2	<5	90	<1	2	1 carb., 1 fat
Cookies, Lemon Drop (1)	93	15	3	<1	9	95	<1	1	1 carb., 1 fat
Cookies, Molasses, Plain (1)	103	18	3	<1	8	145	<1	1	1 carb., 1 fat
Cookies, Oatmeal (1)	110	17	4	<1	<5	90	<1	2	1 carb., 1 fat
Cookies, Oatmeal Pecan (1)	135	16	7	2	5	100	<1	2	1 carb., 1 fat
Cookies, Oatmeal Raisin (1)	110	17	4	<1	<5	100	<1	2	1 carb., 1 fat
Cookies, Oatmeal Raisin, Fat-Free (1)	105	24	0	0	0	165	<1	1	1 1/2 carb.
Cookies, Oatmeal Sugar Free (1)	105	16	5	1	0	75	<1	1	1 carb., 1 fat
Cookies, Old-Fashioned Molasses (1)	105	18	3	<1	8	140	<1	1	1 carb., 1 fat
Cookies, Old-Fashioned Windmill (1)	90	14	4	<1	0	95	<1	1	1 carb., 1 fat
Cookies, Peanut Butter (1)	100	12	5	1	8	85	<1	2	1 carb., 1 fat
Cookies, Peanut Jumble (1)	115	13	6	2	<5	75	<1	2	1 carb., 1 fat
Cookies, Pecan Ice-Box (1)	120	15	6	1	6	75	<1	1	1 carb., 1 fat
Cookies, Pineapple-Filled (1)	110	17	4	1	7	65	<1	1	1 carb., 1 fat
Cookies, Raspberry-Filled (1)	100	16	4	1	7	85	<1	1	1 carb., 1 fat

DESSERTS

Products	Cal.	Carb. (g)	Fat (g)	Sat. Fat (g)	Chol. (mg)	Sod. (mg)	Fib. (g)	Prot. (g)	Servings/Exchanges
Cookies, Raspberry Oatmeal, No-Fat (1)	110	25	0	0	0	165	<1	1	1 1/2 carb.
Cookies, Rocky Road, Sugar Free (1)	100	15	5	1	<1	65	<1	1	1 carb., 1 fat
Cookies, Ruth's Golden Oatmeal (1)	110	17	4	<1	<5	115	<1	2	1 carb., 1 fat
Cookies, Soft Sugar (1)	110	17	3	<1	5	160	<1	1	1 carb., 1 fat
Cookies, Strawberry/Cherry-Filled (1)	100	16	4	1	7	85	<1	1	1 carb., 1 fat
Cookies, Sugar Cookies, Fat-Free (1)	70	17	0	0	0	80	<1	1	1 carb.
BANQUET									
Pie, Apple (1/5)	300	42	13	6	5	370	1	2	3 carb., 3 fat
Pie, Banana (1/3)	350	39	21	5	<5	290	1	2	2 1/2 carb., 4 fat
Pie, Cherry (1/5)	290	39	14	6	10	310	1	2	2 1/2 carb., 3 fat
Pie, Chocolate (1/3)	360	43	20	5	<5	240	1	2	3 carb., 4 fat
Pie, Coconut (1/3)	350	39	20	6	<5	250	1	2	2 1/2 carb., 4 fat
Pie, Lemon (1/3)	360	43	20	5	<5	240	1	2	3 carb., 4 fat
Pie, Peach (1/5)	270	36	13	6	5	340	1	2	2 1/2 carb., 3 fat

BEN & JERRY'S

Frozen Yogurt, Cherry Garcia (1/2 cup)	170	31	3	2	10	70	0	4	2 carb., 1 fat
Frozen Yogurt, Chocolate Cherry Garcia (1/2 cup)	190	35	4	3	15	65	1	5	2 carb., 1 fat
Frozen Yogurt, Chocolate Chip Cookie Dough (1/2 cup)	200	35	5	3	10	120	0	4	2 carb., 1 fat
Frozen Yogurt, Chocolate Fudge Brownie (1/2 cup)	190	35	4	2	10	130	2	6	2 carb., 1 fat
Frozen Yogurt, Chocolate Heath Bar Crunch (1/2 cup)	210	35	6	3	10	115	1	5	2 carb., 1 fat
Frozen Yogurt, Chunky Monkey (1/2 cup)	200	34	6	3	5	65	<1	4	2 carb., 1 fat
Ice Cream, Butter Pecan (1/2 cup)	330	22	25	12	65	140	2	6	1 1/2 carb., 5 fat
Ice Cream, Cherry Garcia (1/2 cup)	260	26	16	11	70	60	0	5	2 carb., 3 fat
Ice Cream, Chocolate Almond Fudge Chip (1/2 cup)	310	24	22	14	40	70	2	5	1 1/2 carb., 4 fat
Ice Cream, Chocolate Chip Cookie Dough (1/2 cup)	300	34	16	10	65	95	0	5	2 carb., 3 fat
Ice Cream, Chocolate Fudge Brownie (1/2 cup)	280	32	15	10	45	90	2	5	2 carb., 3 fat
Ice Cream, Chubby Hubby (1/2 cup)	350	33	21	12	55	250	1	6	2 carb., 5 fat
Ice Cream, Chunky Monkey (1/2 cup)	310	32	19	11	55	55	3	5	1 1/2 carb., 3 fat

DESSERTS

Products	Cal.	Carb. (g)	Fat (g)	Sat. Fat (g)	Chol. (mg)	Sod. (mg)	Fib. (g)	Prot. (g)	Servings/Exchanges
Ice Cream, Coffee Heath Bar Crunch (1/2 cup)	310	32	18	12	65	125	0	4	2 carb., 4 fat
Ice Cream, Low-Fat Blackberry Cobbler (1/2 cup)	180	34	3	2	20	70	<1	3	2 carb., 1 fat
Ice Cream, Low-Fat Chocolate Comfort (1/2 cup)	150	29	2	2	10	85	<1	4	2 carb.
Ice Cream, Mint Chocolate Cookie (1/2 cup)	280	28	17	11	70	130	1	4	2 carb., 3 fat
Ice Cream, New York Super Fudge Chunk (1/2 cup)	220	28	21	12	50	65	4	5	2 carb., 4 fat
Ice Cream, Orange and Cream (1/2 cup)	230	23	14	10	40	50	0	3	1 1/2 carb., 3 fat
Ice Cream, Peanut Butter Cup (1/2 cup)	380	32	25	13	65	130	2	7	2 carb., 5 fat
Ice Cream, S'mores, Low Fat (1/2 cup)	190	35	2	1	15	85	1	5	2 carb.
Ice Cream, Triple Caramel Chunk (1/2 cup)	290	32	17	12	40	105	0	4	2 carb., 3 fat
Ice Cream, Vanilla Caramel Fudge (1/2 cup)	300	33	17	10	70	115	1	4	2 carb., 3 fat
Ice Cream, World's Best Vanilla (1/2 cup)	250	22	16	11	75	60	0	4	1 1/2 carb., 3 fat
Ice Cream, Wavy Gravy (1/2 cup)	340	32	20	10	60	120	2	7	2 carb., 5 fat
Novelty, Cherry Garcia Yogurt Pop (1)	250	32	13	8	15	85	2	6	2 carb., 3 fat
Novelty, Cookie Dough Pop (1)	410	45	24	11	45	140	<1	5	3 carb., 5 fat

Food	Cal.	Carb. (g)	Fat (g)	Sat. Fat (g)	Chol. (mg)	Sod. (mg)	Fiber (g)	Prot. (g)	Exchanges
Novelty, Vanilla Heath Bar Crunch Pop (1)	320	32	21	13	50	105	<1	4	2 carb., 4 fat
Smoothies, Strawberry Banana Manna (12 oz)	290	68	0	0	0	45	5	4	4 1/2 carb.
Smoothies, Tropic of Mango (12 oz)	300	75	<1	0	0	50	5	3	5 carb.
Sorbet, Lemon Swirl (1/2 cup)	120	30	0	0	0	15	0	0	2 carb.
Sorbet, Purple Passion Fruit (1/2 cup)	140	22	0	0	0	25	0	0	1 1/2 carb.
BIRD'S EYE									
Cool Whip Free Whipped Topping (2 Tbsp)	15	3	0	0	0	5	0	0	free
Cool Whip Lite Whipped Topping (2 Tbsp)	20	2	1	1	0	0	0	0	free
Cool Whip Topping, Extra Creamy (2 Tbsp)	30	2	2	2	0	5	0	0	free
Cool Whip Topping, Regular (2 Tbsp)	25	2	2	2	0	0	0	0	free
Dairy Whip Whipped Light Cream (2 Tbsp)	10	<1	1	<1	<5	0	0	0	free
Dream Whip Whipped Topping Mix (2 Tbsp)	20	2	1	<1	0	5	0	0	free
BREYERS									
Ice Cream, Chocolate (1/2 cup)	160	20	8	5	20	30	0	3	1 carb., 2 fat
Ice Cream, Strawberry (1/2 cup)	130	16	6	4	20	40	0	2	1 carb., 1 fat
Ice Cream, Vanilla (1/2 cup)	150	15	8	5	25	50	0	3	1 carb., 2 fat

DESSERTS

Products	Cal.	Carb. (g)	Fat (g)	Sat. Fat (g)	Chol. (mg)	Sod. (mg)	Fib. (g)	Prot. (g)	Servings/Exchanges
Premium Ice Milk, Chocolate Light (1/2 cup)	120	18	4	2	15	55	0	3	1 carb., 1 fat
Premium Ice Milk, Strawberry Light (1/2 cup)	110	18	3	2	15	50	0	3	1 carb., 1 fat
Premium Ice Milk, Vanilla Light (1/2 cup)	120	18	4	2	10	60	0	3	1 carb., 1 fat
DANNON									
Frozen Yogurt, All Flavors, Nonfat (1/2 cup)	80	20	0	0	0	70	0	4	1 carb.
Frozen Yogurt, Chocolate (1/2 cup)	80	19	1	0	0	70	0	4	1 1/2 carb.
Frozen Yogurt, Peach Nonfat (1/2 cup)	80	19	0	0	0	70	0	4	1 carb.
Frozen Yogurt, Strawberry Nonfat (1/2 cup)	80	19	0	0	0	70	0	4	1 carb.
DOLE									
Fruit 'N Cream Bar, Strawberry (1)	90	19	1	0	5	22	0	1	1 carb.
Fruit 'N Juice Bar, Strawberry (1)	70	16	0	0	0	6	NA	<1	1 carb.
Juice Bar, Strawberry, No Sugar Added (1)	25	6	0	0	0	5	0	0	1/2 carb.
Sorbet, Orange, Non-fat (4 oz)	110	28	0	0	0	9	0	<1	2 carb.

DOVE

Ice Cream Bar, Vanilla w/Milk Chocolate (1)	260	24	17	11	30	45	0	3	1 1/2 carb., 3 fat

ENTENMANN'S

Cake, All-Butter French Crumb (1 slice)	210	29	10	6	60	240	0	3	2 carb., 2 fat
Cake, All-Butter Loaf (1 slice)	220	31	10	6	80	290	0	3	2 carb., 2 fat
Cake, Banana Crunch (1 slice)	220	32	9	2	40	280	<1	2	2 carb., 2 fat
Cake, Carrot (1 slice)	290	35	16	4	35	240	<1	3	2 carb., 3 fat
Cake, Chocolate Fudge (1 slice)	310	47	14	5	45	260	2	3	3 carb., 3 fat
Cake, Fat-Free Apple Spice Crumb (1 slice)	130	30	0	0	0	140	2	2	2 carb.
Cake, Fat-Free Banana Crunch (1 slice)	140	33	0	0	0	150	2	2	2 carb.
Cake, Fat-Free Banana Loaf (1 slice)	150	34	0	0	0	190	1	2	2 carb.
Cake, Fat-Free Blueberry Crunch (1 slice)	140	32	0	0	0	200	2	2	2 carb.
Cake, Fat-Free Carrot (1 slice)	170	40	0	0	0	230	NA	3	2 1/2 carb.
Cake, Fat-Free Chocolate Crunch (1 slice)	130	32	0	0	0	170	2	2	2 carb.
Cake, Fat-Free Chocolate Loaf (1 slice)	130	30	0	0	0	250	1	3	2 carb.
Cake, Fat-Free Fudge Chocolate (1 slice)	210	51	0	0	0	270	2	3	3 1/2 carb.

DESSERTS

Products	Cal.	Carb. (g)	Fat (g)	Sat. Fat (g)	Chol. (mg)	Sod. (mg)	Fib. (g)	Prot. (g)	Servings/Exchanges
Cake, Fat-Free Fudge Gold (1 slice)	220	52	0	0	0	200	2	3	3 1/2 carb.
Cake, Fat-Free Gold Chocolate Chip (1 slice)	130	31	0	0	0	220	1	3	2 carb.
Cake, Fat-Free Marble Loaf (1 slice)	130	29	0	0	0	190	1	2	2 carb.
Cake, Fat-Free Raisin Loaf (1 slice)	140	33	0	0	0	150	1	2	2 carb.
Cake, Louisana Crunch (1 slice)	310	45	13	4	50	290	<1	3	3 carb., 3 fat
Cake, Marble Loaf (1 slice)	200	25	10	6	65	230	<1	2	1 1/2 carb., 2 fat
Cake, Marshmallow-Iced Devil's Food (1 slice)	350	45	18	5	45	290	1	3	3 carb., 4 fat
Cake, Raisin Loaf (1 slice)	220	32	9	2	50	200	<1	3	2 carb., 2 fat
Cake, Thick Fudge Golden (1 slice)	330	48	16	4	50	270	2	3	2 carb., 3 fat
Coffee Cake, Cheese (1 slice)	190	24	8	4	30	160	0	4	1 1/2 carb., 2 fat
Coffee Cake, Cheese-Filled Crumb (1 slice)	210	25	10	4	40	190	<1	4	1 1/2 carb., 2 fat
Coffee Cake, Crumb (1 slice)	250	33	12	3	15	210	1	4	2 carb., 2 fat
Coffee Cake, Fat-Free Cinnamon Apple (1 slice)	130	29	0	0	0	110	2	2	2 carb.
Pie, Coconut Custard (1 slice)	340	35	19	8	135	310	1	7	2 carb., 4 fat

Pie, Fat-Free Cherry Behive (1 slice)	270	64	0	0	0	310	1	3	4 carb.
Pie, Homestyle Apple (1 slice)	300	42	14	4	0	300	2	2	3 carb., 3 fat
Pie, Lemon (1 slice)	340	45	17	5	45	420	<1	3	3 carb., 3 fat

ESKIMO PIE

Ice Cream Bar, Original (1)	180	16	12	NA	NA	35	0	2	1 carb., 2 fat
Ice Cream Bar, Sugar Freedom (1)	140	13	11	NA	NA	30	0	2	1 carb., 2 fat
Ice Cream Sandwich, Sugar-Freedom (1)	170	26	6	NA	NA	142	0	4	1 carb., 3 fat

ESTEE

Cookies, No Sucrose Added, Oatmeal Raisin (4)	130	19	5	1	0	25	1	2	1 carb., 1 fat
Cookies, No Sucrose Added Sandwich, Chocolate (3)	160	24	6	2	0	60	1	2	1 1/2 carb., 1 fat
Cookies, No Sucrose Added Sandwich, Original (3)	160	24	6	2	0	45	1	2	1 1/2 carb., 1 fat
Cookies, No Sucrose Added Sandwich, Peanut Butter (3)	160	22	7	1	0	55	1	4	1 1/2 carb., 1 fat
Cookies, No Sucrose Added Sandwich, Vanilla (3)	160	25	5	1	0	35	<1	2	1 1/2 carb., 1 fat
Cookies, No Sucrose Added, Shortbread (4)	130	22	4	1	0	150	<1	2	1 1/2 carb., 1 fat

DESSERTS

Products	Cal.	Carb. (g)	Fat (g)	Sat. Fat (g)	Chol. (mg)	Sod. (mg)	Fib. (g)	Prot. (g)	Servings/Exchanges
Cookies, No Sucrose Added, Vanilla or Lemon Thins (4)	140	19	6	1	0	25	<1	2	1 carb., 1 fat
Cookies, Sugar Free, Chocolate Chip (3)	110	22	4	<1	0	70	1	2	1 1/2 carb., 1 fat
Cookies, Sugar Free, Chocolate Walnut (3)	110	22	4	0	0	95	1	2	1 1/2 carb., 1 fat
Cookies, Sugar Free, Coconut (3)	110	22	4	1	0	110	1	2	1 1/2 carb., 1 fat
Cookies, Sugar Free, Lemon (3)	110	22	3	0	0	90	1	2	1 1/2 carb., 1 fat
Creme Wafer, Sugar Free, Vanilla & Chocolate (5)	150	21	8	2	0	10	0	1	1 1/2 carb., 2 fat
Fig Bars, No Sucrose Added, All Flavors (2 bars)	100	23	1	0	0	20	3	1	1 1/2 carb.
Syrup, Chocolate (2 Tbsp)	15	5	0	0	0	40	0	<1	1 carb.
FROOKIE									
Cookies, Apple Cinnamon Oat Bran (1)	45	7	2	<1	0	35	NA	1	1/2 carb.
Cookies, Fat-Free Banana (1)	45	10	0	0	0	90	1	1	1/2 carb.
Cookies, Fat-Free Cranberry Orange (1)	45	10	0	0	0	75	1	1	1/2 carb.
Cookies, Fat-Free Fruitins Fig (2)	90	21	0	0	0	75	1	1	1 1/2 carb.

Item	Cal.	Carb. (g)	Fat (g)	Sat. Fat (g)	Chol. (mg)	Sod. (mg)	Fiber (g)	Carb Choices	Exchanges
Cookies, Fat-Free Oatmeal Raisin (1)	50	11	0	0	0	75	1	1	1 1/2 carb.
Cookies, Lemon (1)	50	7	2	0	0	30	NA	1	1/2 carb.
Cookies, Sandwich, Chocolate Frookwich (1)	50	7	2	0	0	30	NA	1	1/2 carb.
GRANDMA'S									
Big Chocolate Chip Cookie (1)	190	25	9	3	0	135	<1	2	1 1/2 carb., 2 fat
Big Fudge Chocolate Chip Cookie (1)	170	26	7	3	<5	160	1	1	2 carb., 1 fat
Big Oatmeal Raisin Cookie (1)	160	26	6	2	5	250	1	1	2 carb., 1 fat
Big Old Time Molasses Cookie (1)	160	29	4	2	<5	230	<1	2	2 carb., 1 fat
Big Peanut Butter Chocolate Chip Cookie (1)	190	23	9	3	<5	170	1	4	1 1/2 carb., 2 fat
Big Peanut Butter Cookie (1)	190	22	9	2	5	200	1	2	1 1/2 carb., 2 fat
Mini Fudge Cookies (9)	150	21	7	2	0	180	1	2	1 1/2 carb., 1 fat
Mini Peanut Butter Cookies (9)	150	21	7	2	0	140	1	2	1 1/2 carb., 1 fat
Mini Vanilla Cookies (9)	150	22	7	2	<5	85	<1	2	1 1/2 carb., 1 fat
Peanut Butter Sandwich Cookies (5)	210	28	10	3	0	200	1	3	2 carb., 2 fat
Rich N' Chewy Cookies (1 pkg)	270	39	12	4	10	130	1	2	3 1/2 carb., 2 fat
Vanilla Sandwich Cookies (5)	210	30	10	3	5	125	<1	2	2 carb., 2 fat

DESSERTS

Products	Cal.	Carb. (g)	Fat (g)	Sat. Fat (g)	Chol. (mg)	Sod. (mg)	Fib. (g)	Prot. (g)	Servings/Exchanges
HAAGEN DAZS									
Frozen Yogurt, Chocolate (1/2 cup)	140	28	0	0	<5	45	<1	6	2 carb.
Frozen Yogurt, Coffee (1/2 cup)	140	29	0	0	<5	45	0	6	2 carb.
Frozen Yogurt, Vanilla (1/2 cup)	140	29	0	0	<5	45	0	6	2 carb.
Frozen Yogurt, Vanilla Raspberry Swirl (1/2 cup)	130	28	0	0	<5	30	0	4	2 carb.
Ice Cream Bar, Chocolate & Dark Chocolate (1)	350	28	24	15	85	60	2	5	2 carb., 5 fat
Ice Cream, Chocolate (1/2 cup)	270	22	18	11	115	75	1	5	1 1/2 carb., 4 fat
Ice Cream, Chocolate & Almond (1)	310	23	22	12	<5	50	0	6	1 1/2 carb., 4 fat
Ice Cream, Low-fat Cookies & Fudge (1/2 cup)	180	33	3	2	15	115	<1	7	2 carb., 1 fat
Ice Cream, Low-fat Vanilla (1/2 cup)	170	29	3	2	20	50	0	7	2 carb., 1 fat
Ice Cream, Vanilla (1/2 cup)	270	21	18	11	120	85	0	5	1 1/2 carb., 4 fat
Stick Bars, Raspberry (1)	100	24	<1	0	0	NA	0	<1	1 1/2 carb.
HEALTH VALLEY									
Cookies, Almond Fruit Jumbos (1)	70	10	3	NA	0	30	1	2	1/2 carb., 1 fat

Item									
Cookies, Fat-Free Apple Spice (3)	80	18	0	0	0	80	3	2	1 cart.
Cookies, Fruit Centers Date (1)	70	16	0	0	0	35	4	2	1 carb.
Cookies, Fruit Centers Raspberry (1)	80	17	0	0	0	80	2	2	1 carb.
Cookies, Fruit Centers Strawberry (1)	75	17	0	0	0	60	3	2	1 carb.
Cookies, Oat Bran (1)	70	10	2	NA	0	22	2	1	1/2 carb.
Cookies, Oatmeal Raisin (3)	80	18	0	0	0	80	3	2	1 carb.
Cookies, Peach Apricot Mini Fruit Centers (3)	75	17	0	0	0	60	3	2	1 carb.
Cookies, Peanut (2)	100	14	3	NA	0	585	2	2	1 1/2 carb.
Cookies, Tofu (2)	90	16	3	NA	0	30	1	2	1 1/2 carb.
Granola/Cereal Bar, Blueberry Apple (1)	140	33	0	0	0	10	4	3	2 carb.
Granola/Cereal Bar, Date Almond (1)	140	33	0	0	0	10	4	3	2 carb.
Granola/Cereal Bar, Fat-Free Raspberry (1)	140	33	0	0	0	10	4	3	2 carb.
Snack Bar, Apple (1)	100	16	3	NA	0	27	3	2	1 carb., 1 fat
Snack Bar, Date (1)	100	16	3	NA	0	25	3	3	1 carb., 1 fat
Snack Bar, Fat-Free Apple (1)	140	33	0	0	0	10	4	3	2 carb.
Snack Bar, Fat-Free Apricot (1)	140	33	0	0	0	10	4	3	2 carb.

DESSERTS

Products	Cal.	Carb. (g)	Fat (g)	Sat. Fat (g)	Chol. (mg)	Sod. (mg)	Fib. (g)	Prot. (g)	Servings/Exchanges
Snack Bar, Fat-Free Date (1)	140	33	0	0	0	10	4	3	2 carb.
Snack Bar, Fruit (2)	200	39	3	NA	0	234	5	4	2 1/2 carb., 1 fat
Snack Bar, Fat-Free Raisin (1)	140	33	0	0	0	10	4	3	2 carb.
Snack Bar, Oat Bran, Apricot (1)	100	19	2	NA	0	18	3	2	1 carb.
Snack Bar, Oat Bran, Fig (1)	110	19	3	NA	0	18	3	2	1 carb., 1 fat
Snack Bar, Oat Bran, Fruit Nut (1)	150	29	4	NA	0	11	8	4	2 carb., 1 fat
Snack Bar, Oat Bran, Jumbo Fruit (1)	170	28	5	NA	0	9	7	4	2 carb., 1 fat
Snack Bar, Oat Bran, Raisin & Cinnamon (1)	140	32	2	NA	0	12	6	3	2 carb.
Snack Bar, Raisin (1)	100	16	3	NA	0	19	3	2	1 carb., 1 fat
HEALTHY CHOICE									
Ice Cream, Black Forest (1/2 cup)	120	23	2	1	5	50	1	3	1 1/2 carb.
Ice Cream, Chocolate Chocolate Chunk (1/2 cup)	120	21	2	1	<5	45	2	3	1 1/2 carb.
Ice Cream, Cookies & Cream (1/2 cup)	120	21	2	1	<5	90	<1	3	1 1/2 carb.
Ice Cream, Fudge Brownie (1/2 cup)	120	22	2	1	5	55	<2	3	1 1/2 carb.

	Cal	Carb				Sod			Exchanges
Ice Cream, Low-Fat Praline & Caramel (1/2 cup)	130	25	2	<1	<5	70	<1	3	1 1/2 carb.
Ice Cream, Mint Chocolate Chip (1/2 cup)	120	21	2	1	<5	50	<1	3	1 1/2 carb.
Ice Cream, Old Fashioned Butter Pecan (1/2 cup)	120	22	2	1	<5	60	1	3	1 1/2 carb.
Ice Cream, Old Fashioned Strawberry (1/2 cup)	110	20	2	1	0	35	1	2	1 carb.
Ice Cream, Rocky Road (1/2 cup)	140	28	2	1	<5	60	2	3	1 1/2 carb.
Ice Cream, Vanilla (1/2 cup)	100	18	2	1	5	50	1	3	1 carb.
HEATH									
Ice Cream Bar, English Toffee (1)	205	17	15	12	24	43	<1	2	1 carb., 3 fat
HOSTESS									
Ding Dongs (1)	170	21	9	6	5	115	1	2	1 1/2 carb., 2 fat
Ho Ho's (1)	120	16	6	4	10	70	<1	1	1 carb., 1 fat
Twinkies (1)	150	27	5	2	20	200	<1	2	2 carb., 1 fat
HUNT'S									
Pudding, Snack Pack, Chocolate (4 oz)	161	25	6	2	0	178	0	2	1 1/2 carb., 1 fat
Pudding, Snack Pack, Light Chocolate (4 oz)	100	20	2	NA	0	120	0	3	1 carb.
Pudding, Snack Pack, Tapioca (4 oz)	95	21	<1	0	0	185	0	2	1 1/2 carb.

DESSERTS

Products	Cal.	Carb. (g)	Fat (g)	Sat. Fat (g)	Chol. (mg)	Sod. (mg)	Fib. (g)	Prot. (g)	Servings/Exchanges
Pudding, Snack Pack, Vanilla (4 oz)	158	25	6	2	0	141	0	2	1 1/2 carb., 1 fat
JELL-O									
Cook/Serve Pudding w/2% Milk, Chocolate (1/2 cup)	150	28	3	2	10	170	<1	5	2 carb., 1 fat
Cook/Serve Pudding w/2% Milk, Vanilla (1/2 cup)	140	26	3	2	10	200	0	4	2 carb., 1 fat
Gelatin Dessert, Cherry (1/2 cup)	80	19	0	0	0	100	0	2	1 carb.
Gelatin Dessert, Cherry Sugar-Free (1/2 cup)	10	0	0	0	0	70	0	1	free
Gelatin Snacks, Cherry (1)	70	17	0	0	0	40	0	1	1 carb.
Gelatin Snacks, Sugar Free, Strawberry (1)	10	0	0	0	0	45	0	1	free
Handi-Snacks Pudding, Vanilla (1)	120	22	4	1	0	150	0	1	1 1/2 carb., 1 fat
Instant Pudding w/Skim Milk, Fat Free, Chocolate (1/2 cup)	140	31	0	0	<5	410	<1	5	2 carb.
Instant Pudding w/Skim Milk, Fat Free, Vanilla (1/2 cup)	140	29	0	0	<5	410	0	4	2 carb.

Food	Cal.	Carb. (g)	Fat (g)	Sat. Fat (g)	Chol. (mg)	Sod. (mg)	Fiber (g)		Exchanges
Instant Pudding w/Skim Milk, Fat/Sugar Free, Vanilla (1/2 cup)	70	12	0	0	<5	400	0	4	1 carb.
Instant Pudding w/Skim Milk, Fat/Sugar Free, Chocolate (1/2 cup)	80	14	0	0	<5	390	<1	5	1 carb.
Instant Pudding/Pie Filling w/2% Milk, Chocolate (1/2 cup)	160	31	3	2	10	470	<1	4	2 carb., 1 fat
Instant Pudding/Pie Filling w/2% Milk, Vanilla (1/2 cup)	150	29	3	2	10	410	0	4	2 carb., 1 fat
No-Bake Cherry Cheesecake (1/3)	340	52	12	5	5	400	<1	5	3 1/2 carb., 2 fat
No-Bake Chocolate Silk Pie (1/8)	320	37	16	6	5	490	<1	5	2 1/2 carb., 3 fat
No-Bake Double Layer Lemon (1/8)	260	36	12	4	<5	370	<1	4	2 1/2 carb., 2 fat
Pudding Snacks, Chocolate (1)	160	28	5	2	0	190	0	3	2 carb., 1 fat
Pudding Snacks, Fat-Free, Chocolate (1)	100	23	0	0	0	190	<1	3	1 1/2 carb.
Pudding Snacks, Fat-Free, Chocolate Vanilla Swirl (1)	100	23	0	0	0	210	<1	3	1 1/2 carb.
Pudding Snacks, Tapioca (1)	140	26	4	1.5	0	160	0	2	2 carb., 1 fat

DESSERTS

Products	Cal.	Carb. (g)	Fat (g)	Sat. Fat (g)	Chol. (mg)	Sod. (mg)	Fib. (g)	Prot. (g)	Servings/Exchanges
Pudding Snacks, Vanilla (1)	160	25	5	2	0	170	0	2	2 carb., 1 fat
Pudding Snacks, Vanilla Chocolate Swirl (1)	160	27	5	2	0	180	0	3	2 carb., 1 fat
KEEBLER									
Animal Crackers (10)	130	22	4	1	0	140	<1	2	1 1/2 carb., 1 fat
Chips Deluxe (1)	80	9	5	2	0	60	0	1	1/2 carb., 1 fat
Chips Deluxe, Rainbow (1)	80	10	4	2	<5	45	<1	1	1/2 carb., 1 fat
Chips Deluxe, Soft 'n' Chewy (1)	80	11	4	1	5	60	0	1	1 carb., 1 fat
Chocolate Chip Cookie Stix (4)	130	19	5	2	5	100	<1	2	1 carb., 1 fat
Classic Collection French Vanilla Crème (1)	80	12	4	1	0	65	0	1	1 carb., 1 fat
Deluxe Grahams (3)	140	19	7	5	0	105	<1	1	1 carb., 1 fat
E.L. Fudge, Butter Sandwich Cookies (2)	120	17	6	1	<5	70	<1	1	1 carb., 1 fat
E.L. Fudge, Chocolate Sandwich Cookies (2)	120	17	6	1	0	70	<1	2	1 carb., 1 fat
Fudge Shoppe Fudge Stripes (3)	160	21	8	5	0	140	<1	1	1 1/2 carb., 2 fat
Fudge Shoppe, Reduced-Fat Fudge Stripes (3)	140	21	5	3	0	120	0	1	1 1/2 carb., 1 fat
Ginger Snaps (5)	150	24	6	1	0	120	0	2	1 1/2 carb., 1 fat

Food	Cal.	Carb.				Sod.			Exchanges
Golden Fruit Cranberry Biscuits (1)	80	14	2	0	0	55	<1	1	1 carb.
Golden Vanilla Wafers (8)	150	20	7	2	0	120	<1	1	1 carb., 1 fat
Iced Animal Cookies (6)	150	24	5	1	0	105	0	2	1 1/2 carb., 1 fat
Iced Animal Crackers (6)	130	18	6	2	0	90	0	1	1 carb., 1 fat
Pecan Sandies (1)	80	9	5	1	<5	75	<1	<1	1/2 carb., 1 fat
Sandies, 25% Reduced Fat (1)	80	11	3	<1	0	60	0	<1	1 carb., 1 fat
Soft Batch, Chocolate Chip (1)	80	10	4	1	0	70	<1	<1	1/2 carb., 1 fat
Soft Batch, Oatmeal Raisin (1)	70	10	3	1	0	65	<1	<1	1/2 carb., 1 fat
Vanilla Wafers, 30% Reduced Fat (8)	130	25	4	<1	0	140	<1	2	1 1/2 carb., 1 fat
KLONDIKE									
Ice Cream Bar, Vanilla (1)	280	23	19	14	NA	65	0	4	1 1/2 carb., 4 fat
Ice Cream Bar, Vanilla, Light (1)	140	10	10	NA	10	45	0	3	1/2 carb., 2 fat
Ice Cream Sandwich, Vanilla (1)	230	33	9	NA	NA	220	0	5	2 carb., 2 fat
Ice Cream Sandwich, Vanilla, Light (1)	100	18	2	1	5	110	0	2	1 carb.
KRAFT									
Handi-Snacks Cookie Jammers (1)	130	26	3	0	0	125	<1	1	2 carb., 1 fat

DESSERTS

Products	Cal.	Carb. (g)	Fat (g)	Sat. Fat (g)	Chol. (mg)	Sod. (mg)	Fib. (g)	Prot. (g)	Servings/Exchanges
Handi-Snacks Gel Snacks, Cherry (1)	80	20	0	0	0	45	0	0	1 carb.
Handi-Snacks Pudding, Chocolate (1)	130	23	4	1	0	125	<1	2	1 1/2 carb., 1 fat
Kraft Free Fat Free Whipped Topping (2 Tbsp)	15	2	0	0	0	5	0	0	free
Marshmallow Creme (1 oz)	90	23	0	0	0	20	0	0	1 1/2 carb.
Marshmallows, Jet Puffed (5)	125	30	0	0	0	25	0	0	2 carb.
Marshmallows, Miniature (30)	54	15	0	0	0	15	0	0	1 1/2 carb.
Topping, Butterscotch (2 Tbsp)	130	28	2	1	<5	150	0	<1	2 carb.
Topping, Caramel (2 Tbsp)	120	28	0	0	0	90	0	2	2 carb.
Topping, Chocolate (2 Tbsp)	110	26	0	0	0	30	1	2	2 carb.
Topping, Hot Fudge (2 Tbsp)	140	24	5	2	0	100	<1	1	1 1/2 carb., 1 fat
Topping, Pineapple (2 Tbsp)	110	28	0	0	0	15	0	0	2 carb.
Topping, Strawberry (2 Tbsp)	110	29	0	0	0	15	0	0	2 carb.
LA CHOY									
Cookies, Fortune (4)	112	26	<1	<1	0	11	2	2	2 carb.

LIBBY'S

Pie Filling, Apple (1/3 cup)	80	20	0	0	0	10	0	0	1 carb.
Pie Filling, Blueberry (1/3 cup)	80	19	0	0	0	0	1	0	1 carb.
Pie Filling, Cherry (1/3 cup)	90	22	0	0	0	0	0	0	1 1/2 carb.

MOCHA MIX

Frozen Dessert, Nondairy, Strawberry Swirl (1/2 cup)	140	20	6	2	0	55	0	1	1 carb., 1 fat
Frozen Dessert, Nondairy, Vanilla (1/2 cup)	140	18	7	2	0	70	0	1	1 carb., 1 fat

MR. FREEZE

Freezer Bars, Assorted Flavors (2 bars)	45	11	0	0	0	20	0	0	1 carb.

MRS. SMITH'S

8" Pie Shells (1/8)	80	8	5	1	0	105	NA	1	1/2 strch, 1 fat
Pie, Pie In Minutes 8" Apple (1/8)	210	29	9	2	0	250	NA	2	2 carb., 2 fat
Pie, Pie In Minutes 8" Blueberry (1/8)	220	32	9	2	0	240	NA	2	2 carb., 2 fat
Pie, Pie In Minutes 8" Cherry (1/3)	220	32	9	2	0	200	NA	2	2 carb., 2 fat
Pie, Pie In Minutes 8" Lemon Meringue (1/8)	210	38	5	NA	NA	130	NA	2	2 1/2 carb., 2 fat

DESSERTS

Products	Cal.	Carb. (g)	Fat (g)	Sat. Fat (g)	Chol. (mg)	Sod. (mg)	Fib. (g)	Prot. (g)	Servings/Exchanges
Pie, Pie In Minutes 8" Peach (1/8)	210	29	9	2	0	190	0	2	2 carb., 2 fat
Pie, Pie In Minutes 8" Pecan (1/8)	330	51	13	2	35	200	NA	3	3 1/2 carb., 3 fat
Pie, Pie In Minutes 8" Pumpkin (1/8)	190	30	6	2	35	230	NA	3	2 carb., 1 fat
N A B I S C O									
Bugs Bunny Graham Crackers (10)	120	22	4	0	0	140	NA	2	1 1/2 carb., 1 fat
Cameo w/Creme (1)	70	10	3	0	0	50	0	1	1/2 carb., 1 fat
Chips Ahoy! Chocolate Chip Cookies (3)	160	21	8	3	0	105	1	2	1 1/2 carb., 2 fat
Chips Ahoy! Reduced Fat (3)	140	22	5	2	0	150	<1	2	1 1/2 carb., 1 fat
Ginger Snaps (4)	120	22	3	<1	0	230	0	1	1 1/2 carb., 1 fat
Famous Chocolate Wafers (5)	140	22	4	2	4	110	NA	2	1 1/2 carb., 1 fat
Fat-Free Apple Newtons (2)	90	21	0	0	0	65	<1	1	1 1/2 carb.
Fat-Free Fig Newtons (2)	90	22	0	0	0	115	1	1	1 1/2 carb.
Fat-Free Raspberry Newtons (2)	90	21	0	0	0	100	<1	1	1 1/2 carb.
Fat-Free Strawberry Newtons (2)	90	21	0	0	0	95	0	1	1 1/2 carb.

Fig Newtons (2)	110	22	3	0	0	115	1	1	1 carb., 1 fat
Lorna Doone Shortbread (4)	140	19	7	1	5	130	<1	2	1 carb., 1 fat
Nilla Wafers (8)	140	24	5	1	<5	100	0	1	1 1/2 carb., 1 fat
Nutter Butter Bites (10)	150	20	4	<1	0	125	<1	2	1 carb., 1 fat
Nutter Butters (2)	140	18	6	2	0	50	0	2	1 carb., 1 fat
Old-Fashioned Ginger Snaps (4)	120	24	4	4	0	180	NA	4	1 1/2 strch, 1 fat
Oreo Sandwich Cookies (3)	160	23	7	2	0	220	1	1	1 1/2 carb., 1 fat
Oreo Sandwich Cookies, Reduced-Fat (3)	130	25	4	1	0	190	1	2	1 1/2 carb., 1 fat
Snackwell's Caramel Delights (1)	70	13	2	<1	0	35	0	1	1 carb.
Snackwell's Chocolate Chip Cookies (13)	130	22	4	2	0	160	<1	2	1 1/2 carb., 1 fat
Snackwell's Creme Sandwich Cookies (2)	110	20	3	<1	0	130	0	1	1 carb., 1 fat
Snackwell's Devil's Food Cookie Cakes (1)	50	12	0	0	0	30	0	1	1 carb.
Snackwell's Mint Creame Cookies (1)	110	19	4	1	0	70	<1	1	1 carb., 1 fat
Sweet Crispers Chocolate (18)	130	25	3	<1	0	190	1	2	1 1/2 carb., 1 fat
Teddy Grahams, Chocolate (24)	130	22	5	1	0	170	1	2	1 1/2 carb., 1 fat
Teddy Grahams, Cinnamon (24)	130	23	4	<1	0	150	<1	2	1 1/2 carb., 1 fat

DESSERTS

Products	Cal.	Carb. (g)	Fat (g)	Sat. Fat (g)	Chol. (mg)	Sod. (mg)	Fib. (g)	Prot. (g)	Servings/Exchanges
Teddy Grahams, Honey (24)	130	23	4	<1	0	150	<1	2	1 1/2 carb., 1 fat
Teddy Grahams, Vanilla (24)	130	23	4	<1	0	150	<1	2	1 1/2 carb., 1 fat
Vanilla Wafers, Reduced-Fat (8)	120	24	2	<1	0	105	0	1	1 1/2 carb.
NESTLE									
Crunch Bar (1)	180	30	13	NA	NA	50	2	2	2 carb., 3 fat
Drumstick (1)	340	35	19	11	20	90	2	6	2 carb., 4 fat
ORVAL KENT									
Dessert, Chocolate Chip Amaretto (1/2 cup)	310	31	20	16	10	230	2	3	2 carb., 4 fat
Dessert, Pistachio Creme (1/2 cup)	170	29	5	5	0	135	2	1	2 carb., 1 fat
Parfait, Wild Strawberry (1/2 cup)	130	22	3	3	0	105	1	3	1 1/2 carb., 1 fat
Pudding, Chocolate (1/2 cup)	160	27	4	2	10	110	0	4	2 carb., 1 fat
Pudding, Pearl Tapioca (1/2 cup)	150	25	4	2	35	95	2	4	1 1/2 carb., 1 fat
Pudding, Rice (1/2 cup)	130	21	3	2	15	75	2	4	1 1/2 carb., 1 fat

PEPPERIDGE FARM

Cake, All-Butter Pound (1 slice)	110	13	6	1	0	85	NA	1	1 carb., 1 fat
Cake, Boston Creme (1 slice)	290	39	14	6	50	190	NA	3	2 1/2 carb., 3 fat
Cake, Chocolate Fudge Layer (1 slice)	170	20	9	3	20	140	NA	2	1 carb., 2 fat
Cake, Chocolate Mousse (1 slice)	190	25	9	3	5	260	NA	3	1 1/2 carb., 2 fat
Cake, Coconut Layer (1 slice)	230	31	11	4	20	160	NA	2	2 carb., 2 fat
Cake, Devil's Food Layer (1 slice)	180	24	9	3	20	135	NA	1	1 1/2 carb., 2 fat
Cake, German Chocolate Layer (1 slice)	250	29	13	4	45	230	NA	2	2 carb., 3 fat
Cake, Lemon (1 slice)	170	26	5	1	50	100	NA	4	2 carb., 1 fat
Cake, Old Fashioned Carrot (1 slice)	150	19	9	3	15	160	NA	1	1 carb., 2 fat
Cake, Strawberry Cream (1 slice)	190	30	7	3	20	120	NA	1	2 carb., 1 fat
Cake, Strawberry Stripe Layer (1 slice)	160	21	8	3	20	120	NA	1	1 1/2 carb., 2 fat
Cookies, Beacon Hill Chocolate Chocolate Walnut (1)	120	14	7	2	5	65	1	2	1 carb., 1 fat
Cookies, Chesapeake Chocolate Chunk Pecan (1)	120	14	7	2	5	60	1	1	1 carb., 1 fat
Cookies, Distinctive Bordeaux (2)	70	11	3	1	0	40	NA	1	1/2 carb., 1 fat
Cookies, Distinctive Brussels (2)	110	13	5	2	0	65	NA	1	1 carb., 1 fat

DESSERTS

Products	Cal.	Carb. (g)	Fat (g)	Sat. Fat (g)	Chol. (mg)	Sod. (mg)	Fib. (g)	Prot. (g)	Servings/Exchanges
Cookies, Distinctive Brussels Mint (2)	130	17	7	2	0	40	NA	1	1 carb., 1 fat
Cookies, Distinctive Chessman (2)	90	12	4	2	10	60	NA	2	1 carb.
Cookies, Distinctive Chocolate Chocolate Walnut (1)	130	11	6	2	5	45	NA	1	1 carb., 1 fat
Cookies, Distinctive Double Chocolate Milano (2)	150	18	8	3	10	45	NA	2	1 carb., 2 fat
Cookies, Distinctive Geneva (2)	130	14	6	2	5	50	NA	1	1 carb., 1 fat
Cookies, Distinctive Hazelnut Milano (2)	130	15	8	2	5	30	NA	2	1 carb., 2 fat
Cookies, Distinctive Lido (1)	90	10	5	1	5	30	NA	1	1/2 carb., 1 fat
Cookies, Distinctive Milano (2)	120	15	6	2	5	45	NA	1	1 carb., 1 fat
Cookies, Distinctive Milk Chocolate Macadamia (1)	130	16	7	2	10	45	NA	1	1 carb., 1 fat
Cookies, Distinctive Milk Chocolate Milano (3)	170	21	9	4	10	110	<1	2	1 1/2 carb., 2 fat
Cookies, Distinctive Mint Milano (2)	150	17	7	2	5	60	NA	1	1 carb., 1 fat
Cookies, Distinctive Orange Milano (2)	150	17	7	2	5	60	NA	1	1 carb., 1 fat
Cookies, Mini Chocolate Chip (4)	150	20	8	3	10	70	0	0	1 carb., 2 fat
Cookies, Nantucket Chocolate Chunk (1)	120	15	6	2	5	60	1	1	1 carb., 1 fat

Cookies, Oatmeal Raisin (2)	110	15	5	2	10	115	NA	1	1 carb., 1 fat
Cookies, Old-Fashioned Brownie (2)	110	11	7	2	5	45	NA	1	1/2 carb., 1 fat
Cookies, Old-Fashioned Chocolate Chip (2)	100	12	5	2	5	45	NA	1	1 carb., 1 fat
Cookies, Old-Fashioned Gingerman (2)	70	10	3	0	5	30	NA	1	1/2 carb., 1 fat
Cookies, Old-Fashioned Lemon Nut Crunch (2)	110	13	7	2	5	50	NA	1	1 carb., 1 fat
Cookies, Old-Fashioned Molasses Crisps (2)	70	8	3	0	0	50	NA	1	1/2 carb., 1 fat
Cookies, Old-Fashioned Oatmeal Raisin (2)	90	13	5	1	5	80	NA	1	1 carb., 1 fat
Cookies, Old-Fashioned Pecan Shortbread (1)	70	7	5	2	10	55	NA	1	1/2 carb., 1 fat
Cookies, Old-Fashioned Sugar (2)	100	13	5	2	10	55	NA	1	1 carb., 1 fat
Cookies, Sausalito Milk Chocolate Macadamia (1)	120	14	7	2	5	65	NA	1	1 carb., 1 fat
Cookies, Soft-Baked Chocolate Chunk (1)	130	17	6	2	10	45	NA	2	1 carb., 1 fat
Cookies, Wholesome Choice Raspberry Tart (1)	60	11	1	1	0	35	NA	1	1 carb.
PET									
Topping, Whipped (2 Tbsp)	30	2	2	2	0	0	0	0	free
PILLSBURY									
Bar Mixes, Deluxe Fudge Swirl Cookie (1/20)	180	25	8	2	10	110	<1	1	1 1/2 carb., 2 fat

DESSERTS

Products	Cal.	Carb. (g)	Fat (g)	Sat. Fat (g)	Chol. (mg)	Sod. (mg)	Fib. (g)	Prot. (g)	Servings/Exchanges
Bar Mixes, Deluxe Lemon Cheesecake (1/24)	190	22	10	3	25	105	0	2	1 1/2 carb., 2 fat
Brownie Mix, Chocolate Deluxe (1/20)	180	28	7	2	10	110	<1	2	2 carb., 1 fat
Brownie Mix, Deluxe Fudge (1/16)	150	22	6	1	15	80	<1	2	1 1/2 carb., 1 fat
Cake Mix, Bundt Hot Fudge (1/12)	350	39	20	6	55	280	1	4	2 1/2 carb., 4 fat
Cake Mix, Moist Supreme Chocolate (1/12)	250	35	11	3	35	280	<1	3	2 carb., 2 fat
Cake Mix, Moist Supreme French Vanilla (1/10)	300	42	13	3	45	350	1	3	3 carb., 3 fat
Cake Mix, Moist Supreme Funtetti (1/12)	240	36	9	2	0	290	<1	3	2 1/2 carb., 2 fat
Refrigerated Cookie Dough, Chocolate Chip (1 oz)	130	17	6	3	<5	85	<1	1	1 carb., 1 fat
Refrigerated Cookie Dough, M&M's (1 oz)	130	18	6	2	<5	75	<1	1	1 carb., 1 fat
Refrigerated Cookie Dough, Reduced Fat Chocolate Chip (1 oz)	110	19	3	2	<5	85	<1	1	1 carb., 1 fat
Refrigerated Cookie Dough, Sugar (2)	130	19	5	2	<5	125	0	1	1 carb., 1 fat
Refrigerated One Step Chocolate Chip Pan Cookies (1/8)	130	19	6	2	<5	100	<1	1	1 carb., 1 fat

Refrigerated One Step M&M's Pan Cookies (1/8)	130	19	6	2	<5	85	<1	1	1 carb., 1 fat
Snackwell's Brownie Mix, Devil's Food (1/12)	140	28	3	<1	0	105	<1	2	2 carb., 1 fat
Snackwell's Brownie Mix, Fudge (1/12)	150	29	3	<1	0	115	1	2	2 carb., 1 fat
Snackwell's Cake Mix, Devil's Food (1/6)	200	38	4	2	12	380	2	3	2 1/2 carb., 1 fat
Snackwell's Cake Mix, White (1/6)	210	39	5	2	35	320	1	3	2 1/2 carb., 1 fat
Snackwell's Cake Mix, Yellow (1/6)	210	39	5	2	35	320	1	3	2 1/2 carb., 1 fat
Snackwell's Cookie Mix, Chocolate Chip Reduced Fat (1 oz)	110	19	3	2	<5	85	<1	1	1 carb., 1 fat
Snackwell's Cookie Mix, Chocolate Fudge (1 oz)	90	18	2	0	<5	95	<1	1	1 carb., 1 fat
Snackwell's Frosting, Vanilla (2 Tbsp)	130	25	3	<1	0	65	0	0	1 1/2 carb., 1 fat
Snackwell's Frosting, Chocolate (2 Tbsp)	120	22	3	1	0	65	0	0	1 1/2 carb., 1 fat
Frosting Supreme, Chocolate (2 Tbsp)	140	21	6	2	0	80	0	0	1 1/2 carb., 1 fat
Frosting Supreme, French Vanilla (2 Tbsp)	150	25	6	2	0	80	0	0	1 1/2 carb., 1 fat
SUNSHINE									
Cookies, Lemon Coolers (5)	140	21	6	2	0	100	<1	1	1 1/2 carb., 1 fat
Cookies, Country Style Oatmeal (2)	120	17	5	1	0	115	<1	2	1 carb., 1 fat

DESSERTS

Products	Cal.	Carb. (g)	Fat (g)	Sat. Fat (g)	Chol. (mg)	Sod. (mg)	Fib. (g)	Prot. (g)	Servings/Exchanges
Crackers, Animal (14)	140	24	4	1	0	125	<1	2	1 1/2 carb., 1 fat
Ginger Snaps (7)	130	22	5	1	0	150	<1	2	1 1/2 carb., 1 fat
Hydrox Reduced Fat Sandwich Cookies (3)	140	23	5	2	0	150	1	2	1 1/2 carb., 1 fat
Hydrox Sandwich Cookies (3)	150	21	7	2	0	125	1	2	1 1/2 carb., 1 fat
Vanilla Sugar Wafers (3)	130	18	6	2	0	20	<1	1	1 carb., 1 fat
Vanilla Wafers (7)	150	21	7	2	3	110	<1	2	1 1/2 carb., 1 fat
Vienna Fingers (2)	140	21	6	2	0	105	<1	2	1 1/2 carb., 1 fat
Vienna Fingers 25% Reduced Fat (2)	130	22	5	1	0	105	<1	1	1 1/2 carb., 1 fat
ULTRA SLIM FAST									
Pudding, Butterscotch (4 oz)	100	21	1	NA	0	230	2	2	1 1/2 carb.
Pudding, Chocolate (4 oz)	100	21	1	NA	0	240	2	2	1 1/2 carb.
Pudding, Vanilla (4 oz)	100	21	1	NA	0	230	2	2	1 1/2 carb.
WEIGHT WATCHERS									
Boston Cream Pie (1 slice)	160	34	4	1	5	260	NA	3	2 carb., 1 fat
Brownie, Swiss Mocha Fudge (1)	90	18	2	1	5	140	NA	2	1 carb.

Food								
Chocolate Cookies (3)	80	13	3	NA	0	70	NA	1	1 carb., 1 fat
Chocolate Chip Cookies (2)	90	18	2	1	0	65	NA	1	1 carb.
Chocolate Eclair (1)	150	26	4	2	15	110	NA	3	2 carb., 1 fat
Cookie Bar, Apple Raisin (1)	80	21	1	NA	0	35	NA	1	1 1/2 carb.
Fruit Cookies, Raspberry (1)	80	22	1	NA	0	45	NA	1	1 1/2 carb.
Ice Cream Bar, Sugar Free Chocolate Mousse (1)	35	9	1	0	5	30	NA	2	1/2 carb.
Ice Cream Bar, Sugar Free Orange (1)	30	8	1	0	5	40	NA	2	1/2 carb.
Ice Cream, Chocolate Chip (1/2 cup)	120	19	4	NA	10	80	NA	3	1 cart., 1 fat
Ice Cream, Heavenly Hash (1/2 cup)	130	22	3	2	10	90	NA	4	1 1/2 carb., 1 fat
Ice Cream, Pralines 'n Creme (1/2 cup)	120	19	4	NA	10	110	NA	3	1 carb., 1 fat
Ice Milk, Chocolate (1/2 cup)	120	19	3	2	5	75	NA	3	1 carb., 1 fat
Ice Milk, Neopolitan Reckless Rocky Road (1/2 cup)	110	18	3	1	10	75	NA	3	1 carb., 1 fat
Oatmeal Raisin Cookies (2)	90	20	1	NA	0	75	NA	1	1 carb.
Sandwich Cookies, Chocolate (2)	90	15	3	1	0	90	NA	1	1 carb., 1 fat
Sandwich Cookies, Vanilla (2)	90	15	3	1	0	50	NA	1	1 carb., 1 fat

DESSERTS

Products	Cal.	Carb. (g)	Fat (g)	Sat. Fat (g)	Chol. (mg)	Sod. (mg)	Fib. (g)	Prot. (g)	Servings/Exchanges
YOPLAIT									
Frozen Yogurt Bar, Vanilla Orange Creme (1)	30	8	<1	0	0	25	0	1	1/2 carb.
Frozen Yogurt, Caramel Turtle Fudge (1/2 cup)	120	24	2	1	5	105	0	2	1 1/2 carb.
Frozen Yogurt, Chocolate Fudge Brownie (1/2 cup)	110	24	2	<1	5	75	1	3	1 1/2 carb.
Frozen Yogurt, Vanilla (1/2 cup)	100	20	2	1	5	70	0	3	1 carb.

EGGS AND EGG DISHES

Products	Cal.	Carb. (g)	Fat (g)	Sat. Fat (g)	Chol. (mg)	Sod. (mg)	Fib. (g)	Prot. (g)	Servings/Exchanges
1-Egg Omelet, Plain (1)	93	<1	7	2	214	165	0	6	1 med-fat meat
1-Egg Omelet, Spanish (1)	125	7	9	2	126	251	2	5	1 vegetable, 1 med-fat meat, 1 fat
1-Egg Omelet w/Cheese & Ham (1)	142	<1	11	4	231	368	0	10	1 med-fat meat, 1 fat
1-Egg Omelet w/Chicken (1)	149	<1	10	3	287	222	0	13	2 med-fat meat
1-Egg Omelet w/Fish (1)	132	<1	9	3	267	277	0	10	2 med-fat meat
1-Egg Omelet w/Mushroom (1)	91	1	7	2	204	158	<1	6	1 med-fat meat
1-Egg Omelet w/Onion, Pepper, Tomato, Mushroom (1)	125	7	9	2	126	251	2	5	1 vegetable, 1 med-fat meat, 1 fat
1-Egg Omelet w/Sausage & Mushroom (1)	172	1	13	4	254	454	<1	11	2 med-fat meat, 1 fat
1-Egg Omelet w/Spinach (1)	95	2	7	2	201	201	<1	7	1 med-fat meat
Deviled Egg (1/2 egg + filling)	63	<1	5	1	12	94	0	4	1 med-fat meat

EGGS AND EGG DISHES

Products	Cal.	Carb. (g)	Fat (g)	Sat. Fat (g)	Chol. (mg)	Sod. (mg)	Fib. (g)	Prot. (g)	Servings/Exchanges
Egg, Boiled/Cooked (1 extra large)	90	<1	6	2	246	72	0	7	1 med-fat meat
Egg, Boiled/Cooked (1 jumbo)	99	<1	7	2	271	79	0	8	1 med-fat meat
Egg, Boiled/Cooked (1 large)	78	<1	5	2	212	62	0	6	1 med-fat meat
Egg, Boiled/Cooked (1 medium)	68	<1	5	1	187	55	0	6	1 med-fat meat
Egg, Boiled/Cooked (1 small)	57	<1	4	1	157	46	0	5	1 med-fat meat
Egg, Fried in Margarine (1 large)	92	<1	7	2	211	162	0	6	1 high-fat meat
Egg, Scrambled, Plain (1)	101	1	7	2	215	171	0	7	2 med-fat meat
Egg Substitute (1/4 cup)	35	2	0	0	0	110	0	7	1 very lean meat
Egg Whites (2)	34	<1	0	0	0	110	0	7	1 very lean meat
Souffle, Cheese (1 cup)	197	6	14	6	194	299	<1	12	1/2 reduced-fat milk, 1 med-fat meat, 1 fat
Souffle, Spinach (1 cup)	218	3	18	7	184	763	3	12	1/2 reduced-fat milk, 1 med-fat meat, 2 fat

FLEISCHMANN'S

Egg Beaters (1/4 cup)	25	1	0	0	0	80	0	5	1 very lean meat
Egg Beaters, Vegetable Omelet (1/2 cup)	50	5	0	0	0	170	0	7	1 very lean meat
Egg Beaters w/Cheez (1/2 cup)	110	2	5	2	5	480	0	14	2 lean meat

MORNINGSTAR

Scramblers (1/4 cup)	60	3	3	NA	0	NA	0	6	1 lean meat

SECOND NATURE

Real Egg Product (1/4 cup)	60	3	2	0	0	110	0	6	1 lean meat
Real Egg Product, Non Fat	40	3	0	0	0	115	0	6	1 lean meat

TOFUTTI

Egg Watchers, Egg Substitute (1/4 cup)	50	2	2	NA	0	100	0	7	1 lean meat

ETHNIC FOODS

ALASKA NATIVE

Products	Cal.	Carb. (g)	Fat (g)	Sat. Fat (g)	Chol. (mg)	Sod. (mg)	Fib. (g)	Prot. (g)	Servings/Exchanges
Beach Asparagus (1 cup)	15	2	<1	NA	0	23	NA	1	free
Caribou, Cooked (1 oz)	47	0	1	<1	31	17	0	8	1 very lean meat
Dried Fish/King Salmon (1/2 oz)	60	0	5	NA	NA	NA	0	7	1 med-fat meat
Fiddlehead Fern, Raw (1 cup)	34	5	<1	NA	0	84	NA	3	1 vegetable
Gumboots/Leathery Chiton (2 oz)	46	0	<1	NA	NA	NA	0	10	1 very lean meat
Halibut, Cooked (1 oz)	39	0	<1	<1	12	20	0	8	1 very lean meat
Herring Eggs, Plain (1/2 cup)	48	4	<1	NA	NA	52	0	8	1 very lean meat
Highbush Cranberries (1 1/4 cup)	58	15	<1	NA	0	1	NA	<1	1 fruit
Hooligan, Smoked (1 oz)	86	0	7	NA	NA	NA	0	6	1 high-fat meat
Huckleberries (1 cup)	56	13	<1	NA	0	15	NA	<1	1 fruit
Moose, Cooked (1 oz)	38	0	<1	<1	22	19	0	8	1 very lean meat

Food									Exchanges
Muktuk w/Skin and Fat (1x1x2 inches)	138	0	12	NA	NA	NA	0	8	1 high-fat meat, 1 fat
Muskrat, Cooked (1 oz)	67	0	3	0	34	27	0	9	1 lean meat
Pike, Cooked (1 oz)	33	0	<1	0	14	13	0	7	1 very lean meat
Pilot Bread (1, 4-inch round)	104	18	2	NA	NA	142	NA	2	1 strch
Salmon, Sockeye, Cooked (1 oz)	50	0	3	<1	24	18	0	8	1 lean meat
Salmonberries (1 1/4 cup)	55	13	<1	NA	0	52	NA	1	1 fruit
Seal Meat, Raw (1 oz)	41	0	<1	<1	NA	NA	0	9	1 very lean meat
Seal Oil (1 tsp)	45	0	5	<1	8	NA	0	0	1 fat
Seaweed, Dried Black (1 cup)	39	<1	NA	NA	0	40	NA	4	1 vegetable
Sour Dock, Cooked (1/2 cup)	19	4	<1	NA	0	NA	NA	1	1 vegetable
Venison, Cooked (1 oz)	44	0	<1	<1	31	15	0	9	1 very lean meat
Walrus, Raw (1 oz)	56	0	4	<1	22	NA	0	5	1 lean meat
Whale, Bonehead, Raw (1 oz)	37	0	<1	<1	NA	17	0	7	1 very lean meat
Willow Greens, Cooked (1/2 cup)	23	6	<1	NA	0	NA	NA	2	1 vegetable

ETHNIC FOODS

CHINESE AMERICAN

Products	Cal.	Carb. (g)	Fat (g)	Sat. Fat (g)	Chol. (mg)	Sod. (mg)	Fib. (g)	Prot. (g)	Servings/Exchanges
Amaranth/Chinese Spinach, Cooked (1/2 cup)	14	3	<1	0	0	14	NA	1	1 vegetable
Amaranth/Chinese Spinach, Raw (1 cup)	7	1	<1	0	0	6	NA	<1	1 vegetable
Arrowheads/Fresh Corn, Large (1)	25	5	<1	NA	NA	6	NA	1	1 vegetable
Baby Corn, Canned (1/2 cup)	13	2	<1	NA	0	730	NA	2	1 vegetable
Bamboo Shoots, Canned (1/2 cup)	13	2	<1	0	0	5	<1	1	1 vegetable
Beef Jerky (1/2 oz)	57	2	4	2	7	310	<1	5	1 lean meat
Beef Tongue (1 oz)	81	<1	6	3	30	17	0	6	1 med-fat meat
Bitter Melon/Bitter Gourd/Balsam-Pear Pods (1 cup)	16	3	<1	0	0	5	3	<1	1 vegetable
Bok Choy/Chinese Cabbage/Pakchoi (1/2 cup)	9	2	<1	0	0	46	<1	1	1 vegetable
Carambola/Star Fruit, Medium (2)	60	14	<1	0	0	4	5	1	1 fruit
Cellophane/Mung Bean Noodles, Cooked (1/2 cup)	67	16	NA	0	0	2	<1	NA	1 strch
Cha Shu Bun, Frozen, Steamed (2)	360	50	13	5	20	410	1	8	2 strch, 3 fat

Food									Exchanges
Chayote, Raw (1 cup)	32	7	<1	0	0	5	4	1	1 vegetable
Chinese Banana, Dwarf (1)	72	18	<1	NA	0	18	NA	2	1 fruit
Chinese Celery, Raw (1 cup)	26	5	<1	0	0	116	0	2	1 vegetable
Chinese Eggplant, Purple, Cooked (1/2 cup)	17	4	<1	NA	0	NA	2	<1	1 vegetable
Chinese Eggplant, White, Cooked (1/2 cup)	20	5	<1	NA	0	NA	2	<1	1 vegetable
Chinese Sausage (1 oz)	100	2	8	3	NA	246	NA	6	1 high-fat meat
Chinese/Black Mushrooms, Medium, Dried (2)	21	5	<1	0	0	1	<1	<1	1 vegetable
Chinese/Peking/Pe-tsai/Napa Cabbage, Raw (1 cup)	12	3	<1	0	0	1	<1	<1	1 vegetable
Choy Sum/Chinese Flowering Cabbage (1 cup)	9	2	NA	NA	0	NA	NA	1	1 vegetable
Coconut Milk (1 Tbsp)	35	<1	4	3	0	2	<1	2	1 fat
Coriander, Raw (1 cup)	3	<1	<1	0	0	4	<1	<1	free
Dried Mung Beans/Green Beans, Cooked (1/2 cup)	106	19	<1	<1	0	2	8	7	1 strch, 1 very lean meat
Dried Red Beans, Cooked (1/3 cup)	99	19	<1	0	0	6	1	6	1 strch, 1 very lean meat
Garland Chrysanthemum, Raw (1 cup)	4	1	0	NA	NA	13	NA	<1	free
Ginger Root, Raw (1/4 cup)	17	4	<1	NA	NA	3	NA	<1	free

ETHNIC FOODS

Products	Cal.	Carb. (g)	Fat (g)	Sat. Fat (g)	Chol. (mg)	Sod. (mg)	Fib. (g)	Prot. (g)	Servings/Exchanges
Gingko Seeds, Canned (1/2 cup)	86	17	1	<1	0	238	7	2	1 strch
Guava, Medium (1 1/2)	69	16	<1	<1	0	4	7	1	1 fruit
Hairy Melon/Hairy Cucumber, Raw (1 cup)	22	5	NA	NA	NA	NA	2	1	1 vegetable
Kumquat, Medium (5)	30	16	<1	0	0	6	6	<1	1 fruit
Leeks, Cooked (1/2 cup)	16	4	<1	0	0	5	<1	<1	1 vegetable
Litchi/Lychee, Canned (1/2 cup)	57	15	<1	NA	0	27	<1	<1	1 fruit
Litchi/Lychee, Raw (10)	63	16	<1	<1	0	1	1	<1	1 fruit
Longan, Canned (3/4 cup)	68	18	<1	NA	0	54	NA	<1	1 fruit
Longan, Raw (30)	58	15	<1	0	0	0	1	1	1 fruit
Lotus Root (10 slices)	45	14	<1	<1	0	33	4	2	1 strch
Luffa, Angled, Raw (1 cup)	30	7	<1	NA	0	2	NA	1	1 vegetable
Luffa, Smooth/Sponge, Raw (1 cup)	34	8	<1	NA	0	6	NA	2	1 vegetable
Mango, Small (1/2 cup)	68	18	<1	<1	0	2	2	<1	1 fruit
Moon Cake, Plain Lotus Seed Paste (1/4)	169	24	8	NA	2	NA	<1	2	1 1/2 carb., 2 fat

Mung Bean Sprouts, Seed Attached, Raw (1 cup)	31	6	<1	0	0	6	2	3	1 vegetable
Mustard Greens, Cooked (1/2 cup)	11	2	<1	0	0	11	1	2	1 vegetable
Mustard Greens, Salted (2 Tbsp)	14	4	<1	NA	0	NA	NA	<1	free
Oriental Radish/Daikon, Raw (1 cup)	16	4	<1	0	0	18	1	<1	1 vegetable
Papaya, Medium (1/2)	59	15	<1	<1	0	5	3	<1	1 fruit
Peapods/Sugar Peas, Cooked (1/2 cup)	34	6	<1	0	0	3	2	3	1 vegetable
Pepper, Chili, Raw (1 cup)	60	14	<1	0	0	11	2	3	3 vegetables
Persimmon (1/2)	59	16	<1	0	0	1	3	<1	1 fruit
Pummelo (3/4 cup)	58	14	<1	NA	0	1	<1	1	1 fruit
Rice Noodles, Fresh (1/2 cup)	99	23	<1	0	0	NA	NA	1	1 1/2 strch
Rice Vermicelli, Cooked (1/2 cup)	56	13	0	0	0	NA	NA	1	1 strch
Salted Duck Egg (1)	137	<1	7	NA	NA	NA	0	10	1 high-fat meat
Scallop, Dried, Large (1)	44	1	<1	NA	NA	NA	NA	9	1 very lean meat
Sesame Paste (2 tsp)	60	2	5	1	0	12	<1	2	1 fat
Sesame Seeds, Whole, Dried (1 Tbsp)	52	2	5	<1	0	1	1	2	1 fat
Shrimp, Dried, Medium (10)	40	2	<1	NA	NA	NA	NA	7	1 very lean meat

ETHNIC FOODS

Products	Cal.	Carb. (g)	Fat (g)	Sat. Fat (g)	Chol. (mg)	Sod. (mg)	Fib. (g)	Prot. (g)	Servings/Exchanges
Soybean Milk, Unsweetened (1 cup)	81	4	5	<1	0	29	3	7	1 med-fat meat
Soybean Sprouts, Seed Attached, Raw (1 cup)	86	7	5	<1	0	10	<1	9	1 vegetable, 1 med-fat meat
Soybeans, Cooked (3 Tbsp)	56	3	3	<1	0	0	2	5	1 lean meat
Squid, Raw (2 oz)	52	2	<1	<1	132	26	0	9	1 very lean meat
Straw Mushrooms, Canned (1/2 cup)	20	4	<1	NA	0	172	NA	2	1 vegetable
Sweet Rice Dough Ball (3)	220	29	10	6	0	0	1	3	2 carb., 2 fat
Taro, Cooked (1/2 cup)	94	23	<1	<1	0	10	3	<1	1 1/2 strch
Tofu/Soybean Curd (4 oz, 1/2 cup)	91	2	6	<1	0	8	1	10	1 med-fat meat
Tripe, Beef, Raw (2 oz)	56	0	2	1	54	26	0	8	1 lean meat
Turnip, Raw (1 cup)	35	8	<1	0	0	87	2	1	1 vegetable
Water Chestnuts, Chinese (1/2 cup)	66	15	<1	0	0	9	2	<1	1 strch
Watercress, Raw (1 cup)	4	<1	0	0	0	14	<1	<1	free
Winter Melon/Wax Gourd/Chinese Preserving Melon (1 cup)	17	4	<1	0	0	147	4	<1	1 vegetable

Won Ton, Cantonese Style (5)	83	13	<1	0	0	850	2	6	1 strch
Yard-Long Beans, Cooked (1/2 cup)	24	5	<1	0	0	2	NA	1	1 vegetable
Yard-Long Beans, Raw (1 cup)	43	8	<1	<1	0	4	NA	3	1 vegetable

FILIPINO AMERICAN

Bamboo Shoots, Canned (1/2 cup)	13	2	<1	<1	0	5	1	1	1 vegetable
Banana Squash, Cooked (1/2 cup)	24	6	<1	<1	0	2	1	<1	1 vegetable
Banana Sauce (1 tsp)	11	3	NA	NA	0	NA	0	0	free
Banana, Native, Small (1)	46	12	<1	<1	0	0	<1	<1	1 fruit
Beef Shank, Lean, Cooked (1 oz)	57	0	2	<1	22	18	0	10	1 lean meat
Beef Tongue (1 oz)	80	<1	6	3	30	17	0	6	1 med-fat meat
Bitter Melon, Cooked (1/2 cup)	12	3	<1	NA	0	4	NA	<1	1 vegetable
Bottle Gourd, Cooked (1/2 cup)	9	2	<1	NA	0	NA	<1	<1	free
Caraboa's Milk (1 cup)	62	11	23	11	46	127	0	13	1 whole milk, 3 fat
Cassava Tuber, Cooked (1/2 cup)	60	15	<1	<1	0	4	<1	<1	1 strch
Ceylon Moss Bar, Dried (1/4)	8	2	0	0	0	3	<1	<1	free
Chayote, Cooked (1/2 cup)	19	4	<1	0	0	1	<1	<1	1 vegetable

ETHNIC FOODS

Products	Cal.	Carb. (g)	Fat (g)	Sat. Fat (g)	Chol. (mg)	Sod. (mg)	Fib. (g)	Prot. (g)	Servings/Exchanges
Chicken Gizzard, Cooked (1 oz)	43	<1	1	<1	55	19	0	8	1 lean meat
Chinese Celery, Raw (1 cup)	32	5	2	NA	NA	48	<1	3	1 vegetable
Chinese Sausage (1 oz)	100	2	8	3	30	249	NA	6	1 high-fat meat
Chinese Spinach, Raw (1 cup)	7	1	<1	<1	0	5	NA	<1	free
Clam, Cooked (3, 1 oz)	42	2	<1	<1	19	32	0	7	1 lean meat
Coconut Milk, Canned (1 Tbsp)	35	<1	4	3	0	2	0	<1	1 fat
Corned Beef, Canned (1 oz)	71	0	4	2	24	285	0	8	1 med-fat meat
Cracklings, Crushed (2 Tbsp)	42	0	3	<1	9	3	0	4	1 fat
Fish Sauce (1 Tbsp)	4	0	<1	NA	NA	1088	0	<1	free
Guava, Raw (1 1/2)	61	14	<1	<1	0	3	7	1	1 fruit
Horseradish Leaves, Cooked (1/2 cup)	13	2	<1	NA	0	2	NA	1	1 vegetable
Indian Sardines, Dried (1 oz)	57	0	1	NA	NA	NA	0	11	1 lean meat
Jicama, Cooked (1/2 cup)	19	4	0	0	0	2	<1	<1	1 vegetable
Long-Jawed Anchovy, Dried (2 Tbsp)	64	0	1	NA	NA	26	0	12	1 lean meat

Food									Exchange
Mango, Small (1/2)	61	18	<1	<1	0	2	3	<1	1 fruit
Mung Bean Noodles, Cooked (3/4 cup)	73	18	0	0	0	9	NA	0	1 strch
Mung Beans, Cooked (1/3 cup)	71	13	<1	<1	0	1	NA	5	1 strch
Native Sausage, Raw (1 oz)	167	<1	17	NA	NA	0	3		1 high-fat meat, 1 fat
Oriental Radish/Daikon, Raw (1 cup)	16	2	0	0	0	9	NA	<1	free
Oyster, Cooked, Medium (1)	41	3	1	<1	38	53	0	5	1 lean meat
Papaya, Unripe, Cooked (1/2 cup)	20	5	<1	NA	0	3	<1	1	1 vegetable
Papaya, Yellow, Raw, Cubed (1 cup)	54	14	<1	<1	0	4	2	<1	1 fruit
Peapods, Cooked (1/2 cup)	34	6	<1	<1	0	3	1	3	1 vegetable
Plantain, Cooked, Sliced (1/2 cup)	89	24	<1	NA	0	4	2	<1	1 1/2 strch
Pummelo (3/4 cup)	62	15	<1	NA	0	0	2	1	1 fruit
Rice Sticks/Noodles, Cooked (3/4 cup)	91	19	1	NA	0	1	<1	1	1 strch
Sausage, Simulated (1 oz)	72	3	5	<1	0	251	0	5	1 med-fat meat
Sesame Seeds, Dried (1 Tbsp)	52	2	5	<1	0	1	<1	2	2 fat
Shrimp, Fermented, Small (1 Tbsp)	12	0	<1	<1	0	734	<1	3	free
Soy Bean Curd/Tofu (1/2 cup)	94	2	6	<1	0	9	2	10	1 med-fat meat

ETHNIC FOODS

Products	Cal.	Carb. (g)	Fat (g)	Sat. Fat (g)	Chol. (mg)	Sod. (mg)	Fib. (g)	Prot. (g)	Servings/Exchanges
Spanish Sausage (1 oz)	125	NA	11	4	30	367	0	7	1 high-fat meat, 1 fat
Swamp Cabbage, Cooked (1/2 cup)	9	<1	<1	NA	0	63	<1	1	free
Taro, Cooked (1/3 cup)	62	15	<1	<1	0	6	NA	<1	1 strch
Watermelon Seeds, Dried (1 Tbsp)	38	1	3	<1	0	6	<1	2	1 fat
Yard-Long Beans, Cooked (1/2 cup)	24	5	<1	<1	0	2	NA	1	1 vegetable
HMONG									
Asian Pear (1)	51	13	<1	0	0	0	4	<1	1 fruit
Bamboo Shoots, Canned (1/2 cup)	13	2	<1	<1	0	4	<1	1	1 vegetable
Beef Tallow (1 tsp)	39	0	4	2	5	0	0	0	1 fat
Bitter Melon, Raw (1 cup)	16	3	<1	0	0	5	3	<1	1 vegetable
Cellophane/Mung Bean Noodles, Cooked (1/2 cup)	67	16	NA	0	0	2	<1	NA	1 strch
Chicken Fat (1 tsp)	39	0	4	1	4	0	0	0	1 fat
Chitterlings, Boiled (2 Tbsp)	42	0	4	1	20	6	0	1	1 fat
Coconut Cream, Canned (1 Tbsp)	36	2	3	3	0	10	<1	<1	1 fat

Food									
Coconut Milk, Canned (1 Tbsp)	30	<1	3	3	0	2	0	<1	1 fat
Coconut Milk, Raw (1 Tbsp)	35	<1	4	3	0	2	<1	<1	1 fat
Coconut, Raw (2 Tbsp)	35	2	3	3	0	2	<1	<1	1 fat
Condensed Milk, Sweetened (2 Tbsp)	123	21	3	2	13	46	0	3	1 1/2 carb., 1 fat
Coriander/Chinese Parsley, Raw (1 cup)	3	<1	<1	0	0	4	<1	<1	free
Cucuzzi Squash, Cooked (1/2 cup)	23	5	<1	0	0	14	1	<1	1 vegetable
Fish Sauce (1 Tbsp)	6	<1	0	0	0	1390	0	<1	free
Guava, Medium (1)	69	16	<1	<1	0	4	7	1	1 fruit
Jackfruit (1/2 cup)	78	20	<1	0	0	2	1	1	1 fruit
Leeks, Cooked (1/2 cup)	16	4	<1	0	0	6	NA	<1	1 vegetable
Luffa Gourd/Squash, Raw (1 cup)	30	7	<1	NA	0	6	NA	2	1 vegetable
Mango, Small (1/2)	68	18	<1	<1	0	2	2	<1	1 fruit
Mung Bean Sprouts w/Seeds, Cooked (1/2 cup)	13	3	<1	0	0	6	<1	1	1 vegetable
Mustard Greens (1/2 cup)	10	2	<1	0	0	11	1	2	1 vegetable
Papaya, Medium (1/2)	59	15	<1	<1	9	4	3	<1	1 fruit
Peas, Podded, Cooked (1/2 cup)	24	6	<1	0	0	3	2	3	1 vegetable

ETHNIC FOODS

Products	Cal.	Carb. (g)	Fat (g)	Sat. Fat (g)	Chol. (mg)	Sod. (mg)	Fib. (g)	Prot. (g)	Servings/Exchanges
Peas, Podded, Raw (1/2 cup)	26	5	<1	0	0	3	2	2	1 vegetable
Pheasant, No Skin, Raw (1 oz)	38	0	1	<1	19	10	0	7	1 very lean meat
Pig's Feet (1/2 foot)	68	0	4	1.5	35	11	0	7	1 med-fat meat
Pork Lard (1 tsp)	39	0	4	2	4	0	0	0	1 fat
Pork, Ground (1 oz)	84	0	6	2	27	21	0	7	1 high-fat meat
Pumpkin Blossom, Cooked (1 cup)	20	4	<1	0	0	8	1	2	free
Pumpkin, Cooked (1/2 cup)	24	6	<1	0	0	2	1	<1	1 vegetable
Rice Noodles, Fresh (1/2 cup)	99	23	<1	0	0	NA	<1	1	1 strch
Squirrel, Roasted (1 oz)	49	0	1	<1	34	34	0	9	1 very lean meat
Tofu/Soybean Curd (4 oz, 1/2 cup)	94	2	6	<1	0	9	2	10	1 med-fat meat
Venison (1 oz)	45	0	<1	<1	32	15	0	9	1 very lean meat
Vinespinach, Raw (1 cup)	11	2	<1	0	0	13	0	1	free
Yard-Long Beans, Cooked (1/2 cup)	102	18	<1	<1	0	4	NA	7	1 strch, 1 very lean meat

JEWISH

Food									Exchanges
Bagel (1/2)	78	15	<1	<1	0	151	<1	3	1 strch
Beef Brisket (1 oz)	52	1	2	<1	16	28	0	6	1 lean meat
Beef Tongue (1 oz)	80	<1	6	3	30	17	0	6	1 med-fat meat
Bialy (1/2)	69	16	0	0	0	167	1	7	1 strch
Blintzes (2.25 oz)	80	13	2	<1	118	135	0	6	1 carb.
Borekas (1/2 pie)	114	15	11	5	45	191	<1	5	1 strch, 2 fat
Borscht (1/2 cup)	26	5	<1	<1	0	473	1	2	1 vegetable
Bulgur, Cooked (1/2 cup)	76	17	<1	0	0	5	4	3	1 strch
Bulke Roll (1/2 roll)	78	15	<1	NA	0	137	<1	4	1 strch
Challah (1 oz)	81	14	2	<1	15	139	<1	3	1 strch
Chicken Liver (1 oz)	45	<1	2	<1	179	15	0	7	1 lean meat
Chickpeas (1/2 cup)	135	23	2	<1	0	6	6	7	1 1/2 strch, 1 very lean meat
Corned Beef (1 oz)	71	<1	5	2	28	321	0	5	1 med-fat meat
Couscous (1/2 cup)	88	18	<1	0	0	4	1	3	1 strch
Cream Cheese (1 Tbsp)	51	<1	5	3	16	43	0	1	1 fat

ETHNIC FOODS

Products	Cal.	Carb. (g)	Fat (g)	Sat. Fat (g)	Chol. (mg)	Sod. (mg)	Fib. (g)	Prot. (g)	Servings/Exchanges
Farfel (1/2 cup)	73	15	<1	0	0	0	<1	2	1 strch
Flanken, Raw (1 oz)	51	0	3	1	15	20	0	6	1 lean meat
Gefilte Fish (2 pieces)	71	6	2	<1	25	440	0	8	1/2 carb., 1 very lean meat
Herring in Wine Sauce (1/4 cup)	90	7	4	1	25	420	0	5	1/2 carb., 1 med-fat meat
Herring, Pickled (1 oz)	74	3	5	<1	4	247	0	4	1 med-fat meat
Horseradish, Root (1 Tbsp)	7	2	<1	0	0	47	<1	<1	free
Kasha, Cooked (1/2 cup)	77	17	<1	<1	0	3	2	3	1 strch
Kasha, Dry (2 Tbsp)	71	15	<1	<1	0	2	2	2	1 strch
Kichlach (2–3)	106	15	4	<1	42	13	<1	3	1 carb., 1 fat
Knishes (1 1/2 oz)	114	15	5	<1	35	162	1	3	1 strch, 1 fat
Kreplach (2 oz)	128	13	4	1	62	70	<1	10	1 carb., 1 lean meat
Kugel (1/2 cup)	113	17	2	<1	31	277	<1	7	1 carb.
Leckach (1 oz)	84	16	2	<1	13	43	<1	1	1 strch
Lentils, Cooked (1/2 cup)	115	20	<1	0	0	2	8	9	1 strch, 1 very lean meat

Food									Exchanges
Lox (1 oz)	33	0	1	<1	7	567	0	5	1 very lean meat
Matzoh (3/4 oz)	84	18	<1	C	0	0	<1	2	1 strch
Matzoh Ball (3 balls)	212	16	13	4	127	678	<1	6	1 carb., 2 1/2 fat
Matzoh Meal (2 Tbsp)	65	0	<1	0	0	0	<1	2	1 strch
Pastrami (1 oz)	99	<1	8	3	26	348	0	5	1 high-fat meat
Pickles, Dill, Large (1 1/2)	36	8	<1	<1	0	2596	2	1	1 vegetable
Potato Flour (2 Tbsp)	71	14	<1	<1	0	11	1	1	1 strch
Potato Pancakes, Medium (1)	124	13	7	1	13	232	<1	3	1 strch, 1 fat
Pumpernickel Bread (1 oz)	71	14	<1	<1	0	190	2	3	1 strch
Rye Bread (1 oz)	73	14	<1	<1	0	187	2	2	1 strch
Sablefish (1 oz)	73	0	6	1	18	209	0	5	1 med-fat meat
Salmon, Canned (1 oz)	39	0	2	<1	16	157	0	6	1 lean meat
Sardines, Medium, Canned in Oil, Drained (2)	60	0	3	<1	4	145	0	7	1 lean meat
Schmaltz (1 tsp)	38	0	4	1	4	0	0	0	1 fat
Smelt (1 oz)	35	0	<1	<1	26	22	0	6	1 very lean meat
Sour Cream (2 Tbsp)	52	<1	5	3	11	13	0	<1	1 fat

ETHNIC FOODS

Products	Cal.	Carb. (g)	Fat (g)	Sat. Fat (g)	Chol. (mg)	Sod. (mg)	Fib. (g)	Prot. (g)	Servings/Exchanges
Split Peas, Cooked (1/2 cup)	116	21	<1	0	0	2	8	8	1 1/2 strch, 1 very lean meat
Sweet Wine (4 oz)	173	13	0	0	0	10	0	2	1 carb.
Tzimmes (1/4 cup)	88	21	<1	0	0	118	2	1	1 1/2 strch
Whitefish, Smoked (1 oz)	31	0	<1	<1	9	289	0	7	1 very lean meat
MEXICAN AMERICAN									
Avocado, Medium (1/8)	40	2	4	<1	0	3	<1	<1	1 fat
Bolillo, Large (1/4)	82	16	<1	<1	0	183	<1	3	1 strch
Chayote, Boiled, Drained (1/2 cup)	19	4	<1	0	0	1	2	<1	1 vegetable
Chorizo (1 oz)	129	<1	11	4	25	351	0	7	1 high-fat meat, 1 fat
Corn Tortilla, 6-inch (1)	58	12	<1	<1	0	42	1	2	1 strch
Corn Tortilla, Fat Added, 6-inch (1)	102	12	6	<1	0	42	1	2	1 strch, 1 fat
Flour Tortilla, 6-inch (1)	104	18	2	<1	0	153	1	3	1 strch
Flour Tortilla, Fat Added, 6-inch (1)	148	18	7	1	0	153	1	3	1 strch, 1 fat
Frijoles Cocidos (1/2 cup)	117	22	<1	<1	0	2	7	7	1 strch, 1 very lean meat

Food	Cal	Carb	Fat	Sat Fat	Chol	Sodium	Fiber	Protein	Exchanges
Frijoles Refritos, Fat Added (1/2 cup)	161	22	5.4	<1	0	378	7	7	1 strch, 1 very lean meat, 1 fat
Jicama, Raw (1 cup)	49	12	<1	0	0	5	6	<1	2 vegetable
Mango, Small, Raw (1/2)	68	18	<1	<1	0	2	2	<1	1 fruit
Menudo (1 cup)	170	1	9	4	NA	950	NA	20	3 lean meat
Nopales, Cooked (1/2 cup)	11	3	0	0	0	15	2	1	1 vegetable
Nopales, Raw (1 cup)	14	3	<1	<1	0	19	2	1	1 vegetable
Pan Dulce, 5-inch (1)	458	59	21	NA	NA	389	NA	8	4 carb, 4 fat
Papaya, Raw, Cubed (1 cup)	55	14	<1	<1	0	4	3	<1	1 fruit
Peppers, Hot Green Chili, Chopped, Raw (1 cup)	60	14	<1	0	0	11	2	3	2 vegetable
Queso Anejo (1 oz)	106	1	9	5	30	321	0	6	1 high-fat meat
Queso Asadero (1 oz)	101	<1	8	5	30	186	0	6	1 high-fat meat
Queso Chihuahua (1 oz)	106	2	8	5	30	175	0	6	1 high-fat meat
Queso Fresco (1 oz)	83	NA	7	4	NA	200	0	6	1 med-fat meat
Salsa De Chile (1/4 cup)	14	3	<1	0	0	166	1	<1	free
Taco Shell, 6-inch (2)	122	16	6	<1	0	95	2	2	1 strch, 1 fat

ETHNIC FOODS

Products	Cal.	Carb. (g)	Fat (g)	Sat. Fat (g)	Chol. (mg)	Sod. (mg)	Fib. (g)	Prot. (g)	Servings/Exchanges
Verdolagas, Cooked (1/2 cup)	10	2	<1	0	0	26	1	<1	1 vegetable

NAVAJO

Products	Cal.	Carb. (g)	Fat (g)	Sat. Fat (g)	Chol. (mg)	Sod. (mg)	Fib. (g)	Prot. (g)	Servings/Exchanges
Blue Corn Mush (3/4 cup)	94	21	<1	NA	0	32	NA	3	1 strch
Corn Hominy, Steamed (1/2 cup)	70	13	1	<1	0	18	3	2	1 strch
Four Tortilla, 8-inch (1/4)	87	19	<1	NA	0	211	1	3	1 strch
Mutton, Lean and Fat, Cooked (1 oz)	96	0	9	NA	NA	NA	0	4	1 high-fat meat
Mutton, Lean, Cooked (1 oz)	55	0	3	1	21	10	0	8	1 lean meat
Piñon Nuts, In Shell (1 Tbsp, 25)	60	<1	6	<1	0	7	1	1	1 fat

PLAINS INDIAN

Products	Cal.	Carb. (g)	Fat (g)	Sat. Fat (g)	Chol. (mg)	Sod. (mg)	Fib. (g)	Prot. (g)	Servings/Exchanges
Beans, Dried, Cooked (1/2 cup)	117	22	<1	<1	0	1	7	7	1 1/2 strch, 1 very lean meat
Beef Fat, Raw (1 tsp)	38	0	4	2	5	0	0	0	1 fat
Biscuit Mix, Dry (1/4 cup)	129	19	5	1	19	383	<1	2	1 strch, 1 fat
Buffalo/Bison (1 oz)	40	0	<1	<1	23	16	0	8	1 very lean meat
Chicken w/Skin, Fried (1 oz)	76	<1	4	1	26	24	0	8	1 med-fat meat

Food (serving)									Exchanges
Commodity Meat, Luncheon (1 oz)	97	1	9	NA	NA	420	NA	0	3	1 high-fat meat
Cracklings (1/3 oz)	57	0	5	2	9	18	0	2	1 fat
Dry Meat (1 oz)	47	<1	1	<1	12	984	0	8	1 very lean meat
Eggs, Dried Powdered (3 Tbsp)	81	0	7	2	351	12	0	4	1 med-fat meat
Elk, Roasted (1 oz)	41	0	<1	<1	0	17	0	9	1 very lean meat
Huckleberries (1 cup)	56	13	<1	NA	NA	15	NA	<1	1 fruit
Indian Corn, Dried (1/4 cup)	132	26	2	NA	NA	37	<1	4	2 strch
Kidney, Raw (1 oz)	30	<1	<1	<1	81	51	0	5	1 very lean meat
Lemon, Raw, Peeled (1)	17	5	<1	NA	0	1	0	<1	free
Liver, Beef (1 oz)	46	1	1	<1	110	20	0	7	1 lean meat
Pheasant, Skinless (1 oz)	38	0	1	<1	0	10	0	7	1 very lean meat
Pilot Bread (1, 4-inch piece)	104	18	2	NA	NA	142	NA	2	1 strch
Potatoes, Fried (1/2 cup)	163	17	11	4	NA	19	2	2	1 strch, 2 fat
Short Ribs (1 oz)	83	0	5	2	0	16	0	9	1 med-fat meat
Sweetbreads, Breaded, Fried (1 oz)	108	1	8	3	NA	126	0	7	1 high-fat meat
Venison (1 oz)	45	0	<1	<1	32	15	0	9	1 very lean meat

ETHNIC FOODS

Products	Cal.	Carb. (g)	Fat (g)	Sat. Fat (g)	Chol. (mg)	Sod. (mg)	Fib. (g)	Prot. (g)	Servings/Exchanges
White Fish, Dry Heat Cooked (1 oz)	49	0	2	<1	22	19	0	7	1 lean meat
Wild Rice, Zizania Aquatica (1/2 cup)	82	17	<1	0	0	3	<1	3	1 strch

FAST FOODS

ARBY'S

ROAST BEEF SANDWICHES

Products	Cal.	Carb. (g)	Fat (g)	Sat. Fat (g)	Chol. (mg)	Sod. (mg)	Fib. (g)	Prot. (g)	Servings/Exchanges
Arby's Melt w/Cheddar (1)	368	36	18	6	31	937	2	18	2 1/2 carb., 2 med-fat meat, 1 fat
Beef'n Cheddar (1)	487	40	28	9	50	1216	2	25	2 1/2 carb., 3 med-fat meat, 3 fat
Big Montana Sandwich	686	47	35	15	121	2295	3	48	3 carb., 6 med-fat meat, 1 fat
Roast Beef, Giant (1)	555	43	28	11	71	1561	5	35	3 carb., 4 med-fat meat, 2 fat
Roast Beef, Junior (1)	324	35	14	5	71	779	2	17	2 carb., 2 med-fat meat, 1 fat
Roast Beef, Regular (1)	388	33	19	7	43	1009	3	23	2 carb., 2 med-fat meat, 2 fat
Roast Beef, Super (1)	523	50	27	9	43	1189	5	25	3 carb., 2 med-fat meat, 3 fat

CHICKEN

Products	Cal.	Carb. (g)	Fat (g)	Sat. Fat (g)	Chol. (mg)	Sod. (mg)	Fib. (g)	Prot. (g)	Servings/Exchanges
Chicken Breast Fillet (1)	536	46	28	5	45	1416	5	28	3 carb., 3 med-fat meat, 3 fat

FAST FOODS: ARBY'S (continued)

Products	Cal.	Carb. (g)	Fat (g)	Sat. Fat (g)	Chol. (mg)	Sod. (mg)	Fib. (g)	Prot. (g)	Servings/Exchanges
Chicken Fingers (2)	290	20	16	2	32	677	<1	16	1 1/2 carb., 2 med-fat meat, 1 fat
Chicken Cordon Blue	623	46	33	8	77	1594	5	38	3 carb., 4 med-fat meat, 3 fat
Grilled Chicken Deluxe (1)	430	41	20	4	61	848	3	23	3 carb., 2 med-fat meat, 2 fat
Roast Chicken Deluxe (1)	433	36	22	5	34	763	2	24	2 1/2 carb., 2 med-fat meat, 2 fat
SUB ROLL SANDWICHES									
French Dip (1)	475	40	22	8	55	1411	3	30	2 1/2 carb., 3 med-fat meat, 2 fat
Hot Ham'n Swiss	500	43	23	7	30	1664	2	30	3 carb., 3 med-fat meat, 2 fat
Philly Beef 'n Swiss (1)	755	36	22	15	34	763	2	24	2 1/2 carb., 2 med-fat meat, 2 fat
Sub, Italian (1)	633	46	36	13	83	2089	2	30	3 carb., 3 med-fat meat, 4 fat
Sub, Roast Beef (1)	700	44	42	14	84	2034	4	38	3 carb., 4 med-fat meat, 4 fat

Sub, Turkey (1)	550	47	27	7	65	2084	2	31	3 carb., 3 med-fat meat, 2 fat
Triple Cheese Melt	720	46	45	16	91	1737	2	37	3 carb., 4 med-fat meat, 5 fat
LIGHT MENU									
Light Roast Beef Deluxe (1)	296	33	10	3	42	826	6	18	2 carb., 2 med-fat meat
Light Roast Chicken Deluxe (1)	276	33	6	2	33	777	4	20	2 carb., 2 lean meat
Light Roast Turkey Deluxe (1)	260	33	7	2	33	1262	4	20	2 carb., 2 lean meat
Salad, Garden (1)	61	12	<1	0	0	40	5	3	2 vegetable
Salad, Roast Chicken (1)	149	12	2	<1	29	418	5	20	3 very lean meat, 2 vegetable
Salad, Side (1)	23	4	<1	0	0	15	2	1	1 vegetable
OTHER SANDWICHES									
Fish Fillet (1)	529	50	27	7	43	864	2	23	3 carb., 2 med-fat meat, 3 fat
Ham'n Cheese Melt (1)	329	34	13	4	40	1013	2	20	2 carb., 3 med-fat meat
POTATOES									
Baked Potato, Broccoli 'n Cheddar (1)	571	89	20	5	12	565	9	14	6 carb., 3 fat
Baked Potato, Deluxe (1)	736	86	36	16	59	499	7	19	6 carb., 6 fat
Baked Potato, Margarine & Sour Cream (1)	578	85	24	9	25	209	7	9	5 1/2 carb., 4 fat

FAST FOODS: ARBY'S (continued)

Products	Cal.	Carb. (g)	Fat (g)	Sat. Fat (g)	Chol. (mg)	Sod. (mg)	Fib. (g)	Prot. (g)	Servings/Exchanges
Baked Potato, Plain (1)	355	82	<1	0	0	26	7	7	5 1/2 carb.
Curly Fries (3.5 oz)	300	38	15	3	0	853	0	4	2 1/2 carb., 3 fat
Curly Fries, Cheddar (4.25 oz)	333	40	18	4	3	1016	0	5	2 1/2 carb., 4 fat
Homestyle Fries, Medium	340	46	16	3	0	665	3	4	3 carb., 3 fat
Potato Cakes (3 oz)	204	20	12	2	0	397	0	3	2 carb., 2 fat

DESSERTS

Turnover, Apple (1)	330	48	14	7	0	180	0	4	3 carb., 3 fat
Turnover, Cherry (1)	320	46	13	5	0	190	0	4	3 carb., 3 fat

BOSTON MARKET

ENTREES

1/4 Dark Meat Chicken w/o Skin (1)	190	1	10	3	115	440	0	22	4 lean meat
1/4 Dark Meat Chicken w/Skin (1)	320	2	21	6	155	500	0	30	4 med-fat meat
1/4 Dark Meat Teriyaki Chicken w/Skin (1)	380	17	21	6	155	870	0	30	1 carb., 4 med-fat meat
1/4 White Meat Chicken w/o Skin (1)	170	2	4	1	85	480	0	33	4 very lean meat

Item									Exchanges
1/4 White Meat Chicken w/Skin (1)	280	2	12	4	135	510	0	40	6 lean meat
1/4 White Meat Teriyaki Chicken w/Skin (1)	340	17	12	4	135	890	0	30	1 carb., 5 lean meat
1/2 Chicken w/Skin (1)	590	4	33	10	290	1010	0	70	10 med-fat meat
Chunky Chicken Salad (3/4 cup)	370	3	27	5	120	800	1	28	4 med-fat meat, 2 fat
Hearty Honey Ham (1)	210	9	9	4	75	1490	0	25	1/2 carb., 3 lean meat
Meat Loaf & Brown Gravy (1)	390	19	22	8	120	1040	1	30	1 carb., 4 med-fat meat
Meat Loaf & Chunky Tomato Sauce (1)	370	22	18	8	120	1170	2	30	1 1/2 carb., 4 med-fat meat
Original Chicken Pot Pie (1)	780	61	46	13	135	1480	4	32	4 carb., 3 med-fat meat, 6 fat
Skinless Rotisserie Turkey Breast (1)	170	1	1	<1	100	850	0	36	5 very lean meat
Southwest Savory Chicken (1)	400	26	15	5	100	1670	4	40	2 carb., 5 lean meat
Tabasco BBQ Drumstick (1)	130	4	6	2	50	190	0	14	2 lean meat
Tabasco BBQ Wings (1)	110	4	7	2	30	170	0	9	1 med-fat meat
Triple Topped Chicken (1)	470	20	22	12	155	1350	1	50	1 carb., 7 lean meat

SOUPS, SALADS, AND SANDWICHES

| Salad, Caesar, Entrée (1) | 510 | 17 | 42 | 11 | 35 | 1130 | 3 | 17 | 1 carb., 2 med-fat meat, 6 fat |

FAST FOODS: BOSTON MARKET (continued)

Products	Cal.	Carb. (g)	Fat (g)	Sat. Fat (g)	Chol. (mg)	Sod. (mg)	Fib. (g)	Prot. (g)	Servings/Exchanges
Salad, Caesar w/o Dressing (1)	230	14	12	6	20	500	3	16	2 med-fat meat, 2 vegetable, 1 fat
Salad, Chicken Caesar (1)	650	17	45	12	105	1580	3	43	1 carb., 6 med-fat meat, 3 fat
Salad, Tossed w/Caesar Dressing (1)	380	18	31	5	15	810	3	5	1 carb., 6 fat
Salad, Tossed w/Fat Free Ranch (1)	160	29	3	0	0	940	4	5	2 carb., 1 fat
Sandwich, Chicken, BBQ (1)	540	84	9	3	75	1690	3	30	5 1/2 carb., 2 med-fat meat
Sandwich, Chicken Salad (1)	680	63	30	5	120	1360	4	39	4 carb., 4 med-fat meat, 3 fat
Sandwich, Chicken w/Cheese & Sauce (1)	750	72	33	12	135	1860	5	41	5 carb., 4 med-fat meat, 2 fat
Sandwich, Chicken w/o Sauce & Cheese (1)	430	62	5	1	65	910	4	34	4 carb., 4 very lean meat
Sandwich, Ham w/Cheese & Sauce (1)	750	72	34	12	100	1730	5	38	5 carb., 3 med-fat meat, 4 fat
Sandwich, Ham w/o Cheese & Sauce (1)	440	66	8	3	45	1450	4	25	4 1/2 carb., 2 med-fat meat
Sandwich, Meat Loaf, Open Faced (1)	760	71	35	14	145	2110	4	39	5 carb., 3 med-fat meat, 4 fat
Sandwich, Meat Loaf w/Cheese (1)	860	95	33	16	165	2270	6	46	6 carb., 4 med-fat meat, 3 fat
Sandwich, Meat Loaf w/o Cheese (1)	690	86	21	7	120	1610	6	40	6 carb., 3 med-fat meat, 1 fat

	Calories	Carbohydrate (g)	Fat (g)	Saturated Fat (g)	Cholesterol (mg)	Sodium (mg)	Fiber (g)	Protein (g)	Exchanges/Choices
Sandwich, Pastry—Broccoli, Chicken, Cheddar (1)	690	45	47	13	85	1050	2	21	3 carb., 2 med-fat meat, 7 fat
Sandwich, Pastry—Ham & Cheddar (1)	640	47	41	13	60	1560	1	19	3 carb., 1 med-fat meat, 7 fat
Sandwich, Turkey Club (1)	650	64	26	8	105	1590	4	39	4 carb., 4 med-fat meat, 1 fat
Sandwich, Turkey, Open Faced (1)	500	61	12	2	80	2170	3	37	4 carb., 4 lean meat
Sandwich, Turkey w/Cheese & Sauce (1)	710	68	28	10	110	1390	4	45	4 1/2 carb., 5 med-fat meat, fat
Sandwich, Turkey w/o Cheese & Sauce (1)	400	61	4	1	60	1070	4	45	4 carb., 3 very lean meat
Soup, Chicken Chili (1 cup)	220	21	7	2	40	1000	6	18	1 1/2 carb., 2 lean meat
Soup, Chicken Noodle (1 cup)	130	12	5	1	40	1310	2	11	1 carb., 1 med-fat meat
Soup, Chicken Tortilla (8 oz)	220	19	11	4	35	1410	2	10	1 strch, 1 med-fat meat, 1 fat
Soup, Potato (1 cup)	270	24	16	8	40	1020	2	8	1 1/2 carb., 3 fat
Soup, Tomato Bisque (1 cup)	280	16	23	10	50	1280	2	4	1 carb., 5 fat

HOT SIDE DISHES

	Calories	Carbohydrate (g)	Fat (g)	Saturated Fat (g)	Cholesterol (mg)	Sodium (mg)	Fiber (g)	Protein (g)	Exchanges/Choices
Baked Sweet Potato (1)	460	94	7	1	0	510	10	6	6 carb., 1 fat
BBQ Baked Beans (3/4 cup)	270	48	5	2	0	540	12	8	3 carb., 1 fat
Black Beans and Rice (3/4 cup)	300	45	10	2	0	1050	5	8	3 strch, 2 fat

FAST FOODS: BOSTON MARKET (continued)

Products	Cal.	Carb. (g)	Fat (g)	Sat. Fat (g)	Chol. (mg)	Sod. (mg)	Fib. (g)	Prot. (g)	Servings/Exchanges
Broccoli Cauliflower Au Gratin (3/4 cup)	200	14	11	7	20	600	3	9	1 carb., 1 med-fat meat, 1 fat
Broccoli Rice Casserole (3/4 cup)	240	26	12	8	40	800	2	5	2 carb., 2 fat
Broccoli w/Red Peppers (3/4 cup)	60	5	4	<1	0	130	3	3	1 vegetable, 1 fat
Butternut Squash (3/4 cup)	160	25	6	4	15	580	3	2	1 1/2 carb., 1 fat
Chicken Gravy (1 oz)	15	2	1	0	0	170	0	0	free
Creamed Spinach (3/4 cup)	260	11	20	13	55	740	2	9	1 med-fat meat, 2 vegetable, 3 fat
Green Bean Casserole (3/4 cup)	130	10	9	5	20	440	2	2	1/2 carb., 2 fat
Green Beans (3/4 cup)	80	5	6	1	0	200	3	1	1 vegetable, 1 fat
Homestyle Mashed Potatoes (2/3 cup)	190	24	9	6	25	570	1	3	1 1/2 carb., 2 fat
Homestyle Mashed Potatoes & Gravy (3/4 cup)	210	26	10	6	25	740	1	4	2 carb., 2 fat
Honey-Glazed Carrots (3/4 cup)	280	35	15	3	0	80	4	1	2 carb., 3 fat
Hot Cinnamon Apples (3/4 cup)	250	56	5	<1	0	45	3	0	4 fruit, 1 fat
Macaroni & Cheese (3/4 cup)	280	32	11	6	30	830	1	13	2 carb., 1 med-fat meat, 1 fat

New Potatoes (3/4 cup)	130	25	3	0	0	150	2	3	1 1/2 carb., 1 fat
Oven Roasted Potato Planks (5)	180	32	5	<1	0	370	3	3	2 strch, 1 fat
Red Beans and Rice (1 cup)	260	45	5	0	5	1050	4	8	3 strch, 1 fat
Rice Pilaf (2/3 cup)	180	32	5	1	0	600	2	5	2 carb., 1 fat
Savory Stuffing (3/4 cup)	310	44	12	2	0	1140	3	6	3 strch, 2 fat
Squash Casserole (3/4 cup)	330	20	24	13	70	1110	3	7	1 carb., 5 fat
Steamed Vegetables (2/3 cup)	35	7	<1	0	0	35	3	2	1 vegetable
Sweet Potato Casserole (3/4 cup)	280	39	18	5	10	190	2	3	2 1/2 carb., 4 fat
Whole Kernel Corn (3/4 cup)	180	30	4	<1	0	170	2	5	2 carb., 1 fat
Zucchini Marinara (3/4 cup)	60	7	3	0	0	330	2	1	2 vegetable, 1 fat

COLD SIDE DISHES

Chunky Cinnamon Apple Sauce (3/4 cup)	250	62	0	0	0	30	2	1	4 carb.
Coleslaw (3/4 cup)	300	30	19	3	20	540	3	2	2 carb., 3 fat
Coyote Bean Salad (3/4 cup)	190	24	9	<1	0	210	9	4	1 1/2 carb., 2 fat
Cranberry Relish (3/4 cup)	370	84	5	<1	0	5	5	2	5 1/2 carb., 1 fat
Old-Fashioned Potato Salad (3/4 cup)	340	30	24	4	30	870	2	2	2 carb., 5 fat

FAST FOODS: BOSTON MARKET (continued)

Products	Cal.	Carb. (g)	Fat (g)	Sat. Fat (g)	Chol. (mg)	Sod. (mg)	Fib. (g)	Prot. (g)	Servings/Exchanges
Salad, Caesar Side (1)	200	7	17	5	15	450	1	7	1 med-fat meat, 1 vegetable, 2 fat
Salad, Fruit (3/4 cup)	70	15	<1	0	0	10	1	1	1 fruit
BAKED GOODS									
Cinnamon Apple Pie (1/5)	390	46	23	4	0	250	2	2	3 carb., 5 fat
Brownie (1)	450	47	27	7	80	190	3	6	3 carb., 5 fat
Chocolate Chip Cookie (1)	340	48	17	6	25	240	1	4	3 carb., 3 fat
Corn Bread (1 loaf)	200	33	6	2	25	390	1	3	2 strch, 1 fat

BURGER KING

BURGERS

Products	Cal.	Carb. (g)	Fat (g)	Sat. Fat (g)	Chol. (mg)	Sod. (mg)	Fib. (g)	Prot. (g)	Servings/Exchanges
Bacon Cheeseburger (1)	400	27	22	10	70	940	1	24	2 carb., 3 med-fat meat, 1 fat
Big King Sandwich (1)	640	28	42	18	125	980	1	38	2 carb., 5 med-fat meat, 3 fat
Cheeseburger (1)	360	27	19	9	60	760	1	21	2 carb., 2 med-fat meat, 1 fat
Cheeseburger, Double (1)	580	27	36	17	120	1060	1	38	2 carb., 5 med-fat meat, 2 fat

Cheeseburger, Double w/Bacon (1)	620	28	38	18	125	1230	1	41	2 carb., 5 med-fat meat, 3 fat
Hamburger (1)	320	27	15	6	50	520	1	19	2 carb., 2 med-fat meat, 1 fat
Whopper Jr. Sandwich (1)	400	28	24	8	55	530	2	19	2 carb., 2 med-fat meat, 3 fat
Whopper Jr. Sandwich w/Cheese (1)	450	28	28	10	65	770	2	22	2 carb., 2 med-fat meat, 4 fat
Whopper Sandwich (1)	660	47	40	12	85	900	3	29	3 carb., 3 med-fat meat, 5 fat
Whopper Sandwich, Double (1)	920	47	59	21	155	980	3	49	3 carb., 5 med-fat meat, 6 fat
Whopper Sandwich w/Cheese (1)	760	47	48	17	110	1350	3	35	3 carb., 3 med-fat meat, 6 fat
Whopper Sandwich w/Cheese, Double (1)	1010	47	67	26	180	1460	3	55	3 carb., 7 med-fat meat, 6 fat

SANDWICHES/SIDE ORDERS

Chick 'N Crisp (1)	460	37	27	6	35	890	3	16	2 1/2 carb., 1 med-fat meat, 4 fat
Chicken Tenders (5)	230	11	14	4	40	590	<1	14	1 carb., 2 med-fat meat, 1 fat
French Fries, Salted (1 medium order)	400	50	21	8	0	820	4	3	3 carb., 4 fat
Onion Rings (1 medium order)	380	46	19	4	2	550	4	5	3 carb., 4 fat
Pie, Dutch Apple (1)	300	39	15	3	0	230	2	3	2 1/2 carb., 3 fat
Sandwich, BK Broiler Chicken (1)	530	45	26	5	105	1060	2	29	3 carb., 3 med-fat meat, 2 fat

FAST FOODS: BURGER KING (continued)

Products	Cal.	Carb. (g)	Fat (g)	Sat. Fat (g)	Chol. (mg)	Sod. (mg)	Fib. (g)	Prot. (g)	Servings/Exchanges
Sandwich, BK Big Fish (1)	720	59	43	9	80	1180	3	23	4 carb., 2 med-fat meat, 7 fat
Sandwich, Chicken (1)	710	54	43	9	60	1400	2	26	3 1/2 carb., 2 med-fat meat, 7 fat
DRINKS									
Orange Juice, Tropicana (10 oz)	140	33	0	0	0	0	0	2	2 fruit
Shake, Chocolate (1 medium)	440	75	10	6	30	330	4	12	5 carb., 2 fat
Shake, Chocolate, Syrup Added (1 medium)	570	105	10	6	30	520	3	14	7 carb., 2 fat
Shake, Strawberry, Syrup Added (1 medium)	550	104	9	5	30	350	2	13	7 carb., 2 fat
Shake, Vanilla (1 medium)	430	73	9	5	30	330	2	13	5 carb., 2 fat
BREAKFAST									
Biscuit (1)	300	35	15	3	0	830	1	6	2 carb., 3 fat
Biscuit w/Egg (1)	380	37	21	5	140	1010	<1	11	2 1/2 carb., 1 med-fat meat, 3 fat

	Calories	Carb. (g)	Fat (g)	Sat. Fat (g)	Chol. (mg)	Sod. (mg)	Fiber (g)	Prot. (g)	Exchanges/Choices
Biscuit w/Sausage (1)	490	36	33	10	35	1240	1	13	2 1/2 carb., 1 med-fat meat, 6 fat
Biscuit (1)	300	35	15	3	0	830	1	6	2 carb., 3 fat
Biscuit w/Egg (1)	380	37	21	5	140	1010	<1	11	2 1/2 carb., 1 med-fat meat, 3 fat
Croissan'wich w/Sausage, Egg & Cheese (1)	530	23	41	13	185	1120	1	18	1 1/2 carb., 2 med-fat meat, 6 fat
French Toast Sticks (5 sticks)	440	51	23	5	2	490	3	7	3 1/2 carb., 5 fat
Hash Browns (small)	240	25	15	6	0	440	2	2	2 carb., 3 fat
CONDIMENTS									
a.m. Express Dip (1 pkt)	80	21	0	0	0	20	NA	0	1 1/2 carb.
BBQ Sauce (1 pkt)	35	9	0	0	0	400	NA	0	1/2 carb.
Dipping Sauce, Honey (1 pkt)	90	23	0	0	0	10	NA	0	1 1/2 carb.
Dipping Sauce, Ranch (1 pkt)	170	2	17	3	0	200	NA	0	3 fat
Dipping Sauce, Sweet & Sour (1 pkt)	45	11	0	0	0	50	NA	0	1 carb.
Jam, a.m. Express Grape (1 pkt)	30	7	0	0	0	0	NA	0	1/2 carb.

FAST FOODS: BURGER KING (continued)

Products	Cal.	Carb. (g)	Fat (g)	Sat. Fat (g)	Chol. (mg)	Sod. (mg)	Fib. (g)	Prot. (g)	Servings/Exchanges
Jam, a.m. Express Strawberry (1 pkt)	30	8	0	0	0	0	NA	0	1/2 carb.

CARL'S JR.

SANDWICHES

Products	Cal.	Carb. (g)	Fat (g)	Sat. Fat (g)	Chol. (mg)	Sod. (mg)	Fib. (g)	Prot. (g)	Servings/Exchanges
Carl's Bacon Swiss Crispy Chicken Sandwich (1)	720	66	36	10	75	1610	3	32	4 1/2 carb., 3 med-fat meat, 4 fat
Carl's Catch Fish Sandwich (1)	510	50	27	7	80	1030	1	18	3 carb., 1 med-fat meat, 4 fat
Carl's Famous Star Hamburger (1)	580	49	32	9	70	910	2	25	3 carb., 2 med-fat meat, 4 fat
Carl's Ranch Crispy Chicken Sandwich (1)	620	65	29	6	50	1220	3	25	4 carb., 2 med-fat meat, 4 fat
Charbroiled BBQ Chicken Sandwich (1)	280	37	3	1	60	830	2	25	2 1/2 carb., 2 very lean meat
Charbroiled Chicken Club Sandwich (1)	460	33	22	7	90	1110	2	32	2 carb., 4 med-fat meat
Charbroiled Santa Fe Chicken Sandwich (1)	510	32	31	7	95	1240	2	28	2 carb., 3 med-fat meat, 3 fat
Charbroiled Sirloin Steak Sandwich (1)	580	50	26	5	85	1110	2	33	3 carb., 3 med-fat meat, 2 fat
Double Western Bacon Cheeseburger (1)	900	64	49	21	155	1770	2	51	4 carb., 6 med-fat meat, 4 fat
Jr. Hamburger (1)	330	34	13	5	45	480	1	18	2 carb., 2 med-fat meat, 1 fat

Item	Cal.	Carb. (g)	Fat (g)	Sat. Fat (g)	Chol. (mg)	Sod. (mg)	Fiber (g)	Prot. (g)	Exchanges
Super Star Hamburger (1)	790	50	46	14	130	970	2	42	3 carb., 5 med-fat meat, 4 fat
Western Bacon Cheeseburger (1)	650	63	30	12	80	1430	2	32	4 carb., 3 med-fat meat, 3 fat
GREAT STUFF POTATOES									
Bacon & Cheese (1)	630	76	29	7	35	1700	6	20	5 carb., 1 med-fat meat, 5 fat
Broccoli & Cheese (1)	530	74	21	5	15	950	7	11	5 carb., 4 fat
Plain Potato w/o Margarine (1)	290	68	0	0	0	20	6	6	4 1/2 carb.
Sour Cream & Chives (1)	430	70	14	3	10	135	6	7	4 1/2 carb., 3 fat
SALAD DRESSINGS									
1000 Island Dressing (1 pkt)	230	5	23	4	20	420	0	1	5 fat
Blue Cheese Dressing (1 pkt)	320	1	35	6	25	370	0	2	7 fat
Fat Free French Dressing (1 pkt)	60	16	0	0	0	660	<1	0	1 carb.
Fat Free Italian Dressing (1 pkt)	15	4	0	0	0	770	0	0	free
House Dressing (1 pkt)	220	3	22	4	20	440	0	1	4 fat
SALADS									
Charbroiled Chicken Salad-to-Go (1)	200	12	7	4	75	440	3	25	2 vegetable, 3 lean meat
Garden Salad-to-Go (1)	50	4	3	2	10	60	2	3	1 vegetable, 1 fat

FAST FOODS: CARL'S JR. (continued)

Products	Cal.	Carb. (g)	Fat (g)	Sat. Fat (g)	Chol. (mg)	Sod. (mg)	Fib. (g)	Prot. (g)	Servings/Exchanges
SIDES									
Chicken Stars (6)	280	15	19	5	40	330	0	12	1 carb., 1 med-fat meat, 4 fat
CrissCut Fries (1 order)	410	43	24	5	0	950	4	5	3 carb., 5 fat
French Fries (1 order)	290	37	14	3	0	170	3	5	2 1/2 carb., 3 fat
Hash Brown Nuggets (1 order)	330	32	21	5	0	470	3	3	2 carb., 4 fat
Onion Rings (1 order)	430	53	21	5	0	700	3	7	3 1/2 carb., 4 fat
Zucchini (1 order)	340	37	19	5	0	860	2	5	2 1/2 carb., 4 fat
BREADS/SAUCES									
BBQ Sauce (1 pkt)	50	11	0	0	0	270	0	1	1 carb.
Breadsticks (1)	35	7	<1	0	0	60	1	1	1/2 carb.
Croutons (1 pkg)	35	5	1	0	0	65	0	<1	1/2 carb.
Honey Sauce (1 pkt)	90	22	0	0	0	0	0	0	1 1/2 carb.
Mustard Sauce (1 pkt)	50	11	0	0	0	210	0	0	1 carb.
Salsa (1 pkt)	10	2	0	0	0	160	0	0	free

Sweet n' Sour (1 pkt)	50	12	0	0	0	80	0	0	1 carb.
Table Syrup (1 pkt)	90	21	0	0	0	0	0	0	1 1/2 carb.
BREAKFAST									
Breakfast Burrito (1)	480	26	30	13	465	750	2	27	2 carb., 3 med-fat meat, 3 fat
Breakfast Quesadilla (1)	310	27	16	6	230	670	2	14	2 carb., 1 med-fat meat, 2 fat
English Muffin w/Margarine (1)	210	27	9	1	0	300	2	5	2 carb., 2 fat
French Toast Dips (1 order)	370	42	20	3	0	430	1	6	3 carb., 4 fat
Scrambled Eggs (1 order)	160	1	11	4	425	125	0	13	2 med-fat meat
Sunrise Sandwich w/o Bacon/Sausage (1)	360	28	21	5	225	700	2	14	2 carb., 1 med-fat meat, 3 fat
BAKERY/DESSERTS									
Blueberry Muffin (1)	340	49	14	2	40	340	1	5	3 carb., 3 fat
Bran Raisin Muffin (1)	370	61	13	2	45	410	6	7	4 carb., 3 fat
Cheese Danish (1)	400	49	22	5	15	390	1	5	3 carb., 4 fat
Chocolate Cake (1 slice)	300	49	10	3	23	260	4	3	3 carb., 2 fat
Chocolate Chip Cookie (1)	300	49	10	3	25	350	1	3	3 carb., 2 fat
Strawberry Swirl Cheesecake (1 slice)	290	30	17	9	55	230	0	6	2 carb., 3 fat

FAST FOODS: DAIRY QUEEN/BRAZIER

DAIRY QUEEN/BRAZIER

SANDWICHES

Products	Cal.	Carb. (g)	Fat (g)	Sat. Fat (g)	Chol. (mg)	Sod. (mg)	Fib. (g)	Prot. (g)	Servings/Exchanges
Chicken Strip Basket w/Gravy (1)	100	102	50	13	55	2260	5	35	7 carb., 2 med-fat meat, 8 fat
Chili N' Cheese Dog (1)	330	22	21	9	45	1090	2	14	1 1/2 carb., 1 med-fat meat, 3 fat
Cheeseburger, Homestyle (1)	340	29	17	8	55	850	2	20	2 carb., 2 med-fat meat, 1 fat
Cheeseburger, Homestyle Bacon Double (1)	610	31	36	18	130	1380	2	41	2 carb., 5 med-fat meat, 2 fat
Cheeseburger, Homestyle Double (1)	540	30	31	16	115	1130	2	35	2 carb., 4 med-fat meat, 2 fat
Hamburger, Homestyle (1)	290	29	12	5	45	630	2	17	2 carb., 2 med-fat meat
Hot Dog (1)	240	19	14	5	25	730	1	9	1 carb., 1 med-fat meat, 2 fat
Rib Basket (1)	810	86	25	6	50	2050	3	26	6 carb., 1 med-fat meat, 4 fat
Sandwich, Chicken Breast Fillet (1)	430	37	20	4	25	760	2	24	2 1/2 carb., 2 med-fat meat, 2 fat
Sandwich, Grilled Chicken (1)	310	30	10	3	50	1040	3	24	2 carb., 3 med-fat meat

Ultimate Burger (1)	670	29	43	19	135	1210	2	40	2 carb., 5 med-fat meat, 4 fat

SIDE ITEMS

French Fries (1 medium)	440	53	23	5	0	790	4	5	3 1/2 carb., 5 fat
Onion Rings (1)	320	39	16	4	0	180	3	5	2 1/2 carb., 3 fat

CONES, NOVELTIES, AND TREATS

Banana Split (1)	510	96	12	8	30	180	3	8	6 1/2 carb., 2 fat
Breeze, Heath (1 medium)	710	123	18	11	20	580	1	15	8 carb., 3 fat
Buster Bar (1)	450	41	28	12	15	280	2	10	3 carb., 6 fat
Chocolate Dilly Bar (1)	210	21	13	7	10	75	0	3	1 1/2 carb., 3 fat
Chocolate Rock Treat (1)	730	87	38	18	30	280	3	14	6 carb., 8 fat
DQ Sandwich (1)	150	24	5	2	5	115	1	3	1 1/2 carb., 1 fat
Frozen 8" Round Cake (1/8 cake)	340	53	12	7	25	250	1	7	3 1/2 carb., 2 fat
Fudge Bar-No Sugar Added (1)	50	13	0	0	0	70	0	4	1 carb.
Heath DQ Treatzza Pizza (1/8)	180	28	7	4	5	160	1	3	2 carb., 1 fat
Ice Cream Cone, Chocolate (1 medium)	340	53	11	7	30	160	0	8	3 1/2 carb., 2 fat
Ice Cream Cone, Dipped (1 medium)	490	59	24	13	30	190	1	8	4 carb., 5 fat

FAST FOODS: DAIRY QUEEN/BRAZIER (continued)

Products	Cal.	Carb. (g)	Fat (g)	Sat. Fat (g)	Chol. (mg)	Sod. (mg)	Fib. (g)	Prot. (g)	Servings/Exchanges
Ice Cream Cone, Vanilla (1 medium)	330	53	9	6	30	160	0	8	3 1/2 carb., 2 fat
Ice Cream Sundae, Chocolate (1 medium)	400	71	10	6	30	210	0	8	5 carb., 2 fat
Misty Slush (1 medium)	290	74	0	0	0	30	0	0	5 carb.
Nonfat Frozen Yogurt (1/2 cup)	100	21	0	0	<5	70	9	3	1 1/2 carb.
Peanut Buster Parfait (1)	730	99	31	17	35	400	2	16	6 1/2 carb., 6 fat
Starkiss (1)	80	21	0	0	0	10	0	0	1 1/2 carb.
Vanilla Orange Bar-No Sugar Added (1)	60	17	0	0	0	40	0	2	1 carb
MALTS, SHAKES, AND BLIZZARDS									
Blizzard, Choc. Chip Cookie Dough (1 medium)	950	143	36	19	75	660	2	17	9 1/2 carb., 7 fat
Blizzard, Sandwich Cookie (1medium)	640	97	23	11	45	500	1	12	6 carb., 3 fat
Malt, Chocolate (1 medium)	880	153	22	14	70	500	0	19	10 carb., 4 fat
Malt, Chocolate (1 small)	650	111	16	10	55	370	0	15	7 1/2 carb., 3 fat
Shake, Chocolate (1 medium)	770	130	20	13	70	420	0	17	8 1/2 carb., 4 fat
Shake, Chocolate (1 small)	560	94	15	10	50	310	0	13	6 carb., 3 fat

Smoothy, Strawberry Banana (1)	670	128	14	9	45	250	2	11	8 1/2 carb, 3 fat

NONFAT FROZEN YOGURT

Frozen Yogurt Cone (1 medium)	260	56	1	<1	5	160	0	9	4 carb.
Frozen Yogurt Strawberry Breeze (1 medium)	460	99	1	1	10	270	1	13	6 1/2 carb.
Frozen Yogurt Strawberry Sundae (1 medium)	280	61	<1	0	5	160	1	8	4 1/2 carb.

DOMINO'S

12-INCH HAND-TOSSED PIZZA

Cheese (2 slices)	347	50	11	5	15	723	3	15	3 carb., 1 med-fat meat, 1 fat
Ham (2 slices)	365	50	11	5	22	886	3	17	3 carb., 1 med-fat meat, 1 fat
Italian Sausage (2 slices)	402	51	15	7	26	894	3	17	3 1/2 carb., 1 med-fat meat, 2 fat
Pepperoni (2 slices)	409	50	16	7	28	922	3	17	3 carb., 1 med-fat meat, 1 fat
Veggie (2 slices)	371	52	12	5	15	795	4	15	3 1/2 carb., 1 med-fat meat, 1 fat

12-INCH THIN-CRUST PIZZA

Cheese (1/4)	271	31	12	5	15	809	2	12	2 carb., 1 med-fat meat, 1 fat

FAST FOODS: DOMINO'S (continued)

Products	Cal.	Carb. (g)	Fat (g)	Sat. Fat (g)	Chol. (mg)	Sod. (mg)	Fib. (g)	Prot. (g)	Servings/Exchanges
Ham (1/4)	288	31	13	6	22	972	2	14	2 carb., 1 med-fat meat, 1 fat
Italian Sausage (1/4)	326	32	16	7	26	980	2	14	2 carb., 1 med-fat meat, 2 fat
Pepperoni (1/4)	333	31	17	7	28	1008	2	15	2 carb., 1 med-fat meat, 2 fat
Veggie (1/4)	295	33	13	5	15	882	3	13	2 carb., 1 med-fat meat, 2 fat
12-INCH DEEP-DISH PIZZA									
Cheese (2 slices)	477	55	22	9	19	1085	3	18	4 carb., 1 med-fat meat, 3 fat
Ham (2 slices)	495	56	22	9	26	1248	3	21	4 carb., 1 med-fat meat, 3 fat
Italian Sausage (2 slices)	532	57	26	10	31	1256	4	21	4carb., 1 med-fat meat, 4 fat
Pepperoni (2 slices)	539	56	27	11	32	1258	3	21	4 carb., 2 med-fat meat, 3 fat
Veggie (2 slices)	501	58	23	9	19	1158	4	19	4 carb., 1 med-fat meat, 4 fat
BREADSTICKS									
Breadsticks (1)	78	11	3	<1	0	158	<1	2	1 carb., 1 fat
Cheesy Bread (1)	103	11	5	2	5	187	<1	3	1 carb., 2 fat

BUFFALO WINGS

Barbeque Wings (1)	50	2	2	<1	26	175	<1	6	1 lean meat
Hot Wings (1)	45	<1	2	<1	26	354	<1	6	1 lean meat

SALAD DRESSINGS

Blue Cheese (1 pkt)	220	2	24	4	40	440	0	2	5 fat
Creamy Caesar (1 pkt)	200	2	22	3	10	470	0	1	4 fat
Fat-Free Ranch (1 pkt)	40	10	0	0	0	560	1	0	1/2 carb.
Honey French (1 pkt)	210	14	18	3	0	300	0	0	1 carb., 4 fat
House Italian (1 pkt)	220	1	24	3	0	440	0	0	5 fat
Light Italian (1 pkt)	20	2	1	0	0	780	0	0	free
Thousand Island (1 pkt)	200	5	20	3	25	320	0	0	4 fat

SALADS

Garden Salad, Large (1)	39	8	<1	<1	0	26	3	2	2 vegetable
Garden Salad, Small (1)	22	4	<1	<1	0	14	2	1	1 vegetable

FAST FOODS

HARDEE'S

BREAKFAST

Products	Cal.	Carb. (g)	Fat (g)	Sat. Fat (g)	Chol. (mg)	Sod. (mg)	Fib. (g)	Prot. (g)	Servings/Exchanges
Apple Cinnamon 'N' Raisin Biscuit (1)	200	30	8	2	0	350	NA	2	2 carb., 2 fat
Big Country Breakfast, Bacon (1)	820	62	49	15	535	1870	NA	33	4 carb., 3 med-fat meat, 6 fat
Big Country Breakfast, Sausage (1)	1000	62	66	38	570	2310	NA	41	4 carb., 4 med-fat meat, 9 fat
Biscuit, Bacon & Egg (1)	570	45	33	11	275	1400	NA	22	3 carb., 2 med-fat meat, 5 fat
Biscuit, Bacon, Egg, & Cheese (1)	610	45	37	13	280	1630	NA	24	3 carb., 2 med-fat meat, 5 fat
Biscuit, Country Ham (1)	430	45	22	6	25	1930	NA	15	3 carb., 1 med-fat meat, 3 fat
Biscuit, Ham (1)	400	47	20	6	15	1340	NA	9	3 carb., 1 med-fat meat, 3 fat
Biscuit, Ham, Egg, & Cheese (1)	540	48	30	11	285	1660	NA	20	3 carb., 2 med-fat meat, 4 fat
Biscuit 'N' Gravy (1)	510	55	28	9	15	1500	NA	10	3 1/2 carb., 6 fat
Biscuit, Rise 'N' Shine (1)	390	44	21	6	0	1000	NA	6	3 carb., 4 fat
Biscuit, Sausage & Egg (1)	630	45	40	22	285	1480	NA	23	3 carb., 2 med-fat meat, 6 fat
Biscuit, Sausage (1)	510	44	31	10	25	1360	NA	14	3 carb., 1 med-fat meat, 5 fat

Biscuit, Ultimate Omelet (1)	570	45	33	12	290	1370	NA	22	3 carb., 2 med-fat meat, 5 fat
Frisco Breakfast Sandwich, Ham (1)	500	46	25	9	290	1370	NA	24	3 carb., 2 med-fat meat, 3 fat
Hash Rounds, Regular (16)	230	24	14	3	0	560	NA	3	1 1/2 carb., 3 fat
Jelly Biscuit (1)	440	57	21	6	0	1000	NA	6	4 carb., 4 fat
Three Pancakes (1 order)	280	56	2	1	15	890	NA	8	4 carb.

SANDWICHES

Burger, Frisco (1)	720	43	46	16	95	1340	NA	33	3 carb., 3 med-fat meat, 6 fat
Burger, Mushroom 'N' Swiss (1)	490	39	25	12	80	1100	NA	28	3 1/2 carb., 3 med-fat meat, 2 fat
Burger, The Boss (1)	570	42	33	12	85	910	NA	27	3 carb., 3 med-fat meat, 3 fat
Burger, The Works (1)	530	41	30	12	80	1030	NA	25	3 carb., 2 med-fat meat, 4 fat
Cheeseburger (1)	310	30	14	6	40	890	NA	16	2 carb., 1 med-fat meat, 2 fat
Cheeseburger, Cravin' Bacon (1)	690	38	46	15	95	1150	NA	30	2 1/2 carb., 2 med-fat meat, 7 fat
Cheeseburger, Mesquite Bacon (1)	370	32	18	7	45	970	NA	19	2 carb., 2 med-fat meat, 2 fat
Cheeseburger, Quarter Pound Double (1)	470	31	25	11	80	1290	NA	27	2 carb., 3 med-fat meat, 2 fat

FAST FOODS: HARDEE'S (continued)

Products	Cal.	Carb. (g)	Fat (g)	Sat. Fat (g)	Chol. (mg)	Sod. (mg)	Fib. (g)	Prot. (g)	Servings/Exchanges
Fisherman's Fillet (1)	560	54	27	7	65	1330	NA	26	3 1/2 carb., 2 med-fat meat, 3 fat
Hamburger (1)	270	29	11	3	35	670	NA	14	2 carb., 1 med-fat meat, 1 fat
Hot Ham 'N' Cheese (1)	310	34	12	6	50	1410	NA	16	2 carb., 1 med-fat meat, 1 fat
Sandwich, Big Roast Beef (1)	460	35	24	9	70	1230	NA	26	2 carb., 3 med-fat meat, 2 fat
Sandwich, Chicken Fillet (1)	480	54	18	3	55	1280	NA	26	3 1/2 carb., 2 med-fat meat, 2 fat
Sandwich, Grilled Chicken (1)	350	38	11	2	65	950	NA	25	2 1/2 carb., 3 lean meat
Sandwich, Regular Roast Beef (1)	320	26	16	6	43	820	NA	17	2 carb., 2 med-fat meat, 1 fat
FRIED CHICKEN/SIDES									
Baked Beans (5 oz, small)	170	32	1	0	0	600	NA	8	2 carb.
Chicken Breast (1 serving)	370	29	15	4	75	1190	NA	29	2 carb., 3 med-fat meat
Chicken Leg (1 serving)	170	15	7	2	45	570	NA	13	1 carb., 1 med-fat meat, 1 fat
Chicken Thigh (1 serving)	330	30	15	4	60	1000	NA	19	2 carb., 2 med-fat meat, 1 fat

Food	Cal	Carb	Pro	Fat	Chol	Sod		Fiber	Exchanges
Chicken Wing (1 serving)	200	23	8	2	30	740	NA	10	1 1/2 carb., 1 med-fat meat, 1 fat
Coleslaw (1/2 cup)	240	13	20	3	10	340	NA	2	2 vegetable, 4 fat
Gravy (1 1/2 oz)	20	3	<1	<1	0	260	NA	<1	free
Potatoes, Mashed (1/2 cup)	70	14	<1	<1	0	330	NA	2	1 carb.

SALADS/FRIES

Food	Cal	Carb	Pro	Fat	Chol	Sod		Fiber	Exchanges
French Fries (1 medium order)	350	49	15	4	0	150	NA	5	3 carb., 3 fat
Salad, Garden (1)	220	11	13	9	40	350	NA	12	1 med-fat meat, 2 vegetable, 2 fat
Salad, Grilled Chicken (1)	150	11	3	1	60	610	NA	20	2 very lean meat, 2 vegetable
Salad, Side (1)	25	4	<1	<1	0	45	NA	1	1 vegetable

SHAKES/DESSERTS

Food	Cal	Carb	Pro	Fat	Chol	Sod		Fiber	Exchanges
Big Cookie (1)	280	41	12	4	15	150	NA	4	3 carb., 2 fat
Cool Twist Cone, Vanilla/Chocolate (1)	180	34	2	1	10	120	NA	4	2 carb.
Shake, Strawberry (1)	420	83	4	3	20	270	NA	11	5 1/2 carb., 1 fat

FAST FOODS: HARDEE'S (continued)

Products	Cal.	Carb. (g)	Fat (g)	Sat. Fat (g)	Chol. (mg)	Sod. (mg)	Fib. (g)	Prot. (g)	Servings/Exchanges
Shake, Vanilla (1)	350	65	5	3	20	300	NA	12	4 carb., 1 fat
Sundae, Hot Fudge (1)	290	51	6	3	20	310	NA	7	3 1/2 carb., 1 fat

JACK IN THE BOX

BURGERS

Products	Cal.	Carb. (g)	Fat (g)	Sat. Fat (g)	Chol. (mg)	Sod. (mg)	Fib. (g)	Prot. (g)	Servings/Exchanges
Bacon Ultimate Cheeseburger (1)	1020	37	71	26	210	1740	1	58	2 1/2 carb., 7 med-fat meat, 7 fat
Cheeseburger (1)	320	30	16	6	40	720	2	14	2 carb., 1 med-fat meat, 2 fat
Double Cheeseburger (1)	460	32	27	12	80	1090	2	24	2 carb., 3 med-fat meat, 2 fat
Hamburger (1)	280	30	12	4	30	490	2	12	2 carb., 1 med-fat meat, 1 fat
Jumbo Jack Hamburger (1)	590	39	37	11	90	670	2	27	2 1/2 carb., 3 med-fat meat, 4 fat
Jumbo Jack Hamburger w/Cheese (1)	680	39	45	16	115	1130	2	31	2 1/2 carb., 3 med-fat meat, 6 fat

	Cal.	Carb. (g)	Fat (g)	Sat. Fat (g)	Chol. (mg)	Sod. (mg)	Fiber (g)		Exchanges
Sourdough Jack (1)	690	37	45	15	105	1180	2	34	2 1/2 carb., 4 med-fat meat, 5 fat
Ultimate Cheeseburger (1)	950	37	66	26	195	1370	1	52	2 1/2 carb., 6 med-fat meat, 7 fat

SANDWICHES AND TACOS

	Cal.	Carb. (g)	Fat (g)	Sat. Fat (g)	Chol. (mg)	Sod. (mg)	Fiber (g)		Exchanges
Chicken (1)	420	39	23	4	40	950	2	16	2 1/2 carb., 1 med-fat meat, 4 fat
Chicken Fajita Pita (1)	280	25	9	4	75	840	3	24	1 1/2 carb., 3 lean meat
Chicken Supreme (1)	570	39	37	8	70	1440	3	21	2 1/2 carb., 2 med-fat meat, 5 fat
Grilled Chicken Fillet (1)	480	39	24	6	65	1110	4	27	2 1/2 carb., 3 med-fat meat, 2 fat
Jack's Spicy Chicken (1)	570	52	29	3	50	1020	2	24	3 1/2 carb., 2 med-fat meat, 2 fat
Philly Cheesesteak (1)	580	56	16	8	80	1860	1	33	3 carb., 3 med-fat meat
Taco (1)	170	12	10	4	20	460	2	7	1 carb., 1 med-fat meat, 1 fat

FAST FOODS: JACK IN THE BOX (continued)

Products	Cal.	Carb. (g)	Fat (g)	Sat. Fat (g)	Chol. (mg)	Sod. (mg)	Fib. (g)	Prot. (g)	Servings/Exchanges
Taco, Monster (1)	270	19	17	6	30	670	4	12	1 carb., 1 med-meat meat, 2 fat
SALADS									
Garden Chicken (1)	200	8	9	4	65	420	3	23	3 lean meat, 1 vegetable
Side (1)	50	3	3	2	10	80	1	2	1 vegetable, 1 fat
TERIYAKI BOWLS									
Chicken (1)	670	128	4	1	15	1730	3	26	8 1/2 carb., 1 med-fat meat, 2 vegetable
FINGER FOODS									
Bacon Cheddar Potato Wedges (1)	800	49	58	16	55	1470	4	20	3 carb., 2 med-fat meat, 10 fat
Chicken & Fries (1)	730	79	34	7	65	1690	5	26	5 carb., 2 med-fat meat, 5 fat
Chicken Breast Pieces (5)	360	24	17	3	80	970	1	27	1 1/2 carb., 3 med-fat meat
Egg Rolls (3)	440	40	24	6	35	1020	4	15	2 1/2 carb., 1 med-fat meat, 4 fat

	Calories	Carb. (g)	Fat (g)	Sat. Fat (g)	Chol. (mg)	Sodium (mg)	Fiber (g)	Protein (g)	Exchanges
Fish & Chips (1)	780	86	39	9	45	1740	6	19	6 carb, 1 med-fat meat, 6 fat
Stuffed Jalapeños (7)	530	46	31	12	60	1730	3	14	3 carb, 1 med-fat meat, 5 fat

SIDES AND DESSERTS

	Calories	Carb. (g)	Fat (g)	Sat. Fat (g)	Chol. (mg)	Sodium (mg)	Fiber (g)	Protein (g)	Exchanges
Carrot Cake (1)	370	54	16	3	40	340	2	3	3 1/2 carb., 3 fat
Cheesecake (1)	320	32	18	10	65	220	<1	7	2 carb., 4 fat
Chili Cheese Curly Fries (1)	650	60	41	12	25	1760	4	14	4 carb., 8 fat
Double Fudge Cake (1)	300	50	10	2	50	320	1	3	3 carb., 2 fat
French Fries (1 regular order)	350	46	16	4	0	710	3	4	3 carb., 3 fat
French Fries (1 Super Scoop order)	610	82	28	6	0	1250	5	6	5 1/2 carb., 6 fat
Hot Apple Turnover (1)	340	41	18	4	0	510	2	4	3 carb., 4 fat
Onion Rings (1 order)	410	45	23	5	0	1010	4	6	3 carb., 5 fat
Seasoned Curly Fries (1 regular order)	410	45	23	5	0	1010	4	6	3 carb., 5 fat

BREAKFAST

	Calories	Carb. (g)	Fat (g)	Sat. Fat (g)	Chol. (mg)	Sodium (mg)	Fiber (g)	Protein (g)	Exchanges
Breakfast Jack (1)	280	28	12	5	190	750	1	17	2 carb, 2 med-fat meat
Breakfast Sandwich, Sourdough (1)	450	36	24	8	205	1040	2	21	2 1/2 carb., 2 med-fat meat, 3 fat

FAST FOODS: JACK IN THE BOX (continued)

Products	Cal.	Carb. (g)	Fat (g)	Sat. Fat (g)	Chol. (mg)	Sod. (mg)	Fib. (g)	Prot. (g)	Servings/Exchanges
Breakfast Sandwich, Ultimate (1)	600	39	34	10	400	1470	2	34	2 1/2 carb., 4 med-fat meat, 3 fat
Croissant, Sausage (1)	700	38	51	20	240	1000	0	21	2 1/2 carb., 2 med-fat meat, 7 fat
Croissant, Supreme (1)	530	37	32	13	225	960	0	22	2 1/2 carb., 2 med-fat meat, 4 fat
French Toast Sticks w/Bacon (1)	470	53	23	4	30	700	2	12	3 1/2 carb., 5 fat
Hash Browns (1 order)	170	14	12	2	0	250	1	1	1 carb., 2 fat
Syrup (1 pkt)	130	30	0	0	0	5	0	0	2 carb.

KFC

TENDER ROAST CHICKEN

Products	Cal.	Carb. (g)	Fat (g)	Sat. Fat (g)	Chol. (mg)	Sod. (mg)	Fib. (g)	Prot. (g)	Servings/Exchanges
Breast w/o skin (1)	169	1	4	1	112	797	0	31	4 very lean meat
Breast w/skin (1)	251	1	11	3	151	830	0	37	5 lean meat
Drumstick w/o skin (1)	67	<1	2	<1	63	259	0	11	2 very lean meat

Drumstick w/skin (1)	97	<1	4	1	85	271	0	15	2 lean meat
Thigh w/o skin (1)	106	<1	6	2	84	312	0	13	2 lean meat
Thigh w/skin (1)	207	<2	12	4	120	504	0	18	3 med-fat meat
Wing w/skin (1)	121	1	8	2	74	331	0	12	2 med-fat meat

ORIGINAL RECIPE CHICKEN

Breast (1)	400	16	24	6	135	1116	1	29	1 carb., 4 med-fat meat, 1 fat
Drumstick (1)	140	4	9	2	75	422	0	13	2 med-fat meat
Thigh (1)	250	6	18	5	95	747	1	16	1/2 carb., 2 med-fat meat, 2 fat
Whole Wing (1)	140	5	10	3	55	414	0	9	1 med-fat meat, 1 fat

EXTRA TASTY CRISPY CHICKEN

Breast (1)	470	25	28	7	80	930	1	31	1 1/2 carb., 4 med-fat meat, 2 fat
Drumstick (1)	190	8	11	3	60	260	<1	13	1/2 carb., 2 med-fat meat
Thigh (1)	370	18	25	6	70	540	2	19	1 carb., 2 med-fat meat, 3 fat

FAST FOODS: KFC (continued)

Products	Cal.	Carb. (g)	Fat (g)	Sat. Fat (g)	Chol. (mg)	Sod. (mg)	Fib. (g)	Prot. (g)	Servings/Exchanges
Whole Wing (1)	200	10	13	4	45	290	<1	10	1/2 carb., 1 med-fat meat, 2 fat
HOT AND SPICY CHICKEN									
Breast (1)	530	23	35	8	110	1110	2	32	1 1/2 carb., 4 med-fat meat, 3 fat
Drumstick (1)	190	10	11	3	50	300	<1	13	1/2 carb., 2 med-fat meat
Thigh (1)	370	13	27	7	90	570	1	18	1 carb., 2 med-fat meat, 3 fat
Whole Wing (1)	210	9	15	4	50	340	<1	10	1/2 carb., 1 med-fat meat, 2 fat
OTHER CHICKEN CHOICES									
Chicken Twister (1)	480	51	20	6	60	760	2	25	3 1/2 carb., 2 med-fat meat, 2 fat
Colonel's Crispy Strips (3)	261	10	16	4	40	658	3	20	1/2 carb., 3 med-fat meat
Hot Wings (6)	471	18	33	8	150	1230	2	27	1 carb., 3 med-fat meat, 4 fat

Pot Pie, Chunky Chicken (1)	770	69	42	13	70	2160	5	29	4 1/2 carb., 2 med-fat meat, 6 fat
Sandwich, Original Recipe Chicken (1)	497	46	22	5	52	1213	3	29	3 carb., 3 med-fat meat, 1 fat
Sandwich, Value BBQ-Flavored (1)	256	28	8	1	57	782	2	17	2 carb., 2 med-fat meat
Spicy Buffalo Crispy Strips (3)	350	22	19	4	35	1110	2	22	1 1/2 carb., 3 med-fat meat, 1 fat

SIDE CHOICES

BBQ Baked Beans (1 order)	190	33	3	1	5	760	6	6	2 carb., 1 fat
Biscuit (1)	180	20	10	3	0	560	<1	4	1 carb., 2 fat
Coleslaw (1 order)	180	21	9	2	5	280	3	2	1/2 carb., 2 fat
Corn Bread (1 piece)	228	25	13	2	42	194	1	3	1 1/2 carb., 3 fat
Corn On The Cob (1)	150	35	2	0	0	20	2	5	2 carb.
Green Beans (1 order)	45	7	2	<1	5	730	3	1	1 vegetable
Macaroni & Cheese (1 order)	180	21	8	3	10	860	2	7	1 1/2 carb., 2 fat
Mean Greens (1 order)	70	11	3	1	10	650	5	4	2 vegetables, 1 fat
Potato Salad (1 order)	230	23	14	2	15	540	3	4	1 1/2 carb., 3 fat

FAST FOODS: KFC (continued)

Products	Cal.	Carb. (g)	Fat (g)	Sat. Fat (g)	Chol. (mg)	Sod. (mg)	Fib. (g)	Prot. (g)	Servings/Exchanges
Potato Wedges (1 order)	280	28	13	4	5	750	5	5	2 carb., 3 fat
Potatoes, Mashed, w/Gravy (1 order)	120	17	6	1	<1	440	2	1	1 carb., 1 fat
LITTLE CAESAR'S									
PIZZA AND MORE									
Baby Pan! Pan! (1)	300	31	14	6	30	770	2	13	2 carb., 1 med-fat meat, 2 fat
Cheese (1 slice of 14")	200	25	7	3	20	360	2	10	1 1/2 carb., 1 med-fat meat
Chicken Wings (1)	50	15	14	1	15	710	0	4	1 med-fat meat
Crazy Bread (1 piece)	100	16	3	<1	0	105	1	3	1 carb., 1 fat
Crazy Sauce (4 oz)	60	11	0	0	0	260	4	2	2 vegetable
Italian Cheese Bread (1 piece)	110	11	5	2	10	230	0	5	1 carb., 1 fat
Pan!Pan!, Cheese (1 medium slice)	160	21	6	3	15	410	1	7	1 1/2 carb., 1 med-fat meat
Pan!Pan!, Pepperoni (1 medium slice)	170	21	7	3	20	480	1	8	1 1/2 carb., 1 med-fat meat
Pepperoni (1 slice of 14")	220	25	9	4	25	460	2	11	1 1/2 carb., 1 med-fat meat, 1 fat

Food									Exchanges
Stuffed Crust-Cheese (1 slice)	240	25	11	5	20	470	2	11	1 1/2 carb., 1 med-fat meat, 1 fat
Stuffed Crust-Pepperoni (1 slice)	280	28	13	5	30	580	2	13	2 carb., 1 med-fat meat, 2 fat

SALADS

Food									Exchanges
Salad, Antipasto (1)	80	4	6	3	15	340	1	5	1 med-fat meat, 1 vegetable
Salad, Caesar (1)	80	7	3	2	5	190	1	5	1 med-fat meat, 1 vegetable
Salad, Greek (1)	60	5	3	0	10	330	1	3	1 vegetable, 1 fat
Salad, Tossed (1)	50	9	<1	0	0	60	1	2	2 vegetable

SALAD DRESSINGS

Food									Exchanges
1000 Island (1 pkt)	220	7	21	3	30	360	0	0	1/2 carb., 4 fat
Blue Cheese (1 pkt)	230	2	24	5	30	450	0	2	5 fat
Buttermilk Ranch (1 pkt)	270	1	29	5	4	380	0	0	6 fat
Creamy Caesar (1 pkt)	220	2	23	4	10	540	0	1	5 fat
Golden Italian (1 pkt)	210	2	22	3	0	360	0	2	4 fat
Honey French (1 pkt)	220	14	18	3	0	310	0	0	1 carb., 4 fat
Italian, Fat-Free (1 pkt)	25	5	0	0	0	390	0	0	free

FAST FOODS: LITTLE CAESAR'S (continued)

Products	Cal.	Carb. (g)	Fat (g)	Sat. Fat (g)	Chol. (mg)	Sod. (mg)	Fib. (g)	Prot. (g)	Servings/Exchanges
Italian, Low Calorie (1 pkt)	230	2	25	4	55	360	0	1	5 fat
HOT OVEN-BAKED SANDWICHES									
Cheeser (1)	900	73	48	23	105	2130	5	45	5 carb., 4 med-fat meat, 6 fat
Meatsa (1)	960	72	53	23	115	2240	5	48	5 carb., 6 med-fat meat, 6 fat
Pepperoni (1)	980	71	56	26	125	2290	4	48	5 carb., 5 med-fat meat, 6 fat
Supreme (1)	900	74	49	21	105	2040	5	42	5 carb., 4 med-fat meat, 6 fat
Veggie (1)	760	74	36	17	65	1360	5	38	5 carb., 3 med-fat meat, 4 fat
COLD DELI-STYLE SANDWICHES									
Ham & Cheese (1)	600	68	22	10	55	1410	3	33	4 1/2 carb., 3 med-fat meat, 1 fat
Italian (1)	690	68	31	13	75	1660	3	34	4 1/2 carb., 3 med-fat meat, 3 fat
Tuna (1)	820	71	39	5	80	1330	3	45	5 carb., 4 med-fat meat, 4 fat

	Cal.	Carb.	Fat	Sat. Fat	Chol.	Sod.	Fiber	Prot.	Exchanges
Turkey (1)	600	66	21	10	55	1570	3	38	4 1/2 carb., 2 med-fat meat, 2 fat
Veggie (1)	580	70	24	10	30	940	4	26	4 1/2 carb., 2 med-fat meat, 3 fat

LONG JOHN SILVER'S

SANDWICHES

	Cal.	Carb.	Fat	Sat. Fat	Chol.	Sod.	Fiber	Prot.	Exchanges
Chicken Grab n Go (1)	340	40	14	4	25	840	NA	13	2 1/2 carb., 1 med fat meat, 2 fat
Chicken Grab n Go w/Cheese (1)	390	40	19	9	40	1090	NA	16	2 1/2 carb., 1 med-fat meat, 3 fat
Fish Grab n Go (1)	320	38	14	4	20	850	NA	11	2 1/2 carb., 1 med-fat meat, 2 fat
Fish Grab n Go w/Cheese (1)	370	38	19	9	35	1100	NA	14	2 1/2 carb., 1 med-fat meat, 32 fat
Ultimate Fish (1)	480	46	25	10	50	1400	NA	19	3 carb., 1 med-fat meat, 4 fat

FAST FOODS: LONG JOHN SILVER'S (continued)

Products	Cal.	Carb. (g)	Fat (g)	Sat. Fat (g)	Chol. (mg)	Sod. (mg)	Fib. (g)	Prot. (g)	Servings/Exchanges
MEALS									
Lemon Crumb Fish Meal (1 meal)	730	89	29	6	60	1720	NA	31	6 carb., 2 med-fat meat, 4 fat
FISH, SEAFOOD, AND CHICKEN									
Batter-Dipped Chicken (1 piece)	120	11	6	2	15	400	3	8	1 carb., 1 med-fat meat
Battered Chicken Plank (1 piece)	140	9	8	3	20	400	NA	8	1/2 carb., 1 med-fat meat, 1 fat
Battered Fish Regular (1 piece)	230	16	13	4	30	700	NA	12	1 carb., 1 med-fat meat, 2 fat
Battered Shrimp (1 piece)	45	3	3	1	15	125	NA	2	1 fat
Breaded Clams (1 order)	250	26	14	4	35	560	NA	9	2 carb., 1 med-fat meat, 2 fat
Junior Battered Fish (1 piece)	120	15	8	3	15	410	NA	5	1 carb., 2 fat
Lemon Crumb Fish (2 pieces)	240	10	12	4	55	790	NA	23	1 carb., 3 lean meat
Lemon Crumb Fish a-la-Carte (2 pieces w/rice)	480	52	17	5	55	1490	NA	27	3 1/2 carb., 2 med-fat meat
Lemon Crumb Fish Add-A-Piece (1 piece w/rice)	150	9	7	2	30	450	NA	12	1/2 carb., 1 med-fat meat
Popcorn Shrimp (1 order)	320	33	15	3	85	1440	NA	15	2 carb., 1 med-fat meat, 2 fat

SIDE ITEMS

Broccoli Cheese Soup (1 bowl)	180	13	12	5	15	1240	NA	5	1 carb., 2 fat
Cheese Sticks (5 pieces)	160	12	9	4	10	360	NA	6	1 carb., 2 fat
Coleslaw (4 oz)	170	23	7	0	0	310	0	2	1 1/2 carb., 1 fat
Corn Cobbette w/butter (1)	140	19	8	2	0	0	NA	3	1 carb., 2 fat
Corn Cobbette w/o butter (1)	80	19	<1	0	0	0	NA	3	1 carb.
Fries (1 regular order)	250	28	15	3	0	500	NA	3	2 carb., 3 fat
Hush Puppy (1)	60	9	3	0	0	25	NA	1	1/2 carb., 1 fat
Rice (4 oz)	130	34	4	<1	0	560	NA	3	2 carb., 1 fat
Salad, Side (1)	20	3	0	0	0	10	NA	1	1 vegetable

CONDIMENTS

Malt Vinegar (1 pkt)	0	0	0	0	0	15	NA	0	free
Sauce, Honey Mustard (1 pkt)	20	5	0	0	0	60	NA	0	free
Sauce, Shrimp (1 pkt)	15	3	0	0	0	180	NA	0	free
Sauce, Sweet 'N' Sour (1 pkt)	20	5	0	0	0	45	NA	0	free
Sauce, Tartar (1 pkt)	40	2	4	<1	5	105	NA	0	1 fat

FAST FOODS: LONG JOHN SILVER'S (continued)

Products	Cal.	Carb. (g)	Fat (g)	Sat. Fat (g)	Chol. (mg)	Sod. (mg)	Fib. (g)	Prot. (g)	Servings/Exchanges
SALADS									
Garden Salad (1)	45	9	0	0	0	25	NA	3	2 vegetable
Grilled Chicken Salad (1)	140	10	3	<1	45	260	NA	20	2 vegetable, 2 very lean meat
Ocean Chef Salad (1)	130	15	2	0	60	540	NA	14	3 vegetable, 1 lean meat
SALAD DRESSINGS									
French, Fat-Free (1 pkt)	40	10	0	0	0	240	NA	0	1/2 carb.
Italian (1 pkt)	90	2	9	2	0	290	NA	0	2 fat
Ranch (1 pkt)	170	1	18	3	10	260	NA	0	3 fat
Ranch, Fat-Free (1 pkt)	40	9	0	0	0	290	NA	0	1 carb.
Thousand Island (1 pkt)	120	5	10	2	15	290	NA	0	2 fat
DESSERTS									
Banana Split Sundae Pie (1 piece)	300	34	17	9	15	130	NA	4	2 carb., 3 fat
Chocolate Crème Pie (1 piece)	280	29	17	6	15	125	NA	4	2 carb., 3 fat

Double Lemon Pie (1 piece)	350	41	18	10	40	180	NA	6	3 carb., 4 fat
Pecan Pie (1 piece)	390	53	19	4	40	259	NA	3	3 1/2 carb., 4 fat
Pineapple Crème Cheesecake Pie (1 piece)	310	36	17	9	5	105	NA	4	2 1/2 carb., 3 fat
Strawberries N'Crème Pie (1 piece)	280	32	15	8	15	130	NA	4	2 carb., 3 fat

McDONALD'S

SANDWICHES

Arch Deluxe (1)	550	39	31	11	90	1010	4	28	2 1/2 carb., 3 med-fat meat, 3 fat
Arch Deluxe w/Bacon (1)	590	39	34	12	100	1150	4	32	2 1/2 carb., 3 med-fat meat, 4 fat
Big Mac (1)	560	45	31	10	85	1070	3	26	3 carb., 2 med-fat meat, 4 fat
Cheeseburger (1)	320	35	13	6	40	820	2	15	2 carb., 1 med-fat meat, 2 fat
Crispy Chicken Deluxe (1)	500	43	25	4	55	1100	4	26	3 carb., 3 med-fat meat, 2 fat
Filet-O-Fish (1)	450	42	25	5	50	870	2	16	3 carb., 1 med-fat meat, 4 fat
Fish Filet Deluxe (1)	560	54	28	6	60	1060	4	23	3 1/2 carb., 2 med-fat meat, 4 fat

FAST FOODS: McDONALD'S (continued)

Products	Cal.	Carb. (g)	Fat (g)	Sat. Fat (g)	Chol. (mg)	Sod. (mg)	Fib. (g)	Prot. (g)	Servings/Exchanges
Grilled Chicken Deluxe (1)	440	38	20	3	60	1040	4	27	2 1/2 carb., 3 med-fat meat, 1 fat
Hamburger (1)	260	34	9	4	30	580	2	13	2 carb., 1 med-fat meat, 1 fat
Quarter Pounder (1)	420	37	21	8	70	820	2	23	2 1/2 carb., 2 med-fat meat, 2 fat
Quarter Pounder w/Cheese (1)	530	38	30	13	95	1290	2	28	2 1/2 carb., 3 med-fat meat, 3 fat
FRENCH FRIES									
French Fries (1 large order)	450	57	22	4	0	290	5	6	4 carb., 4 fat
French Fries (1 small order)	210	26	10	2	0	135	2	3	2 carb., 2 fat
French Fries (1 super size order)	540	68	26	5	0	350	6	8	4 1/2 carb., 5 fat
CHICKEN NUGGETS/SAUCES									
Chicken Nuggets (6-piece)	290	15	17	4	60	510	0	18	1 carb., 2 med-fat meat, 3 fat
Honey (1 pkg)	45	12	0	0	0	0	0	0	1 carb

Light Mayonnaise (1 pkg)	40	1	4	<1	5	85	0	0	1 fat
Sauce, Barbecue (1 pkt)	45	10	0	0	0	250	0	0	1/2 carb.
Sauce, Honey Mustard (1 pkt)	50	3	5	<1	10	85	0	0	1 fat
Sauce, Hot Mustard (1 pkt)	60	7	4	0	5	240	<1	1	1/2 carb., 1 fat
Sauce, Sweet 'N Sour (1 pkt)	50	11	0	0	0	140	0	0	1 carb.

SALADS AND SALAD DRESSINGS

Caesar (1 pkg)	50	7	14	3	20	450	0	2	1/2 carb., 3 fat
Croutons (1 pkt)	50	7	2	0	0	80	<1	2	1/2 carb
Fat Free Hot Vinaigrette (1 pkg)	50	11	0	0	0	330	0	2	1 carb.
Garden Salad (1)	35	7	0	0	0	20	3	2	1 vegetable
Grilled Chicken Salad Deluxe (1)	120	7	2	0	45	240	3	21	1 vegetable, 3 very lean meat
Ranch (1 pkg)	230	10	21	3	20	550	0	1	1/2 carb., 4 fat
Red French, Reduced-Calorie (1 pkg)	160	23	8	1	0	490	0	0	1 1/2 carb., 2 fat

BREAKFAST

Biscuit (1)	290	34	15	3	0	780	1	5	2 carb., 3 fat

FAST FOODS: McDONALD'S (continued)

Products	Cal.	Carb. (g)	Fat (g)	Sat. Fat (g)	Chol. (mg)	Sod. (mg)	Fib. (g)	Prot. (g)	Servings/Exchanges
Biscuit, Bacon, Egg, & Cheese (1)	470	36	28	8	235	1250	1	18	2 1/2 carb., 2 med-fat meat, 4 fat
Biscuit, Sausage (1)	470	35	31	9	35	1080	1	11	2 carb., 1 med-fat meat, 5 fat
Biscuit, Sausage w/Egg (1)	550	35	37	10	245	1160	1	18	2 carb., 2 med-fat meat, 5 fat
Breakfast Burrito (1)	320	23	20	7	195	600	2	13	1 1/2 carb., 1 med-fat meat, 3 fat
English Muffin (1)	140	25	2	0	0	210	1	4	1 1/2 carb.
Hash Browns (1)	130	14	8	2	0	330	1	1	1 carb., 2 fat
Hotcakes, Plain (1 order)	240	58	9	2	25	540	2	9	4 carb., 2 fat
McMuffin, Egg (1)	290	27	12	5	235	790	1	17	2 carb., 2 med-fat meat, 1 fat
McMuffin, Sausage (1)	360	26	23	8	45	750	1	13	2 carb., 1 med-fat meat, 3 fat
McMuffin, Sausage w/Egg (1)	440	27	28	10	255	890	1	19	2 carb., 2 med-fat meat, 4 fat
Scrambled Eggs (2)	160	1	11	4	425	170	0	13	2 med-fat meat
Sausage (1)	170	0	16	5	35	290	0	6	1 med-fat meat, 2 fat

MUFFINS/DANISH

Cheese Danish (1)	410	47	22	8	70	340	0	7	3 carb., 4 fat
Cinnamon Roll (1)	390	50	18	5	65	310	2	6	3 carb., 4 fat
Danish, Apple (1)	360	51	16	5	40	290	1	5	3 1/2 carb., 3 fat
Lowfat Apple Bran Muffin (1)	300	61	3	<1	0	380	3	6	4 carb., 1 fat

DESSERTS/SHAKES

Cookies, McDonaldland (1 pkg)	180	32	5	1	0	190	1	3	2 carb., 1 fat
Ice Cream Cone, Reduced Fat Vanilla (1)	150	23	5	3	20	75	0	4	1 1/2 carb., 1 fat
Ice Cream Sundae, Strawberry (1)	290	50	7	5	30	95	<1	7	3 1/2 carb., 1 fat
M&M McFlurry (1)	630	90	23	15	75	210	1	16	6 carb., 5 fat
Oreo McFlurry (1)	570	89	20	12	70	280	<1	15	6 carb., 4 fat
Pie, Apple (1)	260	34	13	4	0	200	<1	3	2 carb., 3 fat
Shake, Vanilla (1 small)	360	59	9	6	40	250	0	11	4 carb., 2 fat

PAPA JOHN'S PIZZA

ORIGINAL CRUST

All The Meats (1 large slice)	410	42	18	7	35	1040	3	21	3 carb., 2 med-fat meat, 2 fat

FAST FOODS: PAPA JOHN'S PIZZA(continued)

Products	Cal.	Carb. (g)	Fat (g)	Sat. Fat (g)	Chol. (mg)	Sod. (mg)	Fib. (g)	Prot. (g)	Servings/Exchanges
Cheese (1 large slice)	286	37	9	3	18	540	2	14	2 1/2 carb., 1 med-fat meat, 1 fat
Garden Special (1 large slice)	298	38	11	4	20	570	3	14	2 1/2 carb., 1 med-fat meat, 1 fat
Pepperoni (1 large slice)	310	35	13	5	25	540	2	15	2 carb., 1 med-fat meat, 2 fat
Sausage (1 large slice)	340	40	13	6	25	910	2	15	2 1/2 carb., 1 med-fat meat, 2 fat
The Works (1 large slice)	369	37	17	6	29	840	3	18	2 1/2 carb., 2 med-fat meat, 1 fat
SIDES									
Breadsticks (1)	170	27	3	0	0	270	<1	6	2 carb., 1 fat
Cheese Sticks (1)	150	21	6	2	10	290	<1	7	1 1/2 carb., 1 fat
Garlic Sauce (1 Tbsp)	75	2	9	2	0	115	<1	0	2 fat
Nacho Cheese (1 Tbsp)	30	0	2	2	8	113	<1	2	1 fat

Pizza Sauce (1 Tbsp)	10	1	<1	0	0	60	<1	0	free

THIN CRUST

All The Meats (1 large slice)	330	23	20	9	39	919	2	15	1 1/2 carb., 2 med-fat meat, 2 fat
Cheese (1 large slice)	220	22	11	5	13	480	2	9	1 1/2 carb., 1 med-fat meat, 1 fat
Garden Special (1 large slice)	238	23	12	6	19	540	3	8	1 1/2 carb., 1 med-fat meat, 1 fat
Pepperoni (1 large slice)	266	22	15	7	24	480	2	11	1 1/2 carb., 1 med-fat meat, 2 fat
Sausage (1 large slice)	270	22	15	7	28	730	2	12	1 1/2 carb., 1 med-fat meat, 2 fat
The Works (1 large slice)	319	24	19	8	35	760	3	14	1 1/2 carb., 1 med-fat meat, 3 fat

FAST FOODS

Products	Cal.	Carb. (g)	Fat (g)	Sat. Fat (g)	Chol. (mg)	Sod. (mg)	Fib. (g)	Prot. (g)	Servings/Exchanges
PIZZA HUT									
APPETIZERS									
Bread Stick (1 serving)	130	20	4	1	0	170	1	3	1 carb., 1 fat
Bread Stick Dipping Sauce (1 serving)	30	5	<1	0	0	170	<1	<1	1 vegetable
Garlic Bread (1 slice)	150	16	8	2	0	240	1	3	1 carb., 2 fat
Hot Wings (4)	210	4	12	3	130	900	<1	22	3 med-fat meat
Mild Wings (5)	200	0	12	4	150	510	0	23	3 med-fat meat
THIN 'N' CRISPY PIZZA									
Beef (1 medium slice)	305	45	15	7	24	814	4	15	3 carb., 1 med-fat meat, 2 fat
Beef Taco (1 medium slice)	260	29	10	5	20	850	2	13	2 carb., 1 med-fat meat, 1 fat
Cheese (1 medium slice)	243	44	10	5	11	653	3	13	3 carb., 1 med-fat meat, 1 fat
Chicken Taco (1 medium slice)	260	26	12	5	20	850	2	11	2 carb., 1 med-fat meat, 1 fat
Ham (1 medium slice)	212	45	7	3	15	662	3	12	3 carb., 1 med-fat meat
Italian Sausage (1 medium slice)	325	45	18	7	32	865	3	15	3 carb., 1 med-fat meat, 3 fat

Meatless Taco (1 medium slice)	230	27	8	4	10	700	2	9	2 carb., 2 fat
Meat Lover's (1 medium slice)	339	45	19	8	35	970	3	16	3 carb., 1 med-fat meat, 3 fat
Pepperoni (1 medium slice)	235	44	10	4	14	627	3	12	3 carb., 1 med-fat meat, 1 fat
Pepperoni Lover's (1 medium slice)	289	28	14	6	22	859	2	13	2 carb., 1 med-fat meat, 2 fat
Pork Topping (1 medium slice)	298	45	15	6	23	875	4	15	3 carb., 1 med-fat meat, 2 fat
Taco (1 medium slice)	260	27	11	5	20	860	2	12	2 carb., 1 med-fat meat, 1 fat
Veggie Lover's (1 medium slice)	222	30	8	3	7	621	3	9	2 carb., 1 med-fat meat, 1 fat

HAND-TOSS PIZZA

Beef (1 medium slice)	347	44	12	5	21	943	4	16	3 carb., 1 med-fat meat, 1 fat
Beef Taco (1 medium slice)	270	35	8	4	15	870	3	13	2 carb., 1 med-fat meat, 1 fat
Cheese (1 medium slice)	309	43	9	5	11	848	3	14	3 carb., 1 med-fat meat, 1 fat
Chicken Supreme (1 medium slice)	291	44	6	3	17	841	4	15	3 carb., 1 med-fat meat
Chicken Taco (1 medium slice)	290	35	11	5	15	940	3	12	2 carb., 1 med-fat meat, 1 fat
Ham (1 medium slice)	279	43	6	3	15	857	3	13	3 carb., 1 med-fat meat
Italian Sausage (1 medium slice)	363	44	14	6	26	975	4	16	3 carb., 1 med-fat meat, 2 fat
Meat Lover's (1 medium slice)	376	44	15	6	30	1077	4	17	3 carb., 1 med-fat meat, 2 fat

FAST FOODS: PIZZA HUT (continued)

Products	Cal.	Carb. (g)	Fat (g)	Sat. Fat (g)	Chol. (mg)	Sod. (mg)	Fib. (g)	Prot. (g)	Servings/Exchanges
Meatless Taco (1 medium slice)	250	35	8	4	10	790	3	14	2 carb., 1 med-fat meat, 1 fat
Pepperoni (1 medium slice)	301	43	8	4	15	867	3	13	3 carb., 1 med-fat meat, 1 fat
Pepperoni Lover's (1 medium slice)	372	43	14	7	26	1123	3	17	3 carb., 1 med-fat meat, 2 fat
Pork Topping (1 medium slice)	342	44	12	5	20	99	4	16	3 carb., 1 med-fat meat, 1 fat
Super Supreme (1 medium slice)	359	45	12	5	23	1024	4	16	3 carb., 1 med-fat meat, 1 fat
Supreme (1 medium slice)	333	44	11	5	18	927	4	15	3 carb., 1 med-fat meat, 1 fat
Taco (1 medium slice)	280	34	11	5	15	870	3	12	2 carb., 1 med-fat meat, 1 fat
Veggie Lover's (1 medium slice)	281	45	6	3	7	771	4	12	3 carb., 1 med-fat meat
PAN PIZZA									
Beef (1 medium slice)	399	45	18	7	20	773	4	15	3 carb., 1 med-fat meat, 3 fat
Beef Taco (1 medium slice)	300	36	12	5	15	770	3	12	2 1/2 carb., 1 med-fat meat, 1 fat
Cheese (1 medium slice)	361	44	15	8	11	678	3	13	2 carb., 1 med-fat meat, 1 fat
Chicken Supreme (1 medium slice)	343	45	12	4	16	671	3	15	3 carb., 1 med-fat meat, 1 fat

Item									Exchanges/Choices
Chicken Taco (1 medium slice)	320	36	15	5	15	830	3	12	2 1/2 carb., 1 med-fat meat, 2 fat
Ham (1 medium slice)	331	44	12	4	15	687	3	12	3 carb., 1 med-fat meat, 1 fat
Italian Sausage (1 medium slice)	415	45	20	7	26	805	3	15	3 carb., 1 med-fat meat, 3 fat
Meat Lover's (1 medium slice)	428	45	21	7	29	607	3	16	3 carb., 1 med-fat meat, 3 fat
Meatless Taco (1 medium slice)	290	36	12	5	15	770	3	10	2 1/2 carb., 1 med-fat meat, 1 fat
Pepperoni (1 medium slice)	353	44	14	5	14	697	3	12	3 carb., 1 med-fat meat, 2 fat
Pepperoni Lover's (1 medium slice)	370	44	16	5	13	767	3	13	3 carb., 1 med-fat meat, 2 fat
Pork Topping (1 medium slice)	394	45	18	6	20	820	4	15	3 carb., 1 med-fat meat, 3 fat
Super Supreme (1 medium slice)	401	46	18	6	22	854	4	15	3 carb., 1 med-fat meat, 3 fat
Supreme (1 medium slice)	385	45	17	6	18	757	4	14	3 carb., 1 med-fat meat, 2 fat
Taco (1 medium slice)	310	36	13	5	15	800	3	12	2 1/2 carb., 1 med-fat meat, 2 fat
Veggie Lover's (1 medium slice)	333	46	12	4	7	601	4	11	3 carb., 1 med-fat meat, 1 fat

FAST FOODS: PIZZA HUT (continued)

Products	Cal.	Carb. (g)	Fat (g)	Sat. Fat (g)	Chol. (mg)	Sod. (mg)	Fib. (g)	Prot. (g)	Servings/Exchanges
PASTA AND SANDWICHES									
Cavatina Supreme (1)	560	73	19	8	10	1400	10	24	5 carb., 1 med-fat meat, 3 fat
Cavatina Pasta (1)	480	66	14	6	8	1170	9	21	4 1/2 carb., 1 med-fat meat, 2 fat
Ham and Cheese Sandwich (1)	550	57	21	7	22	2150	4	33	4 carb., 3 med-fat meat, 1 fat
Spaghetti w/Marina Sauce (1)	490	91	6	1	0	730	8	18	6 carb., 1 fat
Spaghetti w/Meat Sauce (1)	600	98	13	5	8	910	9	23	6 1/2 carb., 1 med-fat meat, 2 fat
Spaghetti w/Meatballs (1)	850	120	24	10	17	1120	10	37	8 carb., 2 med-fat meat, 3 fat
Supreme Sandwich (1)	640	62	28	10	28	2150	4	34	4 carb., 3 med-fat meat, 3 fat
STUFFED CRUST PIZZA									
Beef (1 medium slice)	466	46	22	10	30	1137	3	23	3 carb., 2 med-fat meat, 2 fat
Cheese (1 medium slice)	445	46	19	10	24	1080	3	22	3 carb., 2 med-fat meat, 2 fat
Chicken Supreme (1 medium slice)	532	47	17	8	32	1111	3	24	3 carb., 2 med-fat meat

Item	Cal								Exchanges
Ham (1 medium slice)	404	27	22	12	39	1190	2	24	2 carb., 3 med-fat meat, 1 fat
Meat Lover's (1 medium slice)	543	46	29	13	43	1427	3	26	3 carb., 2 med-fat meat, 4 fat
Pepperoni (1 medium slice)	438	45	19	9	27	1116	2	21	3 carb., 2 med-fat meat, 2 fat
Pepperoni Lover's (1 medium slice)	525	46	26	13	40	1413	3	26	3 carb., 2 med-fat meat, 3 fat
Pork Topping (1 medium slice)	461	46	21	10	29	1176	3	22	3 carb., 2 med-fat meat, 2 fat
Super Supreme (1 medium slice)	505	46	25	11	44	1371	3	25	3 carb., 2 med-fat meat, 3 fat
Supreme (1 medium slice)	487	47	23	11	33	1227	3	24	3 carb., 2 med-fat meat, 3 fat
Veggie Lover's (1 medium slice)	421	48	17	8	19	1029	3	20	3 carb., 2 med-fat meat, 1 fat
THE BIG NEW YORKER									
Cheese (1 slice)	393	42	17	8	19	1099	3	20	3 carb., 2 med-fat meat
Pepperoni (1 slice)	380	42	16	7	22	1115	3	18	3 carb., 1 med-fat meat, 2 fat
Supreme (1 slice)	459	44	22	9	35	1310	4	10	3 carb., 4 fat
THE EDGE PIZZA									
Chicken Veggie (1 slice)	120	16	3	1	10	310	1	6	1 carb., 1 lean meat
Taco (1 slice)	140	17	5	2	10	450	1	6	1 carb., 1 med-fat meat

FAST FOODS

SUBWAY

6-INCH COLD SUBS

Products	Cal.	Carb. (g)	Fat (g)	Sat. Fat (g)	Chol. (mg)	Sod. (mg)	Fib. (g)	Prot. (g)	Servings/Exchanges
Classic Italian B.M.T. (1)	460	45	22	7	56	1664	3	21	3 carb., 2 med-fat meat, 2 fat
Club (1)	312	46	5	1	26	1352	3	21	3 carb., 2 lean meat
Cold Cut Trio (1)	378	46	13	4	64	1412	3	20	3 carb., 2 med-fat meat, 1 fat
Ham (1)	302	45	5	1	28	1319	3	19	3 carb., 1 lean meat
Roast Beef (1)	303	45	5	1	20	939	3	20	3 carb., 2 lean meat
Seafood & Crab w/Light Mayonnaise (1)	347	45	10	2	32	884	3	20	3 carb., 2 med-fat meat
Tun w/Light Mayonnaise (1)	391	46	15	2	32	940	3	19	3 carb., 1 med-fat meat, 2 fat
Turkey Breast (1)	289	46	4	1	19	1403	3	18	3 carb., 1 lean meat
Turkey Breast & Ham (1)	295	46	5	1	24	1361	3	18	3 carb., 1 med-fat meat
Veggie Delite (1)	237	44	3	0	0	593	3	9	3 carb.

6-INCH HOT SUBS

Meatball (1)	419	51	16	6	33	1046	3	19	3 1/2 carb., 1 med-fat meat, 2 fat
Melt (1)	382	46	12	5	42	1746	3	23	3 carb., 2 med-fat meat
Pizza Sub (1)	464	48	22	9	50	1621	3	19	3 carb., 1 med-fat meat, 3 fat
Roasted Chicken Breast (1)	348	47	6	1	48	978	3	27	3 carb., 3 very lean meat
Steak & Cheese (1)	398	47	10	6	70	1117	3	30	3 carb., 2 med-fat meat

SALADS

Classic Italian B.M.T. (1)	274	11	20	7	56	1379	1	14	2 vegetable, 2 med-fat meat, 2 fat
Cold Cut Trio (1)	191	11	11	3	64	1127	1	13	2 vegetable, 1 med-fat meat, 1 fat
Club (1)	126	12	3	1	26	1067	1	14	2 very lean meat, 2 vegetable
Ham (1)	116	11	3	1	23	1034	1	12	2 vegetable, 1 lean meat

FAST FOODS: SUBWAY (continued)

Products	Cal.	Carb. (g)	Fat (g)	Sat. Fat (g)	Chol. (mg)	Sod. (mg)	Fib. (g)	Prot. (g)	Servings/Exchanges
Meatball (1)	233	16	14	5	33	761	2	12	1/2 carb., 2 veg., 1 med-fat meat, 2 fat
Melt (1)	195	12	10	4	42	1461	1	16	2 vegetable, 2 med-fat meat
Pizza (1)	277	13	20	8	50	1336	2	12	2 vegetable, 1 med-fat meat, 3 fat
Roast Beef (1)	117	11	3	1	20	654	1	12	2 vegetable, 1 lean meat
Roasted Chicken Breast (1)	162	13	4	1	48	693	1	20	2 very lean meat, 2 vegetable
Seafood & Crab w/Light Mayonnaise (1)	161	11	8	1	32	599	2	13	1 med-fat meat, 1 fat, 2 vegetable
Steak & Cheese (1)	212	13	8	5	70	832	1	22	2 vegetable, 2 med-fat meat
Tuna w/Light Mayonnaise (1)	205	11	13	2	32	654	1	12	1 med-fat meat, 2 fat, 2 vegetable
Turkey Breast (1)	102	12	2	1	19	1117	1	11	1 lean meat, 2 vegetable

Turkey Breast & Ham (1)	109	11	3	1	24	1076	1	11	2 vegetable, 1 lean meat
Veggie Delite (1)	51	10	1	0	0	308	1	2	2 vegetable
OPTIONAL FIXIN'S									
Bacon (2 slices)	45	0	4	1	8	182	0	2	1 fat
Cheese (2 triangles)	41	0	3	2	10	201	0	2	1 fat
Mayonnaise (1 tsp)	37	0	4	1	3	27	0	0	1 fat
Mayonnaise, Light (1 tsp)	18	0	2	0	2	33	0	0	free
Mustard (2 tsp)	8	1	0	0	0	0	0	0	free
Olive Oil Blend (1 tsp)	45	0	5	1	0	0	1	0	1 fat
Vinegar (1 tsp)	1	0	0	0	0	0	0	0	free
COOKIES									
Chocolate Chip (1)	234	33	10	4	10	148	1	3	2 carb., 2 fat
Oatmeal Raisin (1)	223	32	9	2	12	152	1	3	2 carb., 2 fat
Peanut Butter (1)	231	31	11	2	0	225	1	3	2 carb., 2 fat
Sugar (1)	246	31	13	3	19	179	1	2	2 carb., 3 fat

FAST FOODS: TACO BELL

TACO BELL

TACOS

Products	Cal.	Carb. (g)	Fat (g)	Sat. Fat (g)	Chol. (mg)	Sod. (mg)	Fib. (g)	Prot. (g)	Servings/Exchanges
Double Decker (1)	330	37	15	5	30	740	9	14	2 1/2 carb., 1 med-fat meat, 2 fat
Double Decker Supreme	380	39	18	7	40	760	9	15	2 1/2 carb., 1 med-fat meat, 3 fat
Grilled Chicken Soft (1)	200	20	7	3	35	530	2	14	1 carb., 2 lean meat
Grilled Steak Soft (1)	200	19	7	3	25	570	2	14	1 carb., 2 lean meat
Grilled Steak Soft Supreme (1)	240	21	11	5	35	580	2	15	1 1/2 carb., 1 med-fat meat, 1 fat
Soft (1)	210	20	10	4	30	570	3	11	1 carb., 1 med-fat meat, 1 fat
Soft Supreme (1)	260	22	13	6	40	590	3	11	1 1/2 carb., 1 med-fat meat, 2 fat
Supreme (1)	210	14	14	6	40	350	3	9	1 carb., 1 med-fat meat, 2 fat

Taco	170	12	10	4	30	340	3	9	1 carb., 1 med-fat meat, 1 fat

BURRITOS

7-Layer (1)	520	65	22	7	25	1270	13	16	4 carb., 4 fat
Bean (1)	370	54	12	4	10	1080	12	13	3 1/2 carb., 2 fat
Big Beef (1)	400	43	17	6	50	1320	6	19	3 carb., 1 med-fat meat, 2 fat
Big Beef Supreme (1)	510	52	23	9	60	1500	11	23	3 1/2 carb., 2 med-fat meat, 3 fat
Big Chicken Supreme (1)	460	50	17	6	70	1200	3	27	3 carb., 3 med-fat meat
Chili Cheese (1)	330	40	13	5	25	900	4	13	2 1/2 carb., 1 med-fat meat, 2 fat
Grilled Chicken (1)	390	49	13	4	40	1240	3	19	3 carb., 1 med-fat meat, 2 fat
Supreme (1)	430	50	18	7	40	1210	9	17	3 carb., 1 med-fat meat, 3 fat

SPECIALTIES

Big Beef Meximelt (1)	290	22	15	7	45	830	4	15	1 1/2 carb., 2 med-fat meat, 1 fat
Cheese Quesadilla (1)	350	31	18	9	50	860	3	16	2 carb., 1 med-fat meat, 3 fat

FAST FOODS: TACO BELL (continued)

Products	Cal.	Carb. (g)	Fat (g)	Sat. Fat (g)	Chol. (mg)	Sod. (mg)	Fib. (g)	Prot. (g)	Servings/Exchanges
Chicken Quesadilla (1)	400	33	19	9	75	1050	3	25	2 carb., 3 med-fat meat, 1 fat
Mexican Pizza (1)	540	42	35	10	45	1030	7	20	3 carb., 2 med-fat meat, 5 fat
Mexican Pizza, Chicken (1)	520	41	32	8	50	940	6	23	3 carb., 2 med-fat meat, 4 fat
Mexican Pizza, Steak (1)	530	39	33	9	45	950	6	24	2 1/2 carb., 2 med-fat meat, 5 fat
Taco Salad w/Salsa (1)	850	69	52	14	70	2250	16	30	4 1/2 carb., 3 med-fat meat, 7 fat
Taco Salad w/Salsa w/o Shell (1)	430	36	22	10	70	1990	15	25	2 1/2 carb., 3 med-fat meat, 1 fat
Tostada (1)	250	27	12	5	15	640	11	10	2 carb., 1 med-fat meat, 1 fat
GORDITAS									
Baja Beef (1)	360	29	21	5	35	810	4	13	2 carb., 1 med-fat meat, 3 fat
Baja Chicken (1)	340	28	18	4	40	710	3	16	2 carb., 1 med-fat meat, 3 fat
Baja Steak (1)	340	27	18	4	30	730	3	17	2 carb., 2 med-fat meat, 2 fat

Santa Fe Beef (1)	380	31	23	5	35	700	5	14	2 carb., 1 med-fat meat, 4 fat
Santa Fe Chicken (1)	370	30	20	4	40	610	3	17	2 carb., 2 med-fat meat, 2 fat
Santa Fe Steak (1)	370	29	20	5	35	620	3	17	2 carb., 2 med-fat meat, 2 fat
Supreme Beef (1)	300	27	14	5	35	550	3	17	2 carb., 2 med-fat meat, 1 fat
Supreme Chicken (1)	300	28	13	5	45	530	3	16	2 carb., 1 med-fat meat, 2 fat
Supreme Steak (1)	300	27	14	5	35	550	3	17	2 carb., 2 med-fat meat, 1 fat

CHALUPAS

Baja Beef (1)	420	30	27	7	35	760	3	14	2 carb., 1 med-fat meat, 4 fat
Baja Chicken (1)	400	28	24	5	40	660	2	17	2 carb., 2 med-fat meat, 3 fat
Baja Steak (1)	400	27	24	6	30	680	2	17	2 carb., 2 med-fat meat, 3 fat
Santa Fe Beef (1)	440	31	29	7	35	660	4	14	2 carb., 1 med-fat meat, 5 fat
Santa Fe Chicken (1)	420	30	26	6	40	560	2	17	2 carb., 2 med-fat meat, 3 fat
Santa Fe Steak (1)	430	29	27	6	35	580	2	18	2 carb., 2 med-fat meat, 3 fat
Supreme Beef (1)	380	29	23	8	40	580	3	14	2 carb., 1 med-fat meat, 4 fat
Supreme Chicken (1)	360	28	20	7	45	490	2	17	2 carb., 2 med-fat meat, 2 fat
Supreme Steak (1)	360	27	20	7	35	500	2	17	2 carb., 2 med-fat meat, 2 fat

FAST FOODS: TACO BELL (continued)

Products	Cal.	Carb. (g)	Fat (g)	Sat. Fat (g)	Chol. (mg)	Sod. (mg)	Fib. (g)	Prot. (g)	Servings/Exchanges
NACHOS AND SIDES									
Cinnamon Twists (1 order)	180	25	8	2	0	190	<1	1	1 1/2 carb., 2 fat
Mexican Rice (1 order)	190	23	9	4	15	750	<1	5	1 1/2 carb., 2 fat
Nachos (1 order)	320	34	18	4	<5	560	3	5	2 carb., 4 fat
Nachos BellGrande (1 order)	760	83	39	11	35	1300	17	20	5 1/2 carb., 8 fat
Nachos Supreme, Big Beef (1 order)	440	44	24	7	35	800	9	14	3 carb., 5 fat
Nachos BellGrande, Chicken (1 order)	740	82	36	9	40	1200	15	23	5 1/2 carb., 1 med-fat meat, 6 fat
Nachos BellGrande, Steak (1 order)	740	81	37	9	35	1220	15	24	5 1/2 carb., 1 med-fat meat, 6 fat
Pintos 'N' Cheese (1 order)	180	18	8	4	15	640	10	9	1 carb., 1 med-fat meat, 1 fat

WENDY'S

SANDWICHES

Products	Cal.	Carb. (g)	Fat (g)	Sat. Fat (g)	Chol. (mg)	Sod. (mg)	Fib. (g)	Prot. (g)	Servings/Exchanges
Big Bacon Classic (1)	580	46	30	12	100	1460	3	34	3 carb., 4 med-fat meat, 2 fat

Cheeseburger, Jr. (1)	320	34	13	6	45	830	2	17	2 carb., 2 med-fat meat, 1 fat
Cheeseburger, Jr. Bacon (1)	380	34	19	7	60	850	2	20	2 carb., 2 med-fat meat, 2 fat
Cheeseburger, Jr. Deluxe (1)	360	36	17	6	50	890	3	18	2 1/2 carb., 2 med-fat meat, 1 fat
Cheeseburger, Kid's Meal (1)	320	33	13	6	45	830	2	17	2 carb., 2 med-fat meat, 1 fat
Hamburger, Jr. (1)	270	34	10	4	30	610	2	15	2 carb., 1 med-fat meat, 1 fat
Hamburger, Kid's Meal (1)	270	33	10	4	30	610	2	15	2 carb., 2 med-fat meat
Hamburger, Single, Plain (1)	360	31	16	6	65	580	2	24	2 carb., 3 med-fat meat
Hamburger, Single w/Everything (1)	420	37	20	7	70	920	3	25	2 1/2 carb., 3 med-fat meat, 1 fat
Sandwich, Breaded Chicken (1)	440	44	18	4	60	840	2	28	3 carb., 3 med-fat meat, 1 fat
Sandwich, Chicken Club (1)	470	44	20	4	70	970	2	31	3 carb., 3 med-fat meat, 1 fat
Sandwich, Grilled Chicken (1)	310	35	8	2	65	790	2	27	2 carb., 3 lean meat
Sandwich, Spicy Chicken (1)	410	43	15	3	65	1280	2	28	3 carb., 3 med-fat meat

BAKED POTATOES AND FRENCH FRIES

Baked Potato, Plain (1)	310	71	0	0	0	25	7	7	5 carb.

FAST FOODS: WENDY'S (continued)

Products	Cal.	Carb. (g)	Fat (g)	Sat. Fat (g)	Chol. (mg)	Sod. (mg)	Fib. (g)	Prot. (g)	Servings/Exchanges
Baked Potato w/Bacon & Cheese (1)	530	78	18	4	20	1390	7	17	5 carb., 4 fat
Baked Potato w/Broccoli & Cheese (1)	470	80	14	3	5	470	9	9	5 carb., 3 fat
Baked Potato w/Cheese (1)	570	78	23	8	30	640	7	14	5 carb., 1 med-fat meat, 4 fat
Baked Potato w/Chili & Cheese (1)	630	83	24	9	40	770	9	20	5 1/2 carb., 1 med-fat meat, 4 fat
Baked Potato w/Sour Cream & Chives (1)	380	74	6	4	15	40	8	8	5 carb., 1 fat
French Fries (1 Biggie order)	470	61	23	4	0	150	6	7	4 carb., 5 fat
French Fries (1 medium order)	390	50	19	4	0	120	5	5	3 carb., 4 fat
Sour Cream (1 pkt)	60	1	6	4	10	15	0	1	1 fat
CHILI AND CHICKEN NUGGETS									
Chicken Nuggets (5-piece)	230	11	16	4	30	470	0	11	1/2 carb., 1 med-fat meat, 2 fat
Chicken Nuggets, Kid's Meal (4 pieces)	190	9	13	3	25	380	0	9	1/2 carb., 1 med-fat meat, 2 fat

Chili (1 small)	210	21	7	3	30	800	5	15	1 1/2 carb., 1 med-fat meat
Sauce, Barbeque (1 pkt)	45	10	0	0	0	160	0	1	1 carb.
Sauce, Honey Mustard (1 pkt)	130	6	12	2	10	220	0	0	1/2 carb., 2 fat
Sauce, Sweet & Sour (1 pkt)	50	12	0	0	0	120	0	0	1 carb.

FRESH SALADS TO GO

Salad, Caesar Side w/c Dressing (1)	110	7	5	3	15	650	1	10	1 med-fat meat, 1 vegetable
Salad, Deluxe Garden (1)	110	9	6	1	0	350	3	7	2 vegetable, 1 med-fat meat
Salad, Grilled Chicken w/o Dressing (1)	200	9	8	2	50	720	3	25	3 med-fat meat, 2 vegetables
Salad, Side w/o Dressing (1)	60	5	3	0	0	180	2	4	1 vegetable, 1 fat
Salad, Taco (1)	380	28	19	10	65	1040	7	26	2 carb., 3 med-fat meat, 1 fat
Soft Breadstick (1)	130	23	3	<1	5	250	1	4	1 1/2 carb., 1 fat

SALAD DRESSINGS

Blue Cheese (2 Tbsp)	180	0	19	4	15	180	0	1	4 fat
Caesar Vinaigrette, Reduced Fat (1 Tbsp)	70	1	7	1	0	170	0	0	1 fat
French (2 Tbsp)	120	6	10	2	0	330	0	0	1/2 carb., 2 fat
French, Fat-Free (2 Tbsp)	35	8	0	0	0	150	0	0	1/2 carb.

FAST FOODS: WENDY'S (continued)

Products	Cal.	Carb. (g)	Fat (g)	Sat. Fat (g)	Chol. (mg)	Sod. (mg)	Fib. (g)	Prot. (g)	Servings/Exchanges
Hidden Valley Ranch (2 Tbsp)	100	1	10	2	10	220	0	1	2 fat
Hidden Valley Ranch, Reduced-Fat/Calorie (2 Tbsp)	60	2	5	1	10	240	0	1	1 fat
Italian Caesar (2 Tbsp)	150	1	16	3	20	240	0	1	3 fat
Italian, Reduced-Fat/Calorie (2 Tbsp)	40	2	3	0	0	340	0	0	1 fat
Salad Oil (1 Tbsp)	120	0	14	2	0	0	0	0	3 fat
Thousand Island (2 Tbsp)	90	2	8	2	10	125	0	0	2 fat
FRESH STUFFED PITAS									
Chicken Caesar w/Dressing (1)	490	48	18	5	65	1320	4	34	3 carb., 4 med-fat meat
Classic Greek w/Dressing (1)	440	50	20	8	35	1050	4	15	3 carb., 1 med-fat meat, 3 fat
Garden Ranch Chicken (1)	480	51	18	4	70	1180	5	30	3 1/2 carb., 3 med-fat meat, 1 fat
Garden Ranch Sauce, Reduced Fat (1 Tbsp)	50	1	5	1	10	125	0	0	1 fat
Garden Veggie (1)	400	52	17	4	20	760	5	11	3 1/2 carb., 3 fat

DESSERTS

Cookies, Chocolate Chip (1)	270	36	13	6	30	120	1	3	2 1/2 carb., 3 fat
Frosty Dairy Dessert (1 medium)	440	73	11	7	50	260	0	11	5 carb., 2 fat

WHATABURGER

BAKED POTATOES/SALADS

Baked Potato w/Broccoli/Cheese (1)	453	79	10	NA	17	636	NA	13	5 carb., 2 fat
Baked Potato w/Cheese (1)	510	80	16	NA	22	863	NA	15	5 carb., 3 fat
Garden Salad (1)	56	11	<1	NA	0	32	NA	3	2 vegetable
Grilled Chicken Salad (1)	150	14	1	NA	49	434	NA	23	3 vegetable, 2 very lean meat
Plain Baked Potato (1)	310	72	<1	NA	0	23	NA	7	5 carb.

BREAKFAST

Biscuit w/Bacon (1)	359	37	20	NA	15	730	VA	10	2 1/2 carb., 1 med-fat meat, 3 fat
Biscuit w/Egg and Cheese (1)	434	38	26	NA	202	797	NA	14	2 1/2 carb., 1 med-fat meat, 4 fat

FAST FOODS: WHATABURGER (continued)

Products	Cal.	Carb. (g)	Fat (g)	Sat. Fat (g)	Chol. (mg)	Sod. (mg)	Fib. (g)	Prot. (g)	Servings/Exchanges
Biscuit w/Egg, Cheese & Bacon (1)	511	38	33	NA	213	1010	NA	18	2 1/2 carb., 2 med-fat meat, 5 fat
Biscuit w/Egg, Cheese & Sausage (1)	601	38	42	NA	236	1081	NA	21	2 1/2 carb., 2 med-fat meat, 6 fat
Biscuit w/Gravy (1)	479	48	27	NA	20	1253	NA	9	3 carb., 5 fat
Biscuit w/Sausage (1)	446	37	29	NA	37	794	NA	12	2 1/2 carb., 1 med-fat meat, 5 fat
Blueberry Muffin (1)	239	36	8	NA	0	538	NA	6	2 1/2 carb., 2 fat
Breakfast on a Bun (1)	455	30	28	NA	232	886	NA	20	2 carb., 2 med-fat meat, 4 fat
Breakfast on a Bun w/Bacon (1)	365	29	19	NA	210	815	NA	18	2 carb., 2 med-fat meat, 2 fat
Breakfast Platter w/Bacon (1)	695	54	44	NA	389	1162	NA	22	3 1/2 carb., 2 med-fat meat, 7 fat
Breakfast Platter w/Sausage (1)	785	54	53	NA	412	1234	NA	25	3 1/2 carb., 2 med-fat meat, 9 fat

Food								Exchanges
Buttermilk Biscuit (1)	280	37	13	NA	3	509	NA	5	2 1/2 carb., 3 fat
Egg Omelette Sandwich (1)	288	29	13	NA	193	602	NA	13	2 carb., 1 med-fat meat, 2 fat
Hash Browns (1 order)	150	16	9	NA	0	228	NA	1	1 carb., 2 fat
Pancakes (3)	259	40	6	NA	0	842	NA	11	2 1/2 carb., 1 fat
Pancakes (3) w/Sausage	426	40	21	NA	34	1127	NA	18	2 1/2 carb., 2 med-fat meat, 2 fat
Pecan Danish (1)	270	28	16	NA	11	418	NA	5	2 carb., 3 fat
Scrambled Eggs (2)	189	2	15	NA	374	211	NA	11	2 med-fat meat, 1 fat

BURGERS

Food								Exchanges
Justaburger (1)	276	30	11	NA	34	578	NA	13	2 carb., 1 med-fat meat, 1 fat
Whataburger (1)	598	61	26	NA	84	1096	NA	30	4 carb., 3 med-fat meat, 2 fat
Whataburger Double Meat (1)	823	62	42	NA	168	1298	NA	49	4 carb., 5 med-fat meat, 3 fat
Whataburger Jr. (1)	300	35	12	NA	34	583	NA	14	2 carb., 1 med-fat meat, 1 fat
Whataburger, Small Bun, w/o Oil on Bun (1)	407	34	19	NA	84	839	NA	25	2 carb., 3 med-fat meat, 1 fat

OTHER ENTREES

Food								Exchanges
Beef Fajita (1)	326	34	12	NA	28	670	NA	22	2 carb., 2 med-fat meat

FAST FOODS: WHATABURGER (continued)

Products	Cal.	Carb. (g)	Fat (g)	Sat. Fat (g)	Chol. (mg)	Sod. (mg)	Fib. (g)	Prot. (g)	Servings/Exchanges
Chicken Fajita (1)	272	35	7	NA	33	691	NA	18	2 carb., 2 lean meat
Grilled Chicken Sandwich (1)	442	48	14	NA	66	1103	NA	34	3 carb., 4 lean meat
Grilled Chicken Sandwich w/o Bun Oil or Salad Dressing (1)	358	46	6	NA	66	989	NA	34	3 carb., 4 very lean meat
Taquito, Bacon (1)	335	32	16	NA	286	761	NA	15	2 carb., 1 med-fat meat, 2 fat
Taquito, Potato (1)	446	48	22	NA	281	883	NA	14	3 carb., 1 med-fat meat, 3 fat
Taquito, Sausage (1)	443	32	26	NA	315	790	NA	20	2 carb., 2 med-fat meat, 3 fat
Whatacatch (1)	467	43	25	NA	33	636	NA	18	3 carb., 1 med-fat meat, 4 fat
Whatachicken Sandwich (1)	501	51	23	NA	40	1122	NA	27	3 1/2 carb., 2 med-fat meat, 3 fat
SIDES									
French Fries (1 regular order)	332	37	18	NA	0	208	NA	5	2 1/2 carb., 3 fat
Onion Rings (1 regular order)	329	34	19	NA	0	596	NA	5	2 carb., 4 fat

DESSERTS

Apple Turnover (1)	215	27	11	NA	0	241	NA	2	2 carb., 2 fat
Chocolate Chunk Cookie (1)	247	28	16	NA	36	75	NA	4	2 carb., 3 fat
Oatmeal Raisin (1)	222	37	7	NA	28	70	NA	4	2 1/2 carb., 1 fat

FATS, OILS, AND SALAD DRESSINGS

Products	Cal.	Carb. (g)	Fat (g)	Sat. Fat (g)	Chol. (mg)	Sod. (mg)	Fib. (g)	Prot. (g)	Servings/Exchanges
Butter, Reduced-Fat (1 Tbsp)	50	0	6	4	20	70	0	0	1 fat
Butter, Stick (1 tsp)	36	0	4	3	11	41	0	0	1 fat
Butter, Whipped (2 tsp)	40	0	5	3	13	50	0	0	1 fat
Chitterlings, Boiled (2 Tbsp)	42	0	4	1	20	6	0	1	1 fat
Creamer, Nondairy, Liquid, Regular (1 Tbsp)	18	2	1	1	0	5	0	0	free
Creamer, Nondairy, Powder, Regular (1 tsp)	22	2	1	1	0	7	0	<1	free
Dressing, Oil & Vinegar (2 Tbsp)	144	<1	16	3	0	<1	0	0	3 fat
Dressing, Yogurt (1 Tbsp)	11	1	<1	<1	2	59	<1	<1	free
Lard (1 tsp)	36	0	4	2	4	0	0	0	1 fat
Margarine, Fat-Free/Nonfat (4 Tbsp)	20	0	0	0	0	368	0	0	free
Margarine, Reduced-Calorie (1 Tbsp)	50	0	6	1	0	90	0	0	1 fat
Margarine, Squeeze (1 tsp)	30	0	3	<1	0	37	0	0	1 fat
Margarine, Stick (1 tsp)	34	0	4	<1	0	44	0	0	1 fat

Margarine, Tub (1 tsp)	30	0	4	<1	0	33	0	0	1 fat
Mayonnaise (1 tsp)	33	0	4	<1	3	26	0	0	1 fat
Mayonnaise, Fat-Free (1 Tbsp)	10	2	0	0	NA	105	0	NA	free
Mayonnaise, Light/Reduced-Fat (1 Tbsp)	40	3	3	<1	6	120	0	0	1 fat
Oil, Canola (1 tsp)	41	0	5	<1	0	0	0	0	1 fat
Oil, Cocoa Butter (1 tsp)	40	0	5	3	0	0	0	0	1 fat
Oil, Coconut (1 tsp)	39	0	5	4	0	0	0	0	1 fat
Oil, Cod Liver/Fish (1 tsp)	41	0	5	1	0	26	0	0	1 fat
Oil, Corn (1 tsp)	44	0	5	<1	0	0	0	0	1 fat
Oil, Cottonseed (1 tsp)	40	0	5	1	0	0	0	0	1 fat
Oil, Olive (1 tsp)	40	0	5	<1	0	0	0	0	1 fat
Oil, Palm Kernel (1 tsp)	39	0	5	4	0	0	0	0	1 fat
Oil, Palm (1 tsp)	40	0	5	2	0	0	0	0	1 fat
Oil, Peanut (1 tsp)	40	0	5	<1	0	0	0	0	1 fat
Oil, Safflower (1 tsp)	44	0	5	<1	0	0	0	0	1 fat
Oil, Sardine/Fish (1 tsp)	41	0	5	1	0	32	0	0	1 fat

FATS, OILS, AND SALAD DRESSINGS

Products	Cal.	Carb. (g)	Fat (g)	Sat. Fat (g)	Chol. (mg)	Sod. (mg)	Fib. (g)	Prot. (g)	Servings/Exchanges
Oil, Sesame (1 tsp)	40	0	5	<1	0	0	0	0	1 fat
Oil, Soybean (1 tsp)	44	0	5	<1	0	0	0	0	1 fat
Salad Dressing, Fat-Free (1 Tbsp)	20	5	0	0	0	145	0	0	free
Salad Dressing, Light/Reduced-Calorie/Reduced-Fat (2 Tbsp)	80	5	6	1	NA	307	0	0	1 fat
Salad Dressing, Regular (1 Tbsp)	64	2	6	NA	NA	150	NA	NA	1 fat
Salt Pork, Raw, Cured (1/2 oz)	52	0	6	2	6	100	0	<1	1 fat
Shortening (1 tsp)	35	0	4	1	0	0	0	0	1 fat
Sour Cream, Fat-Free (1 Tbsp)	15	3	0	0	0	20	0	<1	free
Sour Cream, Light (1 Tbsp)	18	2	1	<1	5	15	0	<1	free
Sour Cream, Reduced-Fat (3 Tbsp)	45	2	4	3	15	20	0	1	1 fat
Sour Cream, Regular (2 Tbsp)	52	1	5	3	10	12	0	<1	1 fat
BENECOL									
Margarine Spread (1 Tbsp)	80	0	9	1	0	110	0	0	2 fat

Margarine Spread, Light (1 Tbsp)	30	0	3	0	0	65	0	0	1 fat
Salad Dressing, Creamy Italian (2 Tbsp)	100	3	10	2	0	170	0	0	2 fat
Salad Dressing, French (2 Tbsp)	130	6	11	2	0	170	0	0	1/2 carb., 2 fat
Salad Dressing, Ranch (2 Tbsp)	130	3	13	2	0	250	0	0	3 fat
BLUE BONNET									
Margarine, Soft (1 Tbsp)	100	0	11	2	0	95	0	0	2 fat
Margarine, Whipped (1 Tbsp)	70	0	7	1	0	70	0	0	1 fat
Margarine, Stick (1 Tbsp)	100	0	11	2	0	95	0	0	2 fat
Vegetable Oil Spread, Soft Better Blend (1 Tbsp)	90	0	11	2	0	95	0	0	2 fat
BREAKSTONE									
Sour Cream (2 Tbsp)	60	1	5	4	20	15	0	<1	1 fat
Sour Cream, Fat Free (2 Tbsp)	35	6	0	0	<5	25	0	2	1/2 carb.
Sour Cream, Reduced Fat (2 Tbsp)	45	2	4	3	15	20	0	1	1 fat
BUTTER BUDS									
Butter Replacement, Dry (1 Tbsp)	15	6	0	0	0	360	0	0	free

FATS, OILS, AND SALAD DRESSINGS

Products	Cal.	Carb. (g)	Fat (g)	Sat. Fat (g)	Chol. (mg)	Sod. (mg)	Fib. (g)	Prot. (g)	Servings/Exchanges
CARNATION									
Non-Fat, Nondairy Creamer, Coffee-Mate (1 Tbsp)	10	2	0	0	0	0	0	0	free
Nondairy Creamer, Coffee-Mate (1 Tbsp)	16	2	1	<1	0	5	0	0	free
CREMORA									
Nondairy Powder Creamer (1 tsp)	10	1	1	NA	0	5	0	0	free
Nondairy Powder Creamer, Lite (1 tsp)	8	2	<1	0	0	3	0	0	free
CRISCO									
Vegetable Shortening (1 Tbsp)	110	0	12	3	0	0	0	0	2 fat
ESTEE									
Dressing, Creamy French (2 Tbsp)	10	0	0	0	0	80	0	0	free
Dressing, Italian (2 Tbsp)	5	0	0	0	0	80	0	0	free
FLEISCHMANN'S									
Corn Oil Spread, Extra Light (1 Tbsp)	50	0	6	1	0	5	0	0	1 fat
Corn Oil Spread, Light (1 Tbsp)	80	0	8	1	0	70	0	0	free

	Calories								Exchanges
Margarine, Soft (1 Tbsp)	100	0	11	2	0	95	0	0	2 fat
Margarine, Stick (1 Tbsp)	100	0	11	2	0	95	0	0	2 fat
Margarine, Diet, Reduced Calorie (1 Tbsp)	50	0	6	1	0	50	0	0	1 fat
Margarine, Whipped, Lightly Salted (1 Tbsp)	70	0	7	2	0	60	0	0	1 fat
Margarine, Whipped, Unsalted (1 Tbsp)	70	0	7	2	0	0	0	0	2 fat
Vegetable Oil Spread, Move Over Butter (1 Tbsp)	90	0	10	2	0	100	0	0	2 fat
IMPERIAL									
Margarine, Diet, Reduced Calorie (1 Tbsp)	50	0	6	1	0	140	0	0	1 fat
Margarine, Soft (1 Tbsp)	100	0	11	NA	0	95	0	0	2 fat
Vegetable Oil Spread, Light (1 Tbsp)	60	0	6	NA	0	110	0	0	1 fat
KNUDSEN									
Sour Cream, Fat-Free (2 Tbsp)	35	6	0	0	<5	25	0	2	1/2 carb.
Sour Cream, Light (2 Tbsp)	40	2	3	2	10	20	0	2	1 fat
KRAFT									
Dressing, Bacon & Tomato (2 Tbsp)	140	2	14	3	<5	280	0	<1	3 fat
Dressing, Buttermilk Ranch (2 Tbsp)	150	1	16	3	<5	240	0	0	3 fat

FATS, OILS, AND SALAD DRESSINGS

Products	Cal.	Carb. (g)	Fat (g)	Sat. Fat (g)	Chol. (mg)	Sod. (mg)	Fib. (g)	Prot. (g)	Servings/Exchanges
Dressing, Caesar Italian (2 Tbsp)	100	2	10	2	0	480	0	<1	2 fat
Dressing, Caesar Ranch (2 Tbsp)	110	1	11	2	10	290	0	1	2 fat
Dressing, Catalina French (2 Tbsp)	120	7	10	2	0	390	0	0	1/2 carb., 2 fat
Dressing, Catalina w/Honey (2 Tbsp)	130	7	11	2	0	320	0	0	1/2 carb., 2 fat
Dressing, Coleslaw (2 Tbsp)	130	7	11	2	15	410	0	0	1/2 carb., 2 fat
Dressing, Creamy French (2 Tbsp)	160	5	15	3	0	270	0	0	3 fat
Dressing, Creamy Garlic (2 Tbsp)	110	2	11	2	0	360	0	0	2 fat
Dressing, Creamy Italian (2 Tbsp)	110	2	11	2	0	250	0	0	2 fat
Dressing, Cucumber Ranch (2 Tbsp)	140	2	15	2	0	220	0	0	3 fat
Dressing, Fat-Free Blue Cheese (2 Tbsp)	45	11	0	0	0	360	1	0	1 carb.
Dressing, Fat-Free Caesar Italian (2 Tbsp)	25	4	0	0	0	480	0	<1	free
Dressing, Fat-Free Catalina (2 Tbsp)	35	8	0	0	0	320	<1	0	1/2 carb.
Dressing, Fat-Free French (2 Tbsp)	45	11	0	0	0	300	<1	0	1 carb.
Dressing, Fat-Free Honey Dijon (2 Tbsp)	45	10	0	0	0	330	1	0	1/2 carb.

Dressing, Fat-Free Italian (2 Tbsp)	20	4	0	0	0	430	0	0	free
Dressing, Fat-Free Peppercorn Ranch (2 Tbsp)	45	11	0	0	0	330	<1	0	1 carb.
Dressing, Fat-Free Ranch (2 Tbsp)	50	11	0	0	0	350	1	0	1 carb.
Dressing, Fat-Free Red Wine Vinegar (2 Tbsp)	15	3	0	0	0	410	0	0	free
Dressing, Fat-Free Thousand Island (2 Tbsp)	40	9	0	0	0	280	1	0	1 carb.
Dressing, Honey Dijon (2 Tbsp)	110	6	10	6	2	210	0	0	1/2 carb., 2 fat
Dressing, House Italian (2 Tbsp)	120	2	12	2	2	240	<5	0	2 fat
Dressing, Lightly Done Right, Raspberry Vinaigrette (2 Tbsp)	60	5	4	0	0	270	0	0	1 fat
Dressing, Lightly Done Right, Catalina (2 Tbsp)	80	9	5	0	0	400	0	0	1/2 carb., 1 fat
Dressing, Lightly Done Right, Classic Caesar (2 Tbsp)	70	3	6	1	10	330	0	<1	1 fat
Dressing, Lightly Done Right, Italian (2 Tbsp)	50	2	5	0	0	230	0	0	1 fat
Dressing, Lightly Done Right, Ranch (2 Tbsp)	80	3	7	<1	10	300	0	0	1 fat
Dressing, Lightly Done Right, Red Wine Vinegar (2 Tbsp)	50	3	5	0	0	310	0	0	1 fat

FATS, OILS, AND SALAD DRESSINGS

Products	Cal.	Carb. (g)	Fat (g)	Sat. Fat (g)	Chol. (mg)	Sod. (mg)	Fib. (g)	Prot. (g)	Servings/Exchanges
Dressing, Peppercorn Ranch (2 Tbsp)	170	1	18	3	10	270	0	0	4 fat
Dressing, Presto Italian (2 Tbsp)	90	2	9	2	0	310	0	0	2 fat
Dressing, Ranch (2 Tbsp)	170	1	18	3	10	280	0	0	4 fat
Dressing, Roka Brand Blue Cheese (2 Tbsp)	130	2	13	3	<5	310	<1	<1	3 fat
Dressing, Russian (2 Tbsp)	130	10	10	2	0	310	0	0	1/2 carb., 2 fat
Dressing, Sour Cream & Onion Ranch (2 Tbsp)	170	1	18	3	10	250	0	0	4 fat
Dressing, Taste of Life, Country Ranch (2 Tbsp)	60	4	5	0	0	250	0	0	1 fat
Dressing, Taste of Life, Garden Italian (2 Tbsp)	50	5	5	0	0	300	0	0	1 fat
Dressing, Taste of Life, Honey Catalina (2 Tbsp)	80	8	5	0	0	290	0	0	1/2 carb., 1 fat
Dressing, Taste of Life, Tomato & Garlic (2 Tbsp)	60	4	5	0	0	240	0	0	1 fat
Dressing, Thousand Island & Bacon (2 Tbsp)	130	5	12	2	0	200	0	0	3 fat
Dressing, Thousand Island (2 Tbsp)	110	5	10	2	10	310	0	0	2 fat
Dressing, Zesty Italian (2 Tbsp)	110	2	11	1	0	540	0	0	2 fat
Light Mayonnaise (1 Tbsp)	50	2	5	1	5	90	0	0	1 fat

Margarine, Chiffon Soft (1 Tbsp)	100	0	11	2	0	105	0	0	2 fat
Margarine, Chiffon Whipped (1 Tbsp)	70	0	8	1	0	80	0	0	1 fat
Margarine, Parkay (1 Tbsp)	100	0	11	2	0	105	0	0	2 fat
Margarine, Parkay, Squeeze (1 Tbsp)	90	0	10	2	0	110	0	0	2 fat
Margarine, Parkay Soft. Tub (1 Tbsp)	100	0	11	2	0	105	0	0	2 fat
Margarine, Parkay Soft. Diet (1 Tbsp)	50	0	6	1	0	110	0	0	1 fat
Margarine, Parkay Whipped (1 Tbsp)	70	0	7	1	0	70	0	0	1 fat
Margarine Spread, Touch-Of-Butter (1 Tbsp)	50	0	6	1	0	110	0	0	1 fat
Margarine Spread, Touch-Of-Butter, Stick (1 Tbsp)	90	0	10	2	0	110	0	0	2 fat
Mayonnaise, Fat-Free (1 Tbsp)	10	2	0	0	0	120	0	0	free
Mayonnaise, Real (1 Tbsp)	100	0	11	2	5	75	0	0	2 fat
Miracle Whip Dressing (1 Tbsp)	70	2	7	1	5	95	0	0	1 fat
Miracle Whip Fat-Free Dressing (1 Tbsp)	15	2	0	0	0	125	0	0	free
Miracle Whip Light Dressing (1 Tbsp)	35	2	3	0	<5	130	0	0	1 fat
MARIE'S									
Dressing, Coleslaw (2 Tbsp)	150	6	13	2	10	210	0	0	1/2 carb., 3 fat

FATS, OILS, AND SALAD DRESSINGS

Products	Cal.	Carb. (g)	Fat (g)	Sat. Fat (g)	Chol. (mg)	Sod. (mg)	Fib. (g)	Prot. (g)	Servings/Exchanges
Dressing, Low-Fat Creamy Blue Cheese (2 Tbsp)	45	7	2	0	0	270	<1	0	1/2 carb.
Dressing, Low-Fat Creamy Italian Herb (2 Tbsp)	40	6	2	0	0	290	0	0	1/2 carb.
Dressing, Low-Fat Creamy Parmesan (2 Tbsp)	45	7	2	0	0	270	0	<1	1/2 carb.
Dressing, Low-Fat Zesty Ranch (2 Tbsp)	45	7	2	0	0	330	0	0	1/2 carb.
Dressing/Dip, Buttermilk Ranch (2 Tbsp)	180	4	18	3	15	230	0	0	3 fat
Dressing/Dip, Chunky Blue Cheese (2 Tbsp)	180	3	19	4	15	170	0	1	4 fat
Dressing/Dip, Creamy Ranch (2 Tbsp)	190	3	20	3	15	170	0	<1	4 fat
Dressing/Dip, Honey Mustard (2 Tbsp)	160	8	15	2	5	160	<1	0	1/2 carb., 3 fat
Dressing/Dip, Low-Calorie Blue Cheese (2 Tbsp)	100	7	7	1	10	250	1	1	1/2 carb., 1 fat
Dressing/Dip, Low-Calorie Creamy Ranch (2 Tbsp)	100	7	7	<1	5	240	0	1	1/2 carb., 1 fat
Dressing/Dip, Parmesan Ranch (2 Tbsp)	180	3	19	3	15	160	0	<1	4 fat
Dressing/Dip, Poppyseed (2 Tbsp)	150	8	12	2	10	200	0	0	1/2 carb., 2 fat
Dressing/Dip, Sour Cream & Dill (2 Tbsp)	190	3	20	3	15	160	0	0	4 fat
Dressing/Dip, Tangy French (2 Tbsp)	130	8	11	2	0	260	0	0	1/2 carb., 2 fat

Food	Cal.	Carb.	Fat	Sat. Fat	Chol.	Sod.			Exchanges
Dressing/Dip, Thousand Island (2 Tbsp)	240	7	23	4	20	320	0	0	1/2 carb., 5 fat
Vinaigrette, Fat-Free Honey Dijon (2 Tbsp)	50	11	0	0	0	125	0	0	1 carb.
Vinaigrette, Lite & Zesty Herb (2 Tbsp)	30	8	0	0	0	260	0	0	1/2 carb.
Vinaigrette, Lite & Zesty Italian (2 Tbsp)	35	8	0	0	0	270	0	0	1/2 carb.
Vinaigrette, Lite & Zesty White Wine (2 Tbsp)	40	10	0	0	0	270	0	0	1/2 carb.
NUCOA									
Heart Beat Canola Oil (1 Tbsp)	120	0	14	1	0	0	0	0	3 fat
Heart Beat Margarine (1 Tbsp)	25	0	3	1	0	110	0	0	1 fat
Margarine, Stick (1 Tbsp)	100	0	11	2	0	160	0	0	2 fat
PROMISE									
Margarine Spread, Fat-Free Ultra Tub (1 Tbsp)	5	0	0	0	0	90	0	0	1 fat
Vegetable Oil Spread, Tub (1 Tbsp)	90	0	10	2	0	90	0	0	2 fat
SAFFOLA									
Margarine, Stick (1 Tbsp)	100	0	11	2	0	95	0	0	2 fat
Margarine, Soft, Tub (1 Tbsp)	100	0	11	2	0	95	0	0	2 fat
Margarine, Unsalted, Stick (1 Tbsp)	100	0	11	2	0	0	0	0	2 fat

FATS, OILS, AND SALAD DRESSINGS

Products	Cal.	Carb. (g)	Fat (g)	Sat. Fat (g)	Chol. (mg)	Sod. (mg)	Fib. (g)	Prot. (g)	Servings/Exchanges
SEALTEST									
Sour Cream (2 Tbsp)	60	2	6	4	20	10	0	0	1 fat
Sour Cream, Light (2 Tbsp)	50	2	4	2	10	20	0	2	1 fat
SEVEN SEAS									
Dressing, Chunky Blue Cheese (2 Tbsp)	130	2	13	3	<5	310	<1	<1	3 fat
Dressing, Classic Caesar (2 Tbsp)	100	2	10	2	0	480	0	<1	2 fat
Dressing, Creamy Italian (2 Tbsp)	120	1	12	2	0	510	0	0	3 fat
Dressing, Creamy Italian, Reduced Fat (2 Tbsp)	60	2	5	1	0	500	0	0	1 fat
Dressing, Fat-Free Creamy Italian (2 Tbsp)	50	12	0	0	0	330	<1	0	free
Dressing, Fat-Free Ranch (2 Tbsp)	45	11	0	0	0	330	1	0	1 carb.
Dressing, Fat-Free Red Wine Vinegar (2 Tbsp)	15	3	0	0	0	410	0	0	free
Dressing, Green Goddess (2 Tbsp)	130	1	13	2	0	260	0	0	3 fat
Dressing, Herb Vinaigrette (2 Tbsp)	140	<1	15	2	0	250	0	0	3 fat
Dressing, Herbs & Spices (2 Tbsp)	90	1	9	1	0	290	0	0	2 fat

Dressing, Honey Mustard (2 Tbsp)	110	6	10	2	0	210	0	0	2 fat
Dressing, Italian & Olive Oil, Reduced Fat (2 Tbsp)	45	2	4	0	0	460	0	0	1 fat
Dressing, Ranch (2 Tbsp)	160	2	17	3	<5	260	0	0	3 fat
Dressing, Red Wine Vinegar & Oil (2 Tbsp)	90	2	9	1	0	500	0	0	2 fat
Dressing, Red Wine Vinegar & Oil, Reduced Fat (2 Tbsp)	45	3	4	0	0	320	0	0	1 fat
Dressing, Two-Cheese Italian (2 Tbsp)	70	3	7	1	0	240	0	0	1 fat
Dressing, Viva Italian (2 Tbsp)	90	2	9	1	0	370	0	0	2 fat
Dressing, Viva Italian, Reduced Fat (2 Tbsp)	45	2	4	0	0	320	0	0	1 fat
Dressing, Viva Russian (2 Tbsp)	150	3	16	3	0	210	0	0	3 fat
SHEDD'S SPREAD									
Margarine Spread, Tub (1 Tbsp)	60	0	7	1	0	110	0	0	1 fat
TAKE CONTROL									
Salad Dressing, Blue Cheese (2 Tbsp)	90	8	6	1	15	400	0	1	1/2 carb., 1 fat
Salad Dressing, Italian (2 Tbsp)	50	5	4	0	5	290	0	0	1 fat
Salad Dressing, Reduced Fat Ranch (2 Tbsp)	100	5	8	1	10	290	0	0	2 fat

FATS, OILS, AND SALAD DRESSINGS

Products	Cal.	Carb. (g)	Fat (g)	Sat. Fat (g)	Chol. (mg)	Sod. (mg)	Fib. (g)	Prot. (g)	Servings/Exchanges
Vegetable Spread (1 Tbsp)	50	0	6	<1	<5	110	0	0	1 fat
WEIGHT WATCHERS									
Mayonnaise, Light (1 Tbsp)	50	1	5	1	5	100	?	0	1 fat
Mayonnaise, Low-Sodium Reduced Calorie (1 Tbsp)	50	1	5	1	5	45	0	0	1 fat
Margarine, Reduced-Fat, Stick (1 Tbsp)	60	0	7	1	0	130	0	0	1 fat
Margarine, Sodium-Free Light (1 Tbsp)	50	0	6	1	0	0	0	0	1 fat
Margarine Spread, Extra Light (1 Tbsp)	45	2	4	1	0	75	0	0	1 fat
Margarine Spread, Light (1 Tbsp)	50	2	6	1	0	130	0	0	1 fat
Salad Dressing, Fat-Free Blue Cheese (2 Tbsp)	16	2	0	0	0	110	0	0	free
Salad Dressing, Fat-Free Caesar (2 Tbsp)	8	2	0	0	0	200	0	0	free
Salad Dressing, Fat-Free Creamy Italian (2 Tbsp)	24	6	0	0	0	85	0	0	free
Salad Dressing, Fat-Free French (2 Tbsp)	20	4	0	0	0	170	0	0	free
Salad Dressing, Fat-Free Russian (2 Tbsp)	8	2	0	0	0	120	0	0	free

Food									
Salad Dressing, Fat-Free Tomato Vinaigrette (2 Tbsp)	16	4	0	0	0	150	0	0	free
Salad Dressing, Fat-Free Whipped (1 Tbsp)	12	4	0	0	0	125	0	0	free
WESSON									
Best Blend (1 Tbsp)	120	0	14	1	0	0	0	0	3 fat
Oil, Cottonseed (1 Tbsp)	122	0	14	3	0	0	0	0	3 fat
Oil, Olive (1 Tbsp)	122	0	14	2	0	0	0	0	3 fat
Oil, Peanut (1 Tbsp)	122	0	14	5	0	0	0	0	3 fat
WISH-BONE									
Dressing, Caesar (2 Tbsp)	155	2	16	2	2	496	0	<1	3 fat
Dressing, Chunky Blue Cheese (2 Tbsp)	150	1	16	2	2	300	0	<1	3 fat
Dressing, Creamy Herbal (2 Tbsp)	140	2	14	NA	0	455	0	0	3 fat
Dressing, Creamy Italian (2 Tbsp)	110	3	11	2	2	300	0	<1	1 fat
Dressing, Deluxe French (2 Tbsp)	120	4	11	2	0	165	0	<1	2 fat
Dressing, Dijon Vinaigrette, Lite (2 Tbsp)	60	3	5	1	0	410	0	0	1 fat
Dressing, Fat-Free Blue Cheese (2 Tbsp)	35	7	0	0	0	290	0	0	1/2 carb.

FATS, OILS, AND SALAD DRESSINGS

Products	Cal.	Carb. (g)	Fat (g)	Sat. Fat (g)	Chol. (mg)	Sod. (mg)	Fib. (g)	Prot. (g)	Servings/Exchanges
Dressing, Fat-Free Italian (2 Tbsp)	20	5	0	0	0	390	0	0	free
Dressing, Fat-Free Thousand Island (2 Tbsp)	35	9	0	0	0	290	<1	0	1/2 carb.
Dressing, Healthy Sensations Italian (2 Tbsp)	12	2	0	0	0	280	0	0	free
Dressing, Italian (2 Tbsp)	90	3	5	1	0	560	0	0	1 fat
Dressing, Lite Caeser (2 Tbsp)	60	3	5	1	0	410	0	1	1 fat
Dressing, Lite Dijon Vinaigrette (2 Tbsp)	60	3	5	1	0	410	0	0	1 fat
Dressing, Lite Italian (2 Tbsp)	14	2	<1	0	0	210	0	<1	1/2 carb.
Dressing, Lite Italian (2 Tbsp)	15	2	<1	0	0	500	0	0	free
Dressing, Lite Ranch (2 Tbsp)	100	5	9	4	5	300	0	0	2 fat
Dressing, Lite Sweet Spicy French (2 Tbsp)	36	6	1	0	0	110	0	0	1/2 carb.
Dressing, Lite Thousand Island (2 Tbsp)	72	6	4	<1	20	200	0	<1	1/2 carb., 1 fat
Dressing, Olive Oil Italian (2 Tbsp)	70	3	6	1	0	380	0	0	1 fat
Dressing, Olive Oil Vinaigrette (2 Tbsp)	60	4	4	NA	0	220	0	0	1 fat
Dressing, Ranch (2 Tbsp)	160	2	17	2	4	310	0	<1	3 fat

Dressing, Red Wine Vinegar (2 Tbsp)	90	2	8	2	0	380	0	0	2 fat
Dressing, Robusto Italian (2 Tbsp)	90	4	9	1	0	580	0	<1	2 fat
Dressing, Russian (2 Tbsp)	90	12	5	<1	0	290	0	<1	1 carb., 1 fat
Dressing, Sante Fe (2 Tbsp)	150	3	15	3	5	220	0	0	3 fat
Dressing, Sweet & Spicy French Lite (2 Tbsp)	36	6	1	0	0	110	0	0	1/2 carb.

FRUITS AND FRUIT JUICES

FRUITS

Products	Cal.	Carb. (g)	Fat (g)	Sat. Fat (g)	Chol. (mg)	Sod. (mg)	Fib. (g)	Prot. (g)	Servings/Exchanges
Apple, Unpeeled (1 large)	125	32	<1	0	0	0	6	<1	2 fruit
Apple, Unpeeled (1 small)	63	16	<1	<1	0	0	3	<1	1 fruit
Apples, Dried (4 rings)	63	17	<1	0	0	23	2	<1	1 fruit
Applesauce, Unsweetened (1/2 cup)	52	14	<1	0	0	2	2	<1	1 fruit
Apricots, Canned, Extra Light Syrup (1/2 cup)	60	15	<1	0	0	2	2	<1	1 fruit
Apricots, Canned, Juice Pack (1/2 cup)	60	15	0	0	0	5	2	<1	1 fruit
Apricots, Dried (8 halves)	66	17	<1	0	0	2	3	1	1 fruit
Apricots, Fresh (4)	68	16	1	0	0	1	3	2	1 fruit
Banana (1 small)	64	16	<1	<1	0	1	2	<1	1 fruit
Banana Chips (1/4 cup)	120	14	8	7	0	1	2	<1	1 fruit, 2 fat
Blackberries, Fresh (3/4 cup)	56	14	<1	0	0	0	5	<1	1 fruit
Blackberries, Frozen, Unsweetened (3/4 cup)	73	18	<1	NA	0	2	6	1	1 fruit

Food								
Blueberries, Fresh (3/4 cup)	61	15	<1	0	0	7	3	<1	1 fruit
Blueberries, Frozen, Unsweetened (3/4 cup)	58	14	<1	NA	0	1	3	<1	1 fruit
Cantaloupe, Fresh (1 cup)	56	13	<1	0	0	14	1	1	1 fruit
Cherries, Sweet, Canned, Juice Pack (1/2 cup)	68	17	0	0	0	4	<1	1	1 fruit
Cherries, Sweet, Fresh (12)	59	14	<1	<1	0	0	2	1	1 fruit
Cranberries (1 cup)	47	12	<1	<1	0	<1	4	<1	1 fruit
Cranberry Sauce, Canned (1/4 cup)	105	27	<1	<1	0	20	<1	<1	1 1/2 fruit
Dates (3)	68	18	<1	0	0	0	2	<1	1 fruit
Figs, Dried (1 1/2)	71	18	<1	<1	0	3	3	<1	1 fruit
Figs, Fresh (1 1/2 large)	71	18	<1	<1	0	1	3	<1	1 fruit
Fruit Cocktail, Canned, Extra Light Syrup (1/2 cup)	55	14	<1	0	0	5	1	<1	1 fruit
Fruit Cocktail, Canned, Juice Pack (1/2 cup)	57	15	0	0	0	5	1	<1	1 fruit
Grapefruit, Canned (1/2 cup)	69	17	<1	0	0	13	<1	1	1 fruit
Grapefruit, Fresh (1/2 cup)	51	13	<1	0	0	0	2	1	1 fruit
Grapes, Fresh, Seedless (17)	60	15	<1	<1	0	2	<1	<1	1 fruit
Honeydew Melon, Fresh (1 cup)	59	16	<1	0	0	15	1	<1	1 fruit

FRUITS AND FRUIT JUICES

Products	Cal.	Carb. (g)	Fat (g)	Sat. Fat (g)	Chol. (mg)	Sod. (mg)	Fib. (g)	Prot. (g)	Servings/Exchanges
Kiwi, Fresh (1)	56	14	<1	0	0	5	3	<1	1 fruit
Mango, Fresh (1/2)	68	18	<1	<1	0	2	2	<1	1 fruit
Melon Balls, Mixed, Frozen (1 cup)	57	14	<1	<1	0	54	1	2	1 fruit
Mixed Fruit, Dried (1/4 cup)	83	22	<1	<1	0	6	3	<1	1 1/2 fruit
Nectarine, Fresh (1)	67	16	<1	0	0	0	2	1	1 fruit
Orange, Fresh (1)	62	15	<1	0	0	0	3	1	1 fruit
Oranges, Mandarin, Canned, Juice Pack (3/4 cup)	69	18	<1	0	0	9	1	1	1 fruit
Papaya, Fresh (1/2 medium)	59	15	<1	<1	0	4	3	<1	1 fruit
Peach, Fresh (1 medium)	57	15	<1	0	0	0	3	<1	1 fruit
Peaches, Canned, Extra Light Syrup (1/2 cup)	52	14	<1	0	0	6	1	<1	1 fruit
Peaches, Canned, Juice Pack (1/2 cup)	55	14	0	0	0	5	1	<1	1 fruit
Pear, Fresh (1/2 large)	59	15	<1	0	0	0	2	<1	1 fruit
Pears, Canned (1/2 cup)	62	16	<1	0	0	5	3	<1	1 fruit
Pears, Canned, Light Syrup (1/2 cup)	58	15	<1	0	0	3	3	<1	1 fruit

Pineapple, Canned, Juice Pack (1/2 cup)	74	20	0	0	0	1	<1	<1	1 fruit
Pineapple, Fresh (1/2 cup)	57	14	<1	0	0	1	1	<1	1 fruit
Plums, Canned, Juice Pack (1/2 cup)	73	19	0	0	0	2	1	<1	1 fruit
Plums, Fresh (2 small)	73	17	<1	<1	0	0	2	1	1 fruit
Prunes, Dried, Uncooked (3)	60	16	<1	0	0	1	2	<1	1 fruit
Raisins, Dark, Seedless (2 Tbsp)	54	14	<1	0	0	2	<1	<1	1 fruit
Raspberries, Black, Fresh (1 cup)	60	14	<1	0	0	0	8	1	1 fruit
Rhubarb, Diced (2 cups)	52	12	<1	0	0	10	4	2	1 fruit
Strawberries, Fresh (1 1/2 cups)	56	13	<1	0	0	2	4	1	1 fruit
Strawberries, Frozen, Unsweetened (1 1/2 cups)	65	17	<1	0	0	4	4	<1	1 fruit
Tangerines, Fresh (2 small)	74	19	<1	0	0	2	4	1	1 fruit
Watermelon, Fresh (1 1/2 cups)	64	15	<1	NA	0	4	1	1	1 fruit

JUICES

Apple Juice/Cider, Canned/Bottled (1/2 cup)	58	15	<1	0	0	4	<1	<1	1 fruit
Apricot Nectar, Canned (1/2 cup)	71	18	<1	<1	0	4	<1	<1	1 fruit
Cranberry Juice Cocktail, Bottled (1/3 cup)	48	12	<1	0	0	2	0	0	1 fruit

FRUITS AND FRUIT JUICES

Products	Cal.	Carb. (g)	Fat (g)	Sat. Fat (g)	Chol. (mg)	Sod. (mg)	Fib. (g)	Prot. (g)	Servings/Exchanges
Cranberry Juice Cocktail, Reduced-Calorie (1 cup)	50	11	0	0	0	7	0	0	1 fruit
Fruit Juice Blends, 100% Juice (1/3 cup)	50	12	<1	0	0	10	<1	<1	1 fruit
Grape Juice, Bottled (1/3 cup)	51	13	<1	0	0	3	<1	<1	1 fruit
Grapefruit Juice, Canned (1/2 cup)	47	11	<1	0	0	1	<1	<1	1 fruit
Orange Juice, Canned (1/2 cup)	52	12	<1	<1	0	3	<1	<1	1 fruit
Orange Juice, Fresh (1/2 cup)	56	13	<1	0	0	1	<1	<1	1 fruit
Orange Juice, Frozen, Reconstituted (1/2 cup)	56	13	<1	0	0	1	<1	<1	1 fruit
Pineapple Juice, Canned (1/2 cup)	70	17	<1	0	0	1	<1	<1	1 fruit
Prune Juice, Bottled (1/3 cup)	60	15	0	0	0	3	<1	<1	1 fruit

GRAINS, NOODLES, AND RICE

Products	Cal.	Carb. (g)	Fat (g)	Sat. Fat (g)	Chol. (mg)	Sod. (mg)	Fib. (g)	Prot. (g)	Servings/Exchanges
Barley, Cooked (1/2 cup)	135	30	1	<1	0	<1	7	4	2 strch
Barley, Pearled, Cooked (1/2 cup)	97	22	<1	<1	0	3	3	2	1 1/2 strch
Brown Rice, Long-Grain, Cooked (1/2 cup)	108	23	1	<1	0	5	2	3	1 1/2 strch
Brown Rice, Medium-Grain, Cooked (1/2 cup)	110	23	<1	<1	0	<1	2	2	1 1/2 strch
Bulgur Wheat, Cooked (1/2 cup)	76	17	<1	<1	0	5	4	3	1 strch
Couscous, Cooked (1/2 cup)	88	18	<1	<1	0	4	1	3	1 strch
Noodles, Egg, Cooked (1/2 cup)	107	20	1	<1	26	6	<1	4	1 strch
Grits, Yellow Corn, Cooked (1/2 cup)	73	16	<1	<1	0	0	<1	2	1 strch
Lasagna, Cut, Cooked (1/2 cup)	99	20	<1	<1	0	<1	<1	3	1 strch
Linguine, Cooked (1/2 cup)	99	20	<1	<1	0	<1	2	3	1 strch
Macaroni, Cooked (1/2 cup)	99	20	<1	<1	0	<1	<1	3	1 strch
Macaroni, Vegetable, Cooked (1/2 cup)	86	18	<1	<1	0	4	1	3	1 strch

GRAINS, NOODLES, AND RICE

Products	Cal.	Carb. (g)	Fat (g)	Sat. Fat (g)	Chol. (mg)	Sod. (mg)	Fib. (g)	Prot. (g)	Servings/Exchanges
Macaroni, Whole-Wheat, Cooked (1/2 cup)	87	19	<1	<1	0	2	2	4	1 strch
Millet, Cooked (1/2 cup)	143	28	1	<1	0	2	NA	4	2 strch
Noodles, Chow Mein (1/2 cup)	119	13	7	1	0	99	<1	2	1 strch, 1 fat
Noodles, Ramen, Cooked (1 cup)	156	29	2	<1	38	1349	3	6	2 strch
Noodles, Rice, Cooked (1/2 cup)	80	20	<1	<1	0	5	<1	<1	1 strch
Noodles, Spinach Egg, Cooked (1/2 cup)	106	20	1	<1	27	10	2	4	1 strch
Pasta, Homemade w/o Egg, Cooked (2 oz)	70	14	<1	<1	0	42	<1	3	1 strch
Pasta/Noodles, Egg, Homemade, Cooked (2 oz)	74	13	<1	<1	23	47	2	3	1 strch
Pasta/Noodles, Fresh, Cooked (2 oz)	74	14	<1	<1	19	3	<1	3	1 strch
Pasta/Noodles, Spinach, Fresh, Cooked (2 oz)	74	14	<1	<1	19	3	1	3	1 strch
Pasta/Spirals, Cooked (1/2 cup)	95	19	<1	<1	0	<1	<1	3	1 strch
Pasta/Wagon Wheels, Cooked (1/2 cup)	99	20	<1	<1	0	<1	<1	3	1 strch
Rice Pilaf (1 cup)	268	46	7	1	0	754	1	5	3 strch, 1 fat
Rotini, Cooked (1/2 cup)	99	20	<1	<1	0	<1	<1	3	2 strch

Shells, Jumbo, Cooked (2)	65	13	<1	0	<1	2		1 strch
Shells, Small, Cooked (1/2 cup)	81	17	<1	0	<1	3		1 strch
Shells, Whole-Wheat, Cooked (1/2 cup)	87	19	<1	0	2	4		1 strch
Spaghetti, Cooked (1/2 cup)	99	20	<1	0	2	3		1 strch
Spaghetti, Spinach, Cooked (1/2 cup)	91	19	<1	0	10	3		1 strch
Spaghetti, Whole-Wheat, Cooked (1/2 cup)	87	19	<1	0	2	3		1 strch
Vermicelli, Cooked (1/2 cup)	99	20	<1	0	<1	3		1 strch
Wheat Bran (1/2 cup)	63	19	1	0	<1	12	5	1 strch
Wheat Germ, Toasted (1 Tbsp)	27	4	<1	0	<1	3	6	free
White Flour, All-Purpose (1 Tbsp)	28	6	<1	0	<1	<1		1/2 strch
White Hominy, Canned (1/2 cup)	58	12	<1	0	168	2		1 strch
White Rice, Long-Grain, Cooked (1/2 cup)	134	29	<1	0	1	2		2 strch
White Rice, Long-Grain, Instant, Cooked (1/2 cup)	81	18	<1	0	3	2		1 strch
White Rice, Long-Grain, Parboiled, Cooked (1/2 cup)	100	22	<1	0	3	2		1/2 strch
White Rice, Medium-Grain, Cooked (1/2 cup)	121	27	<1	0	0	<1	2	2 strch

GRAINS, NOODLES, AND RICE

Products	Cal.	Carb. (g)	Fat (g)	Sat. Fat (g)	Chol. (mg)	Sod. (mg)	Fib. (g)	Prot. (g)	Servings/Exchanges
White Rice, Short-Grain, Cooked (1/2 cup)	121	27	<1	<1	0	0	0	2	2 strch
Wild Rice, Cooked (1/2 cup)	83	18	<1	<1	0	3	2	3	1 strch
ALBER'S									
Cornmeal, Yellow (1 Tbsp)	37	8	0	0	0	0	<1	<1	1/2 strch
Grits, Hominy Quick (1/2 cup)	140	31	<1	0	0	0	1	3	2 strch
BETTY CROCKER									
Pasta, Creamy Garlic & Herb Rotini (1 cup)	360	44	16	4	5	840	1	10	3 strch, 3 fat
Pasta, Creamy Homestyle Chicken (1 cup)	210	36	4	1	10	730	1	9	2 1/2 strch, 1 fat
Pasta, Garlic Alfredo Fettuccine (1 cup)	340	45	13	4	10	840	1	11	3 strch, 3 fat
Pasta, Roasted Chicken Vegetable Penne (1 cup)	240	39	7	1	5	860	2	8	2 1/2 strch, 1 fat
Pasta, Three Cheese Gemelli (1 cup)	330	47	12	4	15	930	1	12	3 strch, 2 fat
Pasta, Tomato Parmesan (1 cup)	260	37	10	2	0	840	1	6	2 1/2 strch, 2 fat
Rice & Barley Medley (1/3 cup)	180	39	1	0	0	480	3	6	2 1/2 strch
Rice, Cheddar & Broccoli (1 cup)	310	48	10	3	10	950	1	7	3 strch, 2 fat

Rice, Chicken Herb (1 cup)	270	48	5	1	5	870	1	6	3 strch, 1 fat
Rice, Creamy Herb Risotto (1 cup)	320	49	12	4	5	810	0	5	3 strch, 2 fat
Rice, Garden Vegetable Pilaf (1 cup)	240	43	6	1	<5	840	2	6	3 strch, 1 fat
Rice, Long Grain & Wild Rice Pilaf (1 cup)	220	40	5	1	0	580	1	5	2 1/2 strch, 1 fat
Rice, Southwestern (1 cup)	250	45	6	1	0	950	2	5	3 strch, 1 fat

DI GIORNO

Angel Hair Pasta (2 oz)	160	31	2	0	0	115	2	6	2 strch
Fettuccine Pasta (2.5 oz)	200	38	2	0	0	140	2	8	2 1/2 strch
Herb Linguine Pasta (2.5 oz)	200	38	2	0	0	140	2	8	2 1/2 strch
Red Bell Pepper Fettuccine Pasta (2.5 oz)	200	38	2	0	0	140	2	8	2 1/2 strch
Spinach Fettuccine Pasta (2.5 oz)	200	38	2	0	0	140	2	8	2 1/2 strch

KRAFT

Macaroni & Cheese (1 cup)	410	49	18	5	10	750	1	12	3 strch, 3 fat
Macaroni & Cheese, All Shapes Pastas (1 cup)	410	49	18	5	10	750	1	12	3 strch, 3 fat
Macaroni & Cheese Deluxe, Four Cheese Blend (1 cup)	320	44	10	7	25	910	1	14	3 strch, 1 med-fat meat, 1 fat

GRAINS, NOODLES, AND RICE

Products	Cal.	Carb. (g)	Fat (g)	Sat. Fat (g)	Chol. (mg)	Sod. (mg)	Fib. (g)	Prot. (g)	Servings/Exchanges
Macaroni & Cheese, Deluxe Original (1 cup)	320	44	10	6	25	730	1	14	3 strch, 1 med-fat meat, 1 fat
Macaroni & Cheese, Light (1 cup)	290	48	6	2	10	580	2	12	2 strch, 1 fat
Macaroni & Cheese, Light Deluxe (1 cup)	290	48	5	3	15	810	1	14	3 strch, 1 med-fat meat
Macaroni & Cheese, Thick'n Creamy (1 cup)	420	50	19	5	15	760	2	13	3 strch, 2 fat
Macaroni & Cheese, White Cheddar (1 cup)	410	49	19	4	10	740	1	12	3 strch, 3 fat
Velveeta Rotini & Cheese w/Broccoli (1 cup)	400	47	16	10	50	1230	2	18	3 strch, 1 med-fat meat, 2 fat
Velveeta Shells & Cheese, Bacon (1 cup)	360	43	14	8	40	1140	1	17	3 strch, 1 med-fat meat, 2 fat
Velveeta Shells & Cheese, Original (1 cup)	360	44	13	8	40	1030	1	16	3 strch, 1 med-fat meat, 2 fat
Velveeta Shells & Cheese, Salsa (1 cup)	380	47	14	9	40	1180	2	17	3 strch, 1 med-fat meat, 2 fat
LA CHOY									
Fried Rice (4 oz)	195	44	<1	<1	0	835	2	4	3 strch
Noodles, Chow Mein (1/2 cup)	140	17	6	1	0	210	2	5	1 strch, 1 fat
Noodles, Crispy Wide (1 oz)	150	17	8	2	0	260	1	2	1 strch, 2 fat
Noodles, Rice (1 oz)	125	22	3	<1	0	365	<1	2	1 1/2 strch, 1 fat

LIPTON

Food	Cal								Exchanges
Noodles & Sauce, Alfredo, Dry (2/3 cup)	250	39	7	4	75	940	2	10	2 1/2 strch, 1 fat
Noodles & Sauce, Beef, Dry (1/3 cup)	230	43	4	1	60	840	2	8	3 strch, 1 fat
Noodles & Sauce, Butter Herb, Dry (2/3 cup)	250	42	7	4	65	710	2	9	3 strch, 1 fat
Noodles & Sauce, Chicken Broccoli, Dry (1/2 cup)	230	41	4	2	65	740	2	9	3 strch, 1 fat
Noodles & Sauce, Creamy Tomato Parmesan, Dry (2/3 cup)	240	41	5	3	10	830	2	8	3 strch, 1 fat
Noodles & Sauce, Parmesan, Dry (2/3 cup)	250	37	8	4	70	750	2	10	2 1/2 strch, 2 fat
Noodles & Sauce, Sour Cream & Chives, Dry (1/2 cup)	260	41	8	5	70	800	2	8	3 strch, 2 fat
Pasta & Sauce, Spirals, Roasted Garlic & Olive Oil, Dry (1/2 cup)	220	42	3	<1	0	810	2	8	3 strch, 1 fat
Pasta & Sauce, Zesty Cheddar, Dry (1/2 cup)	240	42	5	2	10	820	2	9	3 strch, 1 fat
Rice & Sauce, Teriyaki, Dry (1/2 cup)	220	45	2	0	0	840	1	5	3 strch
Rice & Sauce, Spanish, Dry (1/2 cup)	220	47	2	0	0	830	2	6	3 strch
Rice & Sauce, Cheddar Broccoli, Dry (1/2 cup)	230	46	3	2	5	940	1	7	3 strch, 1 fat

GRAINS, NOODLES, AND RICE

Products	Cal.	Carb. (g)	Fat (g)	Sat. Fat (g)	Chol. (mg)	Sod. (mg)	Fib. (g)	Prot. (g)	Servings/Exchanges
Rice & Sauce, Chicken Broccoli, Dry (1/2 cup)	230	46	3	1	0	840	2	7	3 strch, 1 fat
Rice & Sauce, Chicken Flavor, Dry (1/2 cup)	230	45	3	1	5	890	1	7	3 strch, 1 fat
Rice & Sauce, Southwestern Chicken, Dry (1/2 cup)	210	47	2	0	0	770	1	5	3 strch
Rice & Sauce, Medley, Dry (1/2 cup)	220	44	3	<1	5	800	2	7	3 strch, 1 fat
MINUTE RICE									
Brown Rice, Whole-Grain, Instant, Cooked (2/3 cup)	170	34	2	0	0	10	2	4	2 strch
Long Grain & Wild Rice, Seasoned (1 cup)	230	50	<1	0	0	950	1	6	3 strch
Rice, Boil-In-Bag, Cooked (1 cup)	190	42	0	0	0	10	<1	4	3 strch
White Rice, Instant, Cooked (3/4 cup)	160	36	0	0	0	5	<1	3	2 1/2 strch
PILLSBURY									
Shake & Blend Flour (1/4 cup)	110	23	0	0	0	0	3	3	1 1/2 strch

RICE-A-RONI

Beef, As Prepared (1 cup)	310	52	9	2	0	1160	2	7	3 1/2 strch, 2 fat
Chicken, As Prepared (1 cup)	310	52	9	2	0	980	2	7	3 1/2 strch, 2 fat
Fried Rice, As Prepared (1 cup)	320	51	11	2	0	1530	2	6	3 1/2 strch, 1 fat

STOVE TOP

Stuffing Mix, Long-Grain & Wild Rice (1/2 cup)	180	22	9	2	0	500	<1	4	1 1/2 strch, 2 fat
Stuffing Mix, Mushroom & Onion (1/2 cup)	180	20	9	2	0	480	<1	4	1 strch, 2 fat

UNCLE BEN'S

Brown Rice, Instant Whole-Grain (1/2 cup)	90	21	1	0	0	11	1	2	1 1/2 strch
Brown Rice, Original (2/3 cup)	130	27	1	0	0	0	1	3	2 strch
Converted Rice (1 cup)	170	38	0	0	0	0	1	4	2 1/2 strch
Converted Rice, Boil-In-Bag (1 cup)	190	44	<1	0	0	0	1	4	3 strch
Long-Grain Rice, Instant (1 cup)	190	43	<1	0	0	15	1	3	3 strch
Long-Grain Rice & Vermicelli, Three Cheese (1 cup)	200	41	3	1	5	770	1	5	3 strch

GRAINS, NOODLES, AND RICE

Products	Cal.	Carb. (g)	Fat (g)	Sat. Fat (g)	Chol. (mg)	Sod. (mg)	Fib. (g)	Prot. (g)	Servings/Exchanges
Long-Grain Rice & Wild Chicken Stock Sauce (1/2 cup)	190	41	1	<1	0	670	1	5	3 strch
Long-Grain Rice & Chicken Vegetable Blend (1/2 cup)	200	42	2	<1	5	620	1	5	3 strch
Pilaf, Specialty Blends (1 cup)	200	44	<1	0	0	630	1	4	3 strch
Risotto, Herb (1 cup)	200	44	<1	0	0	470	0	4	3 strch
Wild Rice, Original Recipe (1 cup)	190	41	<1	0	0	620	1	6	3 strch

Products	Cal.	Carb. (g)	Fat (g)	Sat. Fat (g)	Chol. (mg)	Sod. (mg)	Fib. (g)	Prot. (g)	Servings/Exchanges
LEGUMES									
Baby Lima Beans, Cooked (1/2 cup)	115	21	<1	<1	0	3	7	7	1 1/2 strch
Baked Beans, Homemade (1/2 cup)	190	27	7	3	6	532	7	7	2 strch, 1 fat
Baked Beans, Vegetarian, Canned (1/2 cup)	118	26	<1	<1	0	504	6	6	2 strch
Baked Beans w/Beef, Canned (1/2 cup)	161	23	5	2	29	632	7	9	1 1/2 strch, 1 med-fat meat
Black Beans, Cooked (1/2 cup)	114	21	<1	<1	0	<1	8	8	1 1/2 strch, 1 very lean meat
Black Turtle Soup Beans, Cooked (1/2 cup)	120	22	<1	<1	0	3	5	8	1 1/2 strch, 1 very lean meat
Black-Eyed Cowpeas w/Pork (1/2 cup)	100	20	2	<1	8	420	4	3	1 strch
Fava/Broadbeans, Canned (1/2 cup)	91	16	<1	<1	0	580	5	7	1 strch, 1 very lean meat
French Beans, Cooked (1/2 cup)	114	21	<1	<1	0	5	8	6	1 1/2 strch
Garbanzo Beans/Chickpeas, Cooked (1/2 cup)	135	23	2	<1	0	6	6	7	1 1/2 strch
Great Northern Beans, Cooked (1/2 cup)	105	19	<1	<1	0	2	6	7	1 strch, 1 very lean meat
Hummus (1/2 cup)	210	25	11	2	0	300	6	6	1 1/2 strch, 2 fat

LEGUMES

Products	Cal.	Carb. (g)	Fat (g)	Sat. Fat (g)	Chol. (mg)	Sod. (mg)	Fib. (g)	Prot. (g)	Servings/Exchanges
Kidney Beans, California Red, Cooked (1/2 cup)	109	20	<1	0	4	8	8	1 strch, 1 very lean meat
Kidney Beans, Canned, Not Drained (1/2 cup)	104	19	<1	0	444	5	7	1 strch, 1 very lean meat
Kidney Beans, Red, Cooked (1/2 cup)	112	20	<1	0	2	7	8	1 strch, 1 very lean meat
Kidney Beans, Royal Red, Cooked (1/2 cup)	108	19	<1	0	4	8	8	1 strch, 1 very lean meat
Lentils, Cooked (1/2 cup)	115	20	<1	0	2	9	9	1 strch, 1 very lean meat
Navy Beans, Cooked (1/2 cup)	129	24	<1	0	1	6	8	1 1/2 strch, 1 very lean meat
Pink Beans, Cooked (1/2 cup)	126	24	<1	0	2	5	8	1 1/2 strch, 1 very lean meat
Pinto Beans, Cooked (1/2 cup)	117	22	<1	0	2	7	7	1 1/2 strch
Pork & Beans in Sweet Sauce, Canned (1/2 cup)	140	27	2	<1	9	425	7	7	2 strch
Pork & Beans in Tomato Sauce, Canned (1/2 cup)	124	25	1	<1	9	557	6	7	1 1/2 strch
Refried Beans/Frijoles, Canned (1/2 cup)	118	20	2	<1	10	377	7	7	1 strch, 1 lean meat
Split Peas, Cooked (1/2 cup)	116	21	<1	0	2	8	8	1 1/2 strch, 1 very lean meat
White Beans, Cooked (1/2 cup)	124	23	<1	0	5	6	9	1 1/2 strch, 1 very lean meat
White Beans, Small, Cooked (1/2 cup)	127	23	<1	0	2	9	8	1 1/2 strch, 1 very lean meat

Food	Cal	Carb				Sod			Exchanges
Yellow Beans, Cooked (1/2 cup)	127	22	<1	<1	0	0	4	9	8 — 1 1/2 strch, 1 very lean meat
B & M									
Baked Beans, 99% Fat-Free Vegetarian (1/2 cup)	170	31	1	0	0	220	7	8	2 strch
Baked Beans, Bacon & Onion w/Brown Sugar (1/2 cup)	190	36	2	<1	<5	450	8	8	2 1/2 starch
Baked Beans, Barbeque (1/2 cup)	170	33	1	0	0	460	6	7	2 strch
Baked Beans, Red Kidney (1/2 cup)	170	32	2	<1	<5	440	6	7	2 strch
Baked Beans w/Honey (1/2 cup)	170	30	2	0	0	450	8	8	2 strch
Baked Beans w/Pork (1/2 cup)	180	33	2	<1	<5	430	7	8	2 strch
Baked Beans, Yellow Eye (1/2 cup)	180	30	3	<1	<5	450	8	8	2 strch
CAMPBELL'S									
Chili Beans in Zesty Sauce (1/2 cup)	130	21	3	1	5	490	6	6	1 1/2 strch, 1 fat
New England-Style Baked Beans (1/2 cup)	180	32	3	1	5	460	6	5	2 strch, 1 fat
Old-Fashioned Barbecue Beans (1/2 cup)	170	29	3	<1	5	460	6	7	2 strch, 1 fat
Pork & Beans in Tomato Sauce (1/2 cup)	130	24	2	<1	5	420	6	5	1 1/2 strch

LEGUMES

Products	Cal.	Carb. (g)	Fat (g)	Sat. Fat (g)	Chol. (mg)	Sod. (mg)	Fib. (g)	Prot. (g)	Servings/Exchanges
FRIENDS									
Baked Beans, Original (1/2 cup)	170	32	1	0	<5	390	7	8	2 strch
Baked Beans, Red Kidney (1/2 cup)	170	32	1	0	<5	510	6	7	2 strch
GEBHARDT									
Refried Beans, Jalapeño (1/2 cup)	110	18	2	NA	NA	320	NA	7	1 strch, 1 lean meat
Refried Beans, Traditional (1/2 cup)	130	20	2	0	NA	490	NA	7	1 strch, 1 lean meat
GREEN GIANT									
Baked Beans (1/2 cup)	160	31	2	1	5	580	7	6	2 strch
Barbecue Beans (1/2 cup)	140	28	<1	0	0	460	5	6	2 strch
Beans, Honey Bacon (1/2 cup)	160	34	<1	0	0	490	6	6	2 strch
Black Beans (1/2 cup)	90	21	0	0	0	580	6	7	1 1/2 strch
Black-Eyed Peas (1/2 cup)	90	18	1	0	0	300	4	7	1 strch, 1 very lean meat
Butter Beans, Frozen (1/2 cup)	80	18	0	0	0	170	4	6	1 strch
Chili Beans in Spicy Sauce (1/2 cup)	100	21	1	0	0	580	6	7	1 1/2 strch

Garbanzo Beans (1/2 cup)	110	18	2	0	0	380	5	6	1 strch
Great Northern Beans (1/2 cup)	80	18	1	0	0	290	5	6	1 strch
Italian Beans (1/2 cup)	130	24	1	0	0	480	5	5	1 1/2 strch
Kidney Beans, Dark Red (1/2 cup)	90	20	1	0	0	330	5	7	1 strch, 1 very lean meat
Kidney Beans, Light Red (1/2 cup)	90	20	1	0	0	330	5	7	1 strch, 1 very lean meat
Mexican Beans (1/2 cup)	120	21	2	0	0	530	5	6	1 1/2 strch
Pinto Beans (1/2 cup)	90	20	1	0	0	280	5	6	1 strch
Red Beans (1/2 cup)	90	19	1	0	0	340	5	6	1 strch
HEALTH VALLEY									
Honey-Baked Beans, Fat-Free, Salted (1/2 cup)	110	24	0	0	0	135	7	7	1 1/2 strch
HUNT'S									
Chili Beans (1/2 cup)	87	17	1	0	0	597	6	6	1 strch
Kidney Beans (1/2 cup)	120	21	0	0	0	400	NA	7	1 1/2 strch
Navy Beans w/Ham (9 oz)	239	38	3	<1	10	735	10	16	2 1/2 strch, 1 lean meat
Red Beans, Small (1/2 cup)	91	18	0	0	0	580	NA	6	1 strch

LEGUMES

Products	Cal.	Carb. (g)	Fat (g)	Sat. Fat (g)	Chol. (mg)	Sod. (mg)	Fib. (g)	Prot. (g)	Servings/Exchanges
OLD EL PASO									
Black Beans (1/2 cup)	110	17	1	0	0	400	7	7	1 strch, 1 very lean meat
Garbanzo Beans (1/2 cup)	100	16	2	0	0	340	4	6	1 strch, 1 lean meat
Mexe Beans (1/2 cup)	110	19	0	0	0	630	7	7	1 strch, 1 very lean meat
Pinto Beans (1/2 cup)	100	19	<1	0	0	420	7	6	1 strch, 1 very lean meat
Refried Beans (1/2 cup)	100	17	<1	0	0	570	6	6	1 strch, 1 lean meat
Refried Beans, Fat-Free (1/2 cup)	100	18	0	0	0	480	6	6	1 strch, 1 very lean meat
Refried Beans, Fat-Free, Spicy (1/2 cup)	100	18	0	0	0	720	6	6	1 strch, 1 fat
Refried Beans, Vegetarian (1/2 cup)	100	17	1	0	0	490	6	6	1 strch, 1 very lean meat
Refried Beans & Cheese (1/2 cup)	130	18	4	2	5	500	6	7	1 strch, 1 med-fat meat
Refried Beans w/Green Chili (1/2 cup)	100	17	<1	0	<5	720	6	6	1 strch, 1 very lean meat
Refried Beans w/Sausage (1/2 cup)	200	14	13	5	10	360	4	7	1 strch, 1 med-fat meat, 2 fat
Refried Black Beans (1/2 cup)	110	18	2	0	0	340	6	7	1 strch, 1 lean meat

ORTEGA

Refried Beans/Frijoles (1/2 cup)	140	23	3	<1	0	480	6	8	1 1/2 strch, 1 fat

ORVAL KENT

Barbeque Beans (1/2 cup)	160	34	<1	0	0	700	NA	6	1 strch
Four-Bean Salad (1/2 cup)	100	19	<1	0	0	300	3	4	1 strch

PROGRESSO

Black Beans (1/2 cup)	110	17	1	0	0	400	7	7	1 strch, 1 very lean meat
Cannellini Beans (1/2 cup)	100	18	<1	0	0	270	5	5	1 strch
Chickpeas (1/2 cup)	120	20	3	0	0	280	5	5	1 strch, 1 fat
Fava Beans (1/2 cup)	110	20	<1	0	0	250	5	6	1 strch, 1 very lean meat
Garbanzo Beans (1/2 cup)	110	18	2	0	0	380	5	6	1 starch, 1 very lean meat
Kidney Beans, Red (1/2 cup)	110	20	<1	0	0	280	8	7	1 strch, 1 very lean meat
Pinto Beans (1/2 cup)	110	18	1	0	0	250	7	7	1 strch, 1 very lean meat

ROSARITA

Refried Beans, Bacon (1/2 cup)	110	20	2	<1	14	560	6	7	1 strch, 1 lean meat
Refried Beans, Green Chili (1/2 cup)	90	18	2	<1	0	460	6	6	1 strch

LEGUMES

Products	Cal.	Carb. (g)	Fat (g)	Sat. Fat (g)	Chol. (mg)	Sod. (mg)	Fib. (g)	Prot. (g)	Servings/Exchanges
Refried Beans, Nacho Cheese (1/2 cup)	110	20	2	<1	2	490	6	7	1 strch, 1 lean meat
Refried Beans, No-Fat (1/2 cup)	180	18	0	0	0	490	6	7	1 strch, 1 lean meat
Refried Beans, Onion (1/2 cup)	110	21	2	<1	0	490	6	7	1 1/2 strch
Refried Beans, Spicy (1/2 cup)	120	20	2	1	0	465	6	8	1 strch, 1 lean meat
Refried Beans, Traditional (1/2 cup)	120	19	2	NA	NA	470	6	7	1 strch, 1 lean meat
Refried Beans, Vegetarian (1/2 cup)	100	18	2	0	0	520	2	6	1 strch
Refried Beans w/Green Chiles & Lime, No-Fat (1/2 cup)	90	18	0	0	0	570	5	6	1 strch
Refried Beans w/Zesty Salsa, No-Fat (1/2 cup)	90	18	0	0	0	670	5	6	1 1/2 strch

MEATS, FISH, AND POULTRY

Products	Cal.	Carb. (g)	Fat (g)	Sat. Fat (g)	Chol. (mg)	Sod. (mg)	Fib. (g)	Prot. (g)	Servings/Exchanges
Anchovies in Oil, Canned, Drained (5)	42	0	2	<1	17	734	0	8	1 lean meat
Bacon (3 slices)	105	0	9	3	15	288	0	5	1 high-fat meat
Beef, Chipped, Dried (1 oz)	47	0	1	<1	26	948	0	8	1 very lean meat
Beef, Chuck/Blade Pot Roast (1 oz)	62	0	2	<1	29	19	0	9	1 lean meat
Beef, Corned Brisket (1 oz)	72	<1	5	2	28	323	0	5	1 med-fat meat
Beef, Cubed Steak (1 oz)	58	0	2	<1	27	15	0	9	1 lean meat
Beef, Flank Steak, Lean (1 oz)	59	0	3	1	19	24	0	8	1 lean meat
Beef, Ground, Extra Lean (1 oz)	73	0	5	2	24	20	0	7	1 med-fat meat
Beef, Ground, Lean (1 oz)	78	0	5	2	25	22	0	7	1 med-fat meat
Beef, Ground, Regular (1 oz)	82	0	6	2	26	24	0	7	1 med-fat meat
Beef, Ground Round (1 oz)	56	0	1	<1	26	13	0	10	1 lean meat
Beef, Heart (1 oz)	50	<1	2	<1	55	18	0	8	1 lean meat
Beef, Liver (1 oz)	46	1	1	<1	110	20	0	7	1 lean meat

MEATS, FISH, AND POULTRY

Products	Cal.	Carb. (g)	Fat (g)	Sat. Fat (g)	Chol. (mg)	Sod. (mg)	Fib. (g)	Prot. (g)	Servings/Exchanges
Beef, Prime Rib (1 oz)	83	0	6	2	23	21	0	8	1 med-fat meat
Beef, Rib Roast, Lean (1 oz)	65	0	4	1	23	21	0	8	1 lean meat
Beef, Round Steak, Lean (1 oz)	55	0	2	<1	23	18	0	8	1 lean meat
Beef, Rump Roast, Lean (1 oz)	60	0	2	<1	27	15	0	9	1 lean meat
Beef, Shortribs (1 oz)	83	0	5	2	26	16	0	9	1 med-fat meat
Beef, Sirloin (1 oz)	54	0	2	<1	25	19	0	9	1 lean meat
Beef Jerky (1 oz)	94	4	4	2	14	796	<1	9	1 med-fat meat
Beef Kidney (1 oz)	41	<1	1	<1	110	38	0	7	1 very lean meat
Beef Tenderloin, Lean (1 oz)	67	0	4	1	24	18	0	8	1 lean meat
Beef Tongue (1 oz)	80	<1	6	3	30	17	0	6	1 med-fat meat
Bologna, Beef & Pork (1 oz)	89	<1	8	3	16	289	0	3	1 high-fat meat
Bratwurst, Pork (1 oz)	85	<1	7	3	17	158	0	4	1 high-fat meat
Buffalo (1 oz)	40	0	<1	<1	23	16	0	8	1 very lean meat
Canadian Bacon (1 oz)	53	<1	2	<1	16	441	0	7	1 lean meat

Food									Exchanges
Catfish Fillet (1 oz)	43	0	2	<1	18	23	0	5	1 lean meat
Caviar, Black/Red, Granular (2 Tbsp)	81	1	6	1	188	480	0	8	1 med-fat meat
Chicken, Dark Meat, w/o Skin (1 oz)	58	0	3	<1	26	26	0	8	1 lean meat
Chicken, Dark Meat, w/Skin (1 oz)	72	0	5	1	26	25	0	7	1 med-fat meat
Chicken, Fried, Flour-Coated (1 oz)	76	<1	4	1	26	24	0	8	1 med-fat meat
Chicken, Light Meat, w/Skin (1 oz)	63	0	3	<1	24	21	0	8	1 lean meat
Chicken, Liver (1 oz)	45	<1	2	<1	130	15	0	7	1 lean meat
Chicken, White Meat, w/o Skin (1 oz)	49	0	1	<1	24	22	0	9	1 very lean meat
Chicken Patty, Breaded (1 = 2.7 oz)	213	11	13	4	45	399	<1	12	1 strch, 1 med-fat meat, 2 fat
Clams, Canned, Drained Solids (1 oz)	42	1	<1	<1	19	32	0	7	1 very lean meat
Clams, Fresh, Steamed (1 oz)	42	1	<1	<1	19	32	0	7	1 very lean meat
Clams, Smoked, Canned in Oil, Small (5)	88	1	6	1	19	161	0	7	1 med-fat meat
Cod (1 oz)	30	0	<1	0	16	22	0	7	1 very lean meat
Cornish Hen, w/o Skin (1 oz)	38	0	1	<1	30	18	0	7	1 very lean meat
Crab (1 oz)	38	<1	2	<1	27	151	0	5	1 lean meat
Crab, Canned, Drained Solids (1 oz)	28	0	<1	<1	26	95	0	6	1 very lean meat

MEATS, FISH, AND POULTRY

Products	Cal.	Carb. (g)	Fat (g)	Sat. Fat (g)	Chol. (mg)	Sod. (mg)	Fib. (g)	Prot. (g)	Servings/Exchanges
Duck, Domestic (1 oz)	57	0	3	1	25	19	0	7	1 lean meat
Escargot/Snails (1 oz)	51	1	<1	<1	28	34	0	9	1 very lean meat
Fish, Fried, Cornmeal-Coated (1 oz)	65	2	2	1	23	79	0	5	1 med-fat meat
Fish Sticks, Frozen, Heated (2)	152	13	7	2	63	326	<1	9	1 strch, 1 med-fat meat
Flounder (1 oz)	33	0	<1	<1	19	29	0	7	1 very lean meat
Goose (1 oz)	68	0	4	1	27	22	0	8	1 lean meat
Haddock (1 oz)	32	0	<1	0	21	20	0	7	1 very lean meat
Halibut (1 oz)	40	0	<1	<1	12	20	0	8	1 very lean meat
Ham, Boiled, Lean, Sandwich-Type (1 oz)	46	<1	2	<1	15	362	0	5	1 lean meat
Ham, Canned (1 oz)	48	<1	2	<1	12	304	0	6	1 lean meat
Ham, Cured (1 oz)	45	0	2	<1	16	378	0	7	1 lean meat
Ham, Fresh, Baked (1 oz)	60	0	3	<1	27	18	0	8	1 lean meat
Ham Salad Spread (1/4 cup)	130	6	9	3	22	547	0	5	1 high-fat meat
Herring, Smoked (1 oz)	62	0	4	<1	23	262	0	7	1 lean meat

Food									Exchanges
Hot Dog, Beef & Pork (1)	144	1	13	5	22	504	0	5	1 high-fat meat, 1 fat
Hot Dog, Chicken (1)	116	3	9	3	45	617	0	6	1 high-fat meat
Hot Dog, Fat-Free (1)	30	3	<1	<1	11	286	0	4	1 very ean meat
Hot Dog, Low-Fat (1)	50	<1	2	<1	15	450	0	6	1 lean meat
Hot Dog, Turkey (1)	102	<1	8	2	48	642	0	6	1 high-fat meat
Imitation Shellfish, From Surimi (1 oz)	29	3	<1	<1	6	238	0	3	1 very lean meat
Knockwurst (1 oz)	87	<1	8	3	16	286	0	3	1 high-fat meat
Lamb, Ground (1 oz)	80	<1	6	2	28	23	0	7	1 med-fat meat
Lamb, Rib Roast (1 oz)	67	0	4	1	26	24	0	8	1 med-fat meat
Lamb Leg, Sirloin, Lean (1 oz)	58	0	3	<1	26	20	0	8	1 lean meat
Lamb Loin, Roast/Chop (1 oz)	57	0	3	1	25	19	0	8	1 lean meat
Liver Pate, Canned (2 Tbsp)	52	2	3	1	66	100	0	4	1 lean meat
Liverwurst (1 oz)	92	<1	8	3	45	244	0	4	1 high-fat meat
Lobster, Fresh, Steamed (1 oz)	28	<1	<1	<1	20	108	0	6	1 very lean meat
Mackerel (1 oz)	57	0	3	<1	17	31	0	7	1 lean meat
Meat Loaf (1 oz)	57	<1	4	3	26	186	0	5	1 med-fat meat

MEATS, FISH, AND POULTRY

Products	Cal.	Carb. (g)	Fat (g)	Sat. Fat (g)	Chol. (mg)	Sod. (mg)	Fib. (g)	Prot. (g)	Servings/Exchanges
Meat Sticks, Smoked (1 oz)	153	15	14	6	38	410	NA	6	1 strch, 1 high-fat meat, 1 fat
Meatball, Beef (1 oz)	60	2	4	1	24	107	<1	5	1 med-fat meat
Octopus (1 oz)	46	1	<1	<1	27	130	0	9	1 very lean meat
Orange Roughy (1 oz)	25	0	<1	<1	7	23	0	5	1 very lean meat
Oyster, Medium (6)	58	3	2	<1	44	177	0	6	1 lean meat
Pepperoni Sausage, Beef & Pork (1 oz)	140	<1	13	5	22	578	0	6	1 high-fat meat, 1 fat
Pheasant, w/o Skin (1 oz)	38	0	1	<1	19	10	0	7	1 very lean meat
Pickle & Pimento Loaf (1 oz)	74	2	6	2	10	394	0	3	1 high-fat meat
Pickled Beef Tripe (1 oz)	18	0	<1	<1	19	13	0	3	1 very lean meat
Pork, Boston Blade (1 oz)	66	0	4	2	24	25	0	7	1 med-fat meat
Pork, Ground (1 oz)	84	0	6	2	27	21	0	7	1 high-fat meat
Pork, Spareribs (1 oz)	113	0	9	3	35	27	0	8	1 high-fat meat
Pork Cutlet (1 oz)	50	0	2	<1	23	13	0	8	1 med-fat meat
Pork Loin, Roast/Chop, Center Cut (1 oz)	60	0	3	1	23	16	0	8	1 lean meat

Food									
Pork Sausage, Fresh, Pattie/Link (1 oz)	105	<1	9	3	24	369	0	6	1 high-fat meat
Pork Tenderloin (1 oz)	47	0	1	<1	23	16	0	8	1 lean meat
Rabbit (1 oz)	58	0	2	<1	24	10	0	9	1 lean meat
Rainbow Trout Fillet (1 oz)	42	0	2	<1	20	16	0	7	1 lean meat
Salami, Beef & Pork (1 oz)	71	<1	6	2	18	302	0	4	1 high-fat meat
Salmon, Canned in Water (1 oz)	40	0	2	<1	11	139	0	6	1 lean meat
Salmon Fillet (1 oz)	61	0	3	<1	25	19	0	8	1 lean meat
Sardines, Oil-Packed, Drained (2)	50	0	3	<1	34	121	0	6	1 lean meat
Sausage, Hard, Fat-Free (1 oz)	35	3	<1	<1	12	290	0	5	1 very lean meat
Sausage, Italian, Pork (1 oz)	92	<1	7	3	22	263	0	6	1 high-fat meat
Sausage, Polish (1 oz)	92	<1	8	3	20	248	0	4	1 high-fat meat
Sausage, Smoked (1 oz)	96	<1	9	3	20	269	0	4	1 high-fat meat
Sausage, Vienna, Canned (1 oz)	79	<1	7	3	15	270	0	3	1 high-fat meat
Scallops, Fresh, Steamed (1 oz)	32	0	<1	<1	15	78	0	7	1 very lean meat
Sea Bass (1 oz)	35	0	<1	<1	15	25	0	7	1 very lean meat
Shrimp, Canned, Drained Solids (1 oz)	34	<1	<1	<1	50	48	0	7	1 very lean meat

MEATS, FISH, AND POULTRY

Products	Cal.	Carb. (g)	Fat (g)	Sat. Fat (g)	Chol. (mg)	Sod. (mg)	Fib. (g)	Prot. (g)	Servings/Exchanges
Shrimp, Fresh, Cooked in Water (1 oz)	28	0	<1	<1	56	64	0	6	1 very lean meat
Squid, Pickled (1 oz)	26	1	<1	<1	64	397	0	4	1 very lean meat
Steak, Porterhouse (1 oz)	62	0	3	1	23	19	0	8	1 lean meat
Steak, T-Bone (1 oz)	61	0	3	1	23	19	0	8	1 lean meat
Swordfish (1 oz)	43	0	1	<1	14	32	0	7	1 very lean meat
Tempeh (1/4 cup)	83	7	3	<1	0	2	2	8	1 med-fat meat
Tofu (1/2 cup)	94	2	6	<1	0	9	2	10	1 med-fat meat
Trout (1 oz)	54	0	2	<1	21	19	0	8	1 very lean meat
Tuna, Canned in Oil, Drained (1 oz)	56	0	2	<1	5	100	0	8	1 lean meat
Tuna, Canned, Water-Packed, Solids Only (1 oz)	33	0	<1	<1	9	96	0	7	1 very lean meat
Turkey, Dark Meat, w/o Skin (1 oz)	53	0	2	<1	24	22	0	8	1 lean meat
Turkey, Ground (1 oz)	67	0	4	1	29	30	0	8	1 med-fat meat
Turkey, White Meat, w/o Skin (1 oz)	44	0	<1	<1	20	18	0	9	1 very lean meat
Turkey Ham (1 oz)	36	<1	1	<1	16	282	0	5	1 very lean meat

Turkey Kielbasa, Low-Fat (1 oz)	45	2	3	1	16	300	0	4	1 lean meat
Turkey Pastrami, Low-Fat (1 oz)	40	<1	2	<1	15	296	0	5	1 lean meat
Veal Cutlet, Lean (1 oz)	58	0	6	>1	38	19	0	11	1 med-fat meat
Veal Loin, Chop (1 oz)	50	0	2	<1	30	27	0	8	1 lean meat
Veal Brisket, Lean (1 oz)	47	0	2	<1	31	26	0	7	1 lean meat
Vension (1 oz)	45	0	<1	<1	32	15	0	9	1 very lean meat

BANQUET

Chicken Breast Patties, Grilled Honey Mustard (1)	120	5	5	2	25	500	0	13	2 lean meat
Chicken Breast Patty, Fat Free Baked (1)	100	15	0	0	20	400	1	9	1 strch, 1 very lean meat
Chicken, Country-Fried (3 oz)	270	13	18	5	45	620	1	14	1 strch, 2 med-fat meat, 2 fat
Chicken, Hot'n Spicy Fried (3 oz)	260	13	18	5	65	490	1	14	1 strch, 2 med-fat meat, 2 fat
Chicken, Original Fried (3 oz)	280	15	18	5	65	620	1	14	1 strch, 2 med-fat meat, 2 fat
Chicken, Skinless Fried (3 oz)	210	7	13	3	55	480	2	18	1/2 strch, 2 med-fat meat, 1 fat
Chicken, Southern Fried (3 oz)	260	15	18	5	65	700	1	14	1 strch, 2 med-fat meat, 2 fat
Chicken Breasts, Fried (1)	410	18	26	13	85	60C	4	23	1 strch, 3 med-fat meat, 2 fat

MEATS, FISH, AND POULTRY

Products	Cal.	Carb. (g)	Fat (g)	Sat. Fat (g)	Chol. (mg)	Sod. (mg)	Fib. (g)	Prot. (g)	Servings/Exchanges
Chicken Nuggets, Southern Fried (6)	270	16	18	4	35	570	2	12	1 strch, 1 med-fat meat, 3 fat
Chicken Patties, Boneless (1)	190	10	14	3	30	440	1	7	1/2 strch, 1 med-fat meat, 2 fat
Chicken Patties, Southern Fried (1)	190	10	13	3	25	430	<1	8	1/2 strch, 1 med-fat meat, 2 fat
Chicken Tenders (3)	250	15	15	4	40	480	<1	12	1 strch, 1 med-fat meat, 2 fat
Chicken Tenders, Southern Fried (3)	250	16	16	4	40	460	1	12	1 strch, 2 med-fat meat, 1 fat
Chicken Wings, Hot'n Spicy Breaded (4)	290	9	20	5	90	450	<1	18	1/2 strch, 2 med-fat meat, 2 fat
BRYAN FOODS									
Beef in Broth, Cubed (1 oz)	60	0	1	NA	NA	234	0	7	1 lean meat
Bologna, Beef & Pork (1 oz)	91	<1	9	3	14	298	NA	3	1 high-fat meat
Chicken w/Broth, Boned (1 oz)	74	0	3	NA	NA	153	0	6	1 med-fat meat
Ham, Smoked, 95% Fat-Free (1 oz)	31	<1	1	<1	14	357	0	5	1 very lean meat

Pepperoni (1 oz)	162	1	13	5	23	581	0	6	1 high-fat meat, 1 fat
Salami (2 oz)	70	<1	6	2	20	284	0	4	1 med-fat meat
Turkey Breast, Deli Classics (1 oz)	54	0	2	<1	17	17	0	7	1 lean meat
COUNTRY SKILLET									
Chicken, Fried (3 oz)	270	13	18	5	65	620	1	14	1 strch, 2 med-fat meat, 2 fat
Chicken Chunks (5)	270	18	18	3	20	720	1	12	1 strch, 2 med-fat meat, 2 fat
Chicken Chunks, Southern Fried (5)	270	17	16	4	20	550	1	11	1 strch, 1 med-fat meat, 2 fat
Chicken Nuggets (10)	280	16	17	4	25	610	1	14	1 strch, 2 med-fat meat, 1 fat
Chicken Patties (1)	190	12	11	3	20	490	1	9	1 strch, 1 med-fat meat, 1 fat
Chicken Patties, Southern Fried (1)	190	12	12	3	20	440	1	9	1 strch, 1 med-fat meat, 1 fat
HEALTHY CHOICE									
Franks, Low-Fat (1)	70	7	3	1	15	440	0	6	1/2 carb., 1 lean meat
Ham, Deli Thin Cooked (6 slices)	60	1	2	<1	25	470	0	9	1 lean meat
Turkey Breast, Deli Thin (6 slices)	60	2	2	<1	20	470	0	9	1 lean meat
LIBBY'S									
Chicken Vienna Sausage (2 oz)	130	3	10	NA	NA	560	0	7	1 high-fat meat

MEATS, FISH, AND POULTRY

Products	Cal.	Carb. (g)	Fat (g)	Sat. Fat (g)	Chol. (mg)	Sod. (mg)	Fib. (g)	Prot. (g)	Servings/Exchanges
Potted Meat (1.83 oz)	110	0	9	NA	NA	320	0	7	1 high-fat meat
Vienna Sausage (2 oz)	160	1	15	NA	NA	330	0	6	1 high-fat meat, 1 fat
Vienna Sausage in BBQ Sauce (2.5 oz)	180	2	15	NA	NA	420	0	8	1 high-fat meat, 1 fat
LOUIS RICH									
Chicken, White, Oven-Roasted, Cold Cut (1 slice)	36	<1	2	<1	16	335	0	5	1 lean meat
Chicken Breast, Deluxe Roasted, Cold Cut (1 slice)	30	1	1	NA	15	330	0	5	1 very lean meat
Chicken Breast, Hickory-Smoked, Cold Cut (1 slice)	30	<1	<1	<1	14	356	0	5	1 very lean meat
Franks, Turkey & Chicken (1)	101	1	8	3	42	505	0	6	1 med-fat meat
Franks, Turkey & Chicken, Bun-Length (1)	128	2	10	3	53	640	0	7	1 high-fat meat
Franks, Turkey & Cheese (1)	109	1	9	3	44	523	0	6	1 high-fat meat
Ham, Baked in Juices (2 slices)	44	1	1	<1	12	248	0	8	1 very lean meat
Ham, Dinner Slice, Baked (1 slice)	84	0	2	<1	39	1133	0	16	2 very lean meat
Ham, Honey, Thin-Cut (6 slices)	70	2	2	1	35	760	0	11	1 lean meat
Ham, Honey, Traditional (2 slices)	68	2	2	<1	33	761	0	11	1 lean meat

Food	Cal.							Exchanges
Ham, Smoked (1 oz)	33	0	1	<1	15	372	0	5	1 very lean meat
Turkey, Ground (3 oz)	137	0	8	3	73	109	0	16	3 lean meat
Turkey & Cheddar Smoked Sausage (2 oz)	94	2	6	2	35	540	0	9	2 lean meat
Turkey Bacon (1 slice)	34	<1	3	<1	13	184	0	2	1 fat
Turkey Bologna (1 oz)	51	1	4	1	19	270	0	3	1 med-fat meat
Turkey Bologna, Chunk (1 oz)	51	1	4	1	19	270	0	3	1 med-fat meat
Turkey Breast, Carving Board (2 slices)	40	0	<1	0	20	560	0	9	1 very lean meat
Turkey Breast, Hickory-Smoked, Dinner Slice (1 slice)	80	2	1	0	35	1060	0	16	2 very lean meat
Turkey Breast, Hickory-Smoked, Fat-Free (1 slice)	23	1	<1	<1	10	300	0	4	1 very lean meat
Turkey Breast, Hickory-Smoked, Skinless (2 oz)	53	1	<1	<1	23	746	0	11	2 very lean meat
Turkey Breast, Honey-Roasted, Cold Cut (1 slice)	35	1	1	NA	10	315	0	5	1 very lean meat
Turkey Breast, Honey-Roasted, Dinner Slice (1 slice)	80	3	1	<1	35	940	0	16	2 very lean meat
Turkey Breast, Oven-Roasted, Cold Cut (1 slice)	30	1	1	NA	10	315	0	5	1 very lean meat
Turkey Breast, Oven-Roasted, Dinner Slice (1 slice)	70	NA	1	0	35	910	0	16	2 very lean meat
Turkey Breast, Roasted, Chunk (2 oz)	60	2	2	<1	25	640	0	10	2 very lean meat

MEATS, FISH, AND POULTRY

Products	Cal.	Carb. (g)	Fat (g)	Sat. Fat (g)	Chol. (mg)	Sod. (mg)	Fib. (g)	Prot. (g)	Servings/Exchanges
Turkey Breast, Roasted, Deli Thin (4 slices)	40	4	4	NA	20	500	0	8	1 med-fat meat
Turkey Breast, Roasted, Fat-Free (1 slice)	24	1	<1	<1	9	334	0	4	1 very lean meat
Turkey Breast, Smoked, Carving Board (2 slices)	42	<1	<1	<1	18	544	0	9	1 very lean meat
Turkey Breast, Smoked, Cold Cut (1 slice)	21	<1	<1	<1	9	211	0	5	1 very lean meat
Turkey Breast, Smoked, Deli Thin (4 slices)	40	4	4	0	20	440	0	8	1 med-fat meat
Turkey Cotto Salami (1 slice)	42	<1	3	<1	22	285	0	4	1 lean meat
Turkey Ham (1 slice)	32	<1	1	<1	19	316	0	5	1 very lean meat
Turkey Ham, Chopped (1 slice)	46	<1	3	<1	19	289	0	5	1 lean meat
Turkey Ham, Chunk (2 oz)	68	<1	2	1	38	600	0	10	1 lean meat
Turkey Ham, Deli Thin (4 slices)	48	<1	2	<1	28	444	0	8	1 lean meat
Turkey Ham, Honey-Cured (1 slice)	25	1	1	<1	15	215	0	4	1 lean meat
Turkey Nuggets, Breaded (4)	308	16	18	4	44	760	<1	16	1 strch, 2 med-fat meat, 2 fat
Turkey Pastrami, Chunk (2 oz)	64	<1	2	<1	36	576	0	10	1 lean meat
Turkey Patties (1)	115	0	6	2	70	338	0	19	2 lean meat

Turkey Polska Kielbasa Sausage (2 oz)	80	<1	4	2	38	494	0	9	1 med-fat
Turkey Salami (1 slice)	41	<1	3	<1	21	281	0	4	1 lean meat
Turkey Salami, Chunk (2 oz)	111	2	8	3	40	530	0	8	1 med-fat meat
Turkey Sausage Links (2)	92	<1	6	6	36	468	0	11	2 lean meat
Turkey Sausage, Ground, Cooked (1 oz)	56	<1	35	2	22	215	0	6	1 med-fat meat
Turkey Sausage, Smoked (2 oz)	90	2	5	2	36	515	0	8	1 med-fat meat
Turkey Sticks, Breaded (3)	230	12	15	3	35	580	0	12	1 strch, 1 med-fat meat, 2 fat
MRS. PAUL'S									
Deviled Crabs (3 oz)	180	19	9	3	24	540	<1	7	2 carb, 2 fat
Fish Portions, Battered (2)	250	20	16	5	30	430	2	9	1 strch, 1 med-fat meat, 2 fat
Fish Portions, Breaded (2)	190	16	10	3	15	280	1	9	1 strch, 1 med-fat meat, 1 fat
Fish Shapes, Sea Pals Breaded (5)	190	18	9	3	20	320	1	9	1 strch, 1 med-fat meat, 1 fat
Fish Sticks, Breaded (6)	210	19	11	2	20	370	1	9	1 strch, 1 med-fat meat, 1 fat
Fish Sticks, Breaded Minis (12)	220	20	11	3	30	330	2	11	1 strch, 1 med-fat meat, 1 fat
Fish Sticks, Healthy Treasure, Breaded (4)	170	20	3	2	20	350	2	10	1 strch, 1 lean meat
Premium Fillets, Haddock (1)	230	18	11	3	35	450	2	16	1 strch, 2 med-fat meat

MEATS, FISH, AND POULTRY

Products	Cal.	Carb. (g)	Fat (g)	Sat. Fat (g)	Chol. (mg)	Sod. (mg)	Fib. (g)	Prot. (g)	Servings/Exchanges
Premium Fillets, Sole (1)	250	22	13	4	40	510	2	14	1 1/2 strch, 2 med-fat meat, 1 fat
Shrimp, Breaded, Garlic & Herb (1)	340	33	15	3	110	910	3	19	2 strch, 2 med-fat meat, 1 fat
Shrimp, Breaded, Special Recipe (1)	350	32	16	3	95	720	2	20	2 strch, 2 med-fat meat, 1 fat
OSCAR MAYER									
Bacon (2 slices)	70	0	6	2	15	290	0	4	1 med-fat meat
Bacon, 1/8-inch Thick Cut (1 slice)	60	0	5	2	10	250	0	4	1 med-fat meat
Bacon, Canadian-Style (2 slices)	50	0	2	1	25	620	0	8	1 lean meat
Bacon, Lower Sodium (2 slices)	70	0	5	2	15	200	0	5	1 med-fat meat
Bacon Bits, Real (1 Tbsp)	25	0	2	<1	5	220	0	3	1 fat
Bologna (1 slice)	90	1	8	3	30	290	0	3	1 high-fat meat
Bologna, Beef (1 slice)	90	1	8	4	20	310	0	3	1 high-fat meat
Bologna, Beef, Light (1 slice)	60	2	4	2	15	310	0	3	1 med-fat meat
Bologna, Fat-Free (1 slice)	20	2	0	0	5	280	0	4	1 very lean meat

Food									Exchanges
Bologna, Garlic (1 slice)	130	1	12	5	40	420	0	4	1 high-fat meat, 1 fat
Bologna, Light (1 slice)	60	2	4	2	15	310	0	3	1 med-fat meat
Bologna, Wisconsin-Made Ring (2 oz)	180	2	16	6	35	460	0	6	1 high-fat meat, 2 fat
Chicken Breast, Oven-Roasted, Fat-Free (4 slices)	45	1	0	0	25	650	0	10	1 very lean meat
Franks, Beef (1)	140	1	13	6	30	460	0	5	1 high-fat meat, 1 fat
Franks, Beef, Bun-Length (1)	180	2	17	7	35	580	0	6	1 high-fat meat, 2 fat
Franks, Beef, Fat-Free (1)	40	3	0	0	15	460	0	7	1 very lean meat
Franks, Beef, Light (1)	110	2	8	4	30	620	0	6	1 high-fat meat
Franks, Big & Juicy Deli-Style (1)	230	1	22	10	50	680	0	9	2 high-fat meat, 1 fat
Franks, Big & Juicy Original Beef (1)	240	1	22	9	45	700	0	9	2 high-fat meat, 1 fat
Franks, Big & Juicy Quarter Pound Beef (1)	350	2	33	13	65	1050	0	13	2 high-fat meat, 3 fat
Ham, Baked (3 slices)	70	2	3	1	30	790	0	11	1 lean meat
Ham, Baked, Fat-Free (3 slices)	35	1	0	0	15	520	0	7	1 very lean meat
Ham, Boiled (3 slices)	60	0	3	1	30	820	0	10	1 lean meat
Ham, Chopped w/Natural Juices (1 slice)	50	1	3	2	15	340	0	4	1 lean meat
Ham, Honey (3 slices)	70	2	3	1	30	760	0	10	1 lean meat

MEATS, FISH, AND POULTRY

Products	Cal.	Carb. (g)	Fat (g)	Sat. Fat (g)	Chol. (mg)	Sod. (mg)	Fib. (g)	Prot. (g)	Servings/Exchanges
Ham, Honey, Fat-Free (3 slices)	35	2	0	0	15	580	0	7	1 very lean meat
Ham, Lower Sodium (3 slices)	70	2	3	1	30	520	0	10	1 lean meat
Ham, Smoked (3 slices)	60	0	2	1	30	760	0	11	1 lean meat
Ham, Smoked, Fat-Free (3 slices)	35	1	0	0	15	550	0	7	1 very lean meat
Ham & Cheese Loaf (1 slice)	70	1	5	3	20	350	0	4	1 med-fat meat
Head Cheese (1 slice)	50	0	4	2	25	360	0	5	1 med-fat meat
Hot Dogs, Cheese (1)	140	1	13	5	1	510	0	5	1 high-fat meat, 1 fat
Hot Dogs, Fat-Free (1)	50	2	0	0	15	490	0	6	1 very lean meat
Liver Cheese (1 slice)	120	1	10	4	80	420	0	6	1 high-fat meat
Luncheon Loaf, Spiced (1 slice)	70	2	5	2	20	340	0	4	1 med-fat meat
Old-Fashioned Loaf (1 slice)	70	2	5	2	15	330	0	4	1 med-fat meat
Olive Loaf (1 slice)	70	2	6	2	20	370	0	3	1 med-fat meat
Pepperoni (15 slices)	140	0	13	5	25	550	0	6	1 high-fat meat, 1 fat
Pickle & Pimento Loaf (1 slice)	80	3	6	2	20	360	0	3	1 med-fat meat

Salami for Beer (2 slices)	110	1	9	3	30	580	0	6	1 high-fat meat
Salami, Hard (3 slices)	100	0	9	3	25	510	0	6	1 high-fat meat
Salami, Cotto (1 slice)	70	1	5	2	25	280	0	3	1 med-fat meat
Salami, Cotto, Beef (1 slice)	60	1	5	2	25	370	0	4	1 med-fat meat
Salami, Genoa (3 slices)	100	0	9	3	25	490	0	5	1 high-fat meat
Sandwich Spread (2 oz)	130	8	10	4	25	460	0	4	1/2 strch, 1 high-fat meat
Sausage, Liver, Braunschweiger (1 slice)	100	1	9	3	50	320	0	4	1 high-fat meat
Sausage, Liver, Braunschweiger Spread (2 oz)	190	2	17	6	90	630	0	8	1 high-fat meat, 2 fat
Sausage, New England Brand (2 slices)	60	1	3	1	25	570	0	8	1 lean meat
Sausage, Pork Links (2)	170	1	15	5	40	410	0	9	2 high-fat meat
Sausage, Smokie Links (1)	130	1	12	4	25	430	0	5	1 high-fat meat, 1 fat
Sausage, Smokies Little (6)	170	1	15	6	35	570	0	7	1 high-fat meat, 2 fat
Sausage, Smokies Little Cheese (6)	180	1	16	6	40	590	0	7	1 high-fat meat, 2 fat
Sausage, Summer (2 slices)	140	0	13	5	40	650	0	7	1 high-fat meat, 1 fat
Sausage, Summer, Beef (2 slices)	140	1	12	5	35	640	0	7	1 high-fat meat, 1 fat
Turkey, White, Oven-Roasted (1 slice)	30	1	1	0	10	300	0	4	1 very lean meat

MEATS, FISH, AND POULTRYS

Products	Cal.	Carb. (g)	Fat (g)	Sat. Fat (g)	Chol. (mg)	Sod. (mg)	Fib. (g)	Prot. (g)	Servings/Exchanges
Turkey, White, Smoked (1 slice)	30	1	1	0	10	310	0	4	1 very lean meat
Turkey Breast, Oven-Roasted, Fat-Free (4 slices)	40	2	0	0	15	670	0	8	1 very lean meat
Turkey Breast, Smoked, Fat-Free (4 slices)	40	2	0	0	15	570	0	8	1 very lean meat
Wieners (1)	150	1	13	5	35	430	0	5	1 high-fat meat, 1 fat
Wieners, Big & Juicy Hot 'N Spicy (1)	220	1	20	8	45	750	0	10	2 high-fat meat, 1 fat
Wieners, Big & Juicy Original (1)	240	1	22	9	45	690	0	9	2 high-fat meat, 1 fat
Wieners, Big & Juicy Smokie Links (1)	220	1	19	7	50	770	0	10	2 high-fat meat, 1 fat
Wieners, Bun-Length (1)	190	2	17	6	40	550	0	6	1 high-fat meat, 2 fat
Wieners, Light (1)	110	2	8	3	35	590	0	7	1 high-fat meat
Wieners, Little (6)	180	2	17	6	35	570	0	6	1 high-fat meat, 2 fat
PROGRESSO									
Clams, Minced (1/4 cup)	25	2	0	0	10	250	0	4	1 very lean meat
Tuna, Solid in Olive Oil (1/4 cup)	160	0	12	2	30	250	0	13	2 med-fat meat

RED DEVIL

Food	Cal	Carb (g)	Fat (g)	Sat. Fat (g)	Chol (mg)	Sod (mg)	Fiber (g)	Pro (g)	Exchanges
Snackers, Chunky Chicken (1/4 cup)	140	2	10	3	30	400	0	10	1 strch, 1 high-fat meat
Snackers, Deviled Ham (1/4 cup)	140	3	11	4	30	410	0	7	1 strch, 2 high-fat meat

SLIM JIM

Food	Cal	Carb (g)	Fat (g)	Sat. Fat (g)	Chol (mg)	Sod (mg)	Fiber (g)	Pro (g)	Exchanges
Beef Jerky, Big Jerk (.25 oz)	25	1	1	0	NA	220	0	3	1 very lean meat
Beef Jerky, Giant Jerk (.63 oz)	60	2	2	NA	NA	510	0	7	1 very lean meat

SWANSON

Food	Cal	Carb (g)	Fat (g)	Sat. Fat (g)	Chol (mg)	Sod (mg)	Fiber (g)	Pro (g)	Exchanges
Chicken, Chunk (2.5 oz)	130	1	8	NA	NA	230	0	13	2 med-fat meat
Chicken, Chunk White, in Water (2.5 oz)	100	0	4	NA	35	240	0	15	2 lean meat
Chicken, Chunk, White/Dark (2.5 oz)	100	0	4	NA	40	240	0	16	2 lean meat
Turkey, Chunk White, in Water (2.5 oz)	80	1	1	<1	NA	260	0	17	2 very lean meat

TYSON

Food	Cal	Carb (g)	Fat (g)	Sat. Fat (g)	Chol (mg)	Sod (mg)	Fiber (g)	Pro (g)	Exchanges
Chicken Breast, Baked (3 oz)	116	0	2	NA	72	63	0	24	3 very lean meat
Chicken Nuggets (3 oz)	207	9	14	4	49	383	<1	11	1/2 strch, 1 med-fat meat, 2 fat
Cornish Hen (3.5 oz)	240	0	14	NA	75	70	0	28	4 lean meat

MEATS, FISH, AND POULTRY

Products	Cal.	Carb. (g)	Fat (g)	Sat. Fat (g)	Chol. (mg)	Sod. (mg)	Fib. (g)	Prot. (g)	Servings/Exchanges
UNDERWOOD									
Chicken Spread, Chunky (1/4 cup)	120	2	8	3	40	390	0	9	1 high-fat meat
Ham Spread, Deviled (1/4 cup)	160	0	14	5	45	440	0	8	1 high-fat meat, 1 fat
Ham Spread, Honey (1/4 cup)	140	5	11	4	30	370	0	6	1 med-fat meat, 1 fat
Liverwurst Spread (1/4 cup)	170	3	14	5	65	380	1	7	1 high-fat meat, 1 fat
Roast Beef Spread (1/4 cup)	140	0	11	5	45	390	0	9	1 high-fat meat, 1 fat
Sardines in Mustard Sauce (3.8-oz can)	180	2	12	3	105	820	1	17	2 med-fat meat
Sardines in Soy Oil, Drained (3.8-oz can)	220	1	16	4	100	310	0	18	2 high-fat meat
Sardines in Tomato Sauce (3.8-oz can)	180	4	11	3	115	960	1	16	2 med-fat meat
Tuna Spread, Lightly Seasoned (1/4 cup)	50	2	1	0	30	480	0	9	1 very lean meat
VAN DE KAMP'S									
Battered Fish Portions (2)	350	26	22	4	20	710	0	6	2 carb., 1 med-fat meat, 3 fat
Cheese & Crab Poppers (4)	320	27	16	7	35	800	<1	17	2 strch, 2 med-fat meat, 1 fat
Cod Fillets, Premium Breaded (1)	230	18	11	2	35	400	0	14	1 strch, 2 med-fat meat

Food								Exchanges
Crab Cakes (1)	170	17	9	2	15	460	<1	6	1 strch, 2 fat
Fillets, Breaded, Garlic & Herb Crisp & Healthy (2)	170	25	3	<1	25	450	0	11	1 1/2 strch, 1 med-fat meat
Fillets, Breaded, Lemon Pepper Crisp & Healthy (2)	170	24	3	<1	25	450	0	11	1 1/2 strch, 1 med-fat meat, 1 fat
Fillets, Grilled Garlic Butter (1)	120	0	6	1	60	210	0	17	2 lean meat
Fillets, Grilled Lemon Butter (1)	120	0	6	1	60	190	0	17	2 lean meat
Fish Fillet, Battered (1)	170	13	10	2	20	390	0	8	1 strch, 1 med-fat meat, 1 fat
Fish Fillets, Breaded (2)	260	17	17	3	25	380	0	10	1 strch, 1 med-fat meat, 2 fat
Fish Sticks, Breaded (6)	290	22	17	3	30	420	0	12	1 1/2 strch, 1 med-fat meat, 2 fat
Fish Sticks, Mini, Breaded (13)	250	19	14	2	30	330	0	11	1 strch, 1 med-fat meat, 2 fat
Fish Sticks Snack Pack (6)	260	20	15	3	25	360	0	11	1 strch, 1 med-fat meat, 2 fat
Fish Tenders, Battered (4)	290	24	17	3	25	590	0	11	1 1/2 strch, 1 med-fat meat, 2 fat
Flounder Fillet, Premium Breaded (1)	230	18	11	2	40	390	0	14	1 strch, 2 lean meat
Haddock Fillets, Battered (2)	240	19	12	2	25	530	0	12	1 strch, 1 med-fat meat, 1 fat

MEATS, FISH, AND POULTRY

Products	Cal.	Carb. (g)	Fat (g)	Sat. Fat (g)	Chol. (mg)	Sod. (mg)	Fib. (g)	Prot. (g)	Servings/Exchanges
Haddock Fillets, Premium Breaded (2)	230	18	11	2	35	410	0	14	1 strch, 2 med-fat meat
Halibut Fillets, Battered (3)	220	19	10	2	25	530	0	13	1 strch, 1 med-fat meat, 1 fat
Ocean Perch Fillets, Battered (2)	240	20	13	3	25	510	0	11	1 strch, 1 med-fat meat, 2 fat
Shrimp, Butterfly, Breaded (7)	300	30	15	3	80	610	3	10	2 strch, 1 med-fat meat, 2 fat
Shrimp, Popcorn, Breaded (20)	270	30	12	2	80	850	2	10	2 strch, 1 med-fat meat, 2 fat
Shrimp, Stuffed (3)	290	32	13	5	70	720	<1	12	2 strch, 1 med-fat meat, 1 fat

MILK AND YOGURT

Products	Cal.	Carb. (g)	Fat (g)	Sat. Fat (g)	Chol. (mg)	Sod. (mg)	Fib. (g)	Prot. (g)	Servings/Exchanges
Buttermilk, Skim, Cultured (1 cup)	99	12	2	1	9	257	0	8	1 skim milk
Carob Flavor Beverage Mix w/Milk (1 cup)	195	23	8	5	33	133	1	9	1 whole milk, 1 carb.
Carob Flavor Beverage Mix, Powder (1 Tbsp)	45	11	<1	<1	0	12	<1	<1	1 carb.
Chocolate Drink, Syrup w/Reduced-Fat Milk (1 cup)	181	30	5	3	16	140	<1	8	1 reduced-fat milk, 1 carb.
Chocolate Malted Milk Drink (1 cup)	228	30	9	5	35	172	<1	9	1 whole milk, 1 carb.
Cocoa, Sugar-Free, Mix w/Water, (1 pkt)	48	9	<1	<1	1	168	<1	4	1/2 skim milk
Cocoa/Hot Chocolate Mix w/Water (1 pkt)	102	22	1	<1	1	143	<1	3	1/2 skim milk, 1 carb.
Cocoa/Hot Chocolate Mix w/Whole Milk (1 cup)	193	30	6	4	20	128	2	10	1 whole milk, 1 carb.
Cocoa Mix, Sugar-Free, w/Reduced-Fat Milk (1 cup)	136	15	6	3	18	160	2	9	1 reduced-fat milk
Cocoa Mix, Sugar-Free w/Water (1 cup)	63	11	<1	<1	3	230	<1	5	1 skim milk
Eggnog (1 cup)	343	34	19	11	149	138	0	10	1 whole milk, 1 1/2 carb., 2 fat

MILK AND YOGURT

Products	Cal.	Carb. (g)	Fat (g)	Sat. Fat (g)	Chol. (mg)	Sod. (mg)	Fib. (g)	Prot. (g)	Servings/Exchanges
Eggnog, 2% Reduced-Fat (1 cup)	189	17	8	4	194	155	0	12	1 whole milk
Instant Breakfast Powder (1 pkt)	131	25	<1	<1	4	142	<1	7	1 skim milk, 1 carb.
Milk, 1%, Low-Fat (1 cup)	102	12	3	2	10	123	0	8	1 skim milk
Milk, 1%, Low-Fat , Acidophilus (1 cup)	102	12	3	2	10	123	0	8	1 skim milk
Milk, 1%, Low-Fat, Chocolate (1 cup)	158	26	3	2	7	152	1	9	1 skim milk, 1 carb.
Milk, 1%, Low-Fat, Protein-Fortified (1 cup)	119	14	3	2	10	143	0	10	1 skim milk
Milk, 2%, Reduced-Fat (1 cup)	121	12	5	3	18	122	0	8	1 reduced-fat milk
Milk, 2%, Reduced-Fat, Chocolate (1 cup)	179	26	5	3	17	151	1	9	1 reduced-fat milk, 1 carb.
Milk, 2%, Reduced-Fat, Protein-Fortified (1 cup)	137	14	5	3	19	145	0	10	1 reduced-fat milk
Milk, Evaporated Skim (1 cup)	199	29	<1	<1	9	293	0	19	2 skim milk
Milk, Evaporated Whole (1 cup)	338	25	19	12	74	267	0	17	2 whole milk
Milk, Fat-Free Chocolate (1 cup)	144	27	1	<1	4	121	2	9	1 skim milk, 1 carb.
Milk, Fat-Free Powder w/Water (1 cup)	82	12	<1	<1	4	131	0	8	1 skim milk
Milk, Fat-Free (1 cup)	86	12	<1	<1	4	126	0	8	1 skim milk

Food	Cal								Exchanges
Milk, Fat-Free, Lactose-Reduced (1 cup)	86	12	<1	<1	4	126	0	9	1 skim milk
Milk, Fat-Free, Protein-Fortified (1 cup)	100	14	<1	<1	5	144	0	10	1 skim milk
Milk, Goat (1 cup)	168	11	10	7	28	122	0	9	1 whole milk
Milk, Soy (1 cup)	81	4	5	<1	0	29	3	7	1 reduced-fat milk
Milk, Sweetened Condensed, Canned (1 cup)	982	166	27	17	104	389	0	24	3 whole milk, 9 carb.
Milk, Whole (1 cup)	150	11	8	5	33	120	8	8	1 whole milk
Milk, Whole, Chocolate (1 cup)	209	26	9	5	3*	149	2	8	1 whole milk, 1 carb.
Yogurt, Low-Fat, Custard-Style, Fruit (1 cup)	253	43	5	4	20	127	0	9	1 reduced-fat milk, 2 carb.
Yogurt, Low-Fat, Fruit & Nuts (1 cup)	290	47	7	2	10	139	<1	11	1 1/2 ow-fat milk, 2 carb.
Yogurt, Low-Fat, Fruit (1 cup)	250	47	3	2	10	143	<1	11	1 1/2 skim milk, 2 carb.
Yogurt, Low-Fat, Plain (1 cup)	155	17	4	3	15	172	0	13	1 reduced-fat milk
Yogurt, Nonfat, Fruit w/LoCal Sweetener (1 cup)	122	19	<1	<1	3	139	1	12	1 skim milk, 1/2 carb.
Yogurt, Nonfat, Plain (1 cup)	137	19	<1	<1	4	187	0	15	1 1/2 skim milk
Yogurt, Whole-Milk, Plain (1 cup)	150	11	8	5	31	114	0	9	1 whole milk

ALBA

Food	Cal								Exchanges
Cocoa Mix, Powder (1 pkt)	62	10	<1	NA	4	134	NA	5	1 skim milk

MILK AND YOGURT

Products	Cal.	Carb. (g)	Fat (g)	Sat. Fat (g)	Chol. (mg)	Sod. (mg)	Fib. (g)	Prot. (g)	Servings/Exchanges
Shake Mix, Chocolate, w/Water (1 pkt)	60	10	0	0	0	160	NA	6	1 skim milk
Shake Mix, Vanilla, w/Water (1 pkt)	70	12	0	0	0	150	NA	5	1 skim milk
BREYERS									
Yogurt, 1% Lowfat Blended, Blueberry (4.4 oz)	130	25	1	<1	10	60	0	4	1/2 skim milk, 1 carb.
Yogurt, 1% Lowfat Strawberry (4.4 oz)	130	26	1	<1	10	60	0	4	1/2 skim milk, 1 carb.
Yogurt, 1% Lowfat, Blueberry (8 oz)	230	43	3	2	15	125	0	9	1 skim milk, 2 carb.
Yogurt, 1% Lowfat, Strawberry (8 oz)	230	43	3	2	15	125	0	9	1 skim milk, 2 carb.
Yogurt, 1% Smooth & Creamy Classic Strawberry (8 oz)	230	45	2	1	20	125	0	9	1 skim milk, 2 carb.
Yogurt, 1% Smooth & Creamy, Blueberries 'N Cream (8 oz)	240	46	2	1	20	125	0	9	1 skim milk, 2 carb.
Yogurt, Nonfat Blueberries N' Cream (8 oz)	120	23	0	0	10	100	0	8	1 skim milk, 1 carb.
Yogurt, Nonfat Classic Strawberry (8 oz)	120	22	0	0	10	100	0	8	1 skim milk, 1 carb.

CARNATION

Cocoa Mix w/Marshmallow (1 pkt)	120	23	3	2	<5	170	<1	1	1 1/2 carb., 1 fat
Cocoa Mix, No Sugar Added (1 pkt)	50	9	<1	0	0	170	<1	4	1/2 carb.
Cocoa Mix, Rich Chocolate (1 pkt)	120	23	3	2	<5	180	<1	1	1 1/2 carb., 1 fat
Instant Breakfast, Cafe Mocha (1 pkt)	130	28	<1	0	3	100	<1	5	2 carb.
Instant Breakfast, Chocolate Malt, No Sugar Added (1 pkg)	70	11	2	1	3	115	1	5	1 carb.
Instant Breakfast, French Vanilla (1 pkt)	130	27	0	0	3	110	0	5	2 carb.
Instant Breakfast, Milk Chocolate (1 pkt)	130	28	1	<1	<5	100	1	4	2 carb.
Instant Breakfast, Milk Chocolate, No Sugar Added (1 pkt)	70	12	1	<1	<5	95	1	4	1 carb.
Instant Breakfast, Strawberry Cream (1 pkt)	130	28	0	0	NA	160	0	5	2 carb.
Instant Breakfast, Vanilla, No Sugar Added (1 pkt)	70	12	0	0	<5	95	0	4	1 carb.
Milk, Evaporated Low-Fat (2 Tbsp)	25	3	<1	0	5	35	0	2	free
Milk, Evaporated (2 Tbsp)	40	3	2	2	10	30	0	2	2 whole milk
Milk, Sweetened Condensed (2 Tbsp)	130	22	3	2	10	45	0	3	1 1/2 carb., 1 fat

MILK AND YOGURT

Products	Cal.	Carb. (g)	Fat (g)	Sat. Fat (g)	Chol. (mg)	Sod. (mg)	Fib. (g)	Prot. (g)	Servings/Exchanges
Sweet Success Creamy Milk Chocolate Powder (1 scoop)	90	24	<1	<1	2	125	6	3	1 1/2 carb.
Sweet Success Creamy Milk Chocolate Shake (10 oz)	200	32	3	<1	5	230	6	11	1 skim milk, 1 1/2 carb.
Sweet Success Creamy Vanilla Delight (10 oz)	200	32	3	<1	NA	230	6	11	1 skim milk, 1 1/2 carb.
Sweet Success Drink, Chocolate Chip (1 scoop)	90	12	2	NA	NA	300	6	7	1 low-fat milk
Sweet Success Drink, Chocolate Fudge (10 oz)	200	32	3	NA	NA	210	6	11	1 skim milk, 1 carb., 1 fat
Sweet Success Shake, Chocolate Mocha (10 oz)	200	32	3	0	NA	230	6	11	1 skim milk, 2 carb.
COLOMBO									
Yogurt, Fat Free, Banana/Strawberry (8 oz)	220	47	0	0	5	90	0	7	1 skim milk, 2 carb.
Yogurt, Fat Free, Fruited Flavors (8 oz)	200	42	0	0	5	105	0	7	1 skim milk, 2 carb.
Yogurt, Fat Free, Lemon & Vanilla (8 oz)	160	32	0	0	5	120	0	8	1 skim milk, 1 carb.
Yogurt, Fat Free, Plain (8 oz)	100	16	0	0	0	125	0	10	1 skim milk
Yogurt, Light, All Flavors (8 oz)	100	17	0	0	<5	110	0	7	1 skim milk

DANNON

Danimals, Lowfat Wild Raspberry (4 oz)	110	20	<1	0	5	85	0	5	1/2 skim milk, 1/2 carb.
Danimals, Lowfat Tropical Punch (4 oz)	120	22	<1	0	5	85	0	5	1/2 skim milk, 1/2 carb.
Double Delights, Blueberry French Vanilla (6 oz)	180	36	1	<1	5	105	0	7	1 skim milk, 1 1/2 carb.
Double Delights, Chocolate Cheesecake (6 oz)	220	46	1	<1	5	160	0	8	1 skim milk, 2 carb.
Double Delights, Lemon Meringue Pie (6 oz)	180	37	1	<1	5	190	0	7	1 skim milk, 1 1/2 carb.
Double Delights, Strawberry Cheesecake (6 oz)	170	33	1	<1	5	115	0	7	1 skim milk, 1 carb.
Yogurt, Fat-Free Blenced, Raspberry (4 oz)	100	21	0	0	<5	75	0	5	1 skim milk, 1/2 carb.
Yogurt, Fat-Free Blended, Strawberry Banana (4 oz)	100	21	0	0	<5	75	0	5	1 skim milk, 1/2 carb.
Yogurt, Fruit-On-The-Bottom, Blueberry (8 oz)	220	41	2	1	10	210	<1	9	1 skim milk, 2 carb.
Yogurt, Fruit-On-The-Bottom, Peach (8 oz)	210	40	2	1	10	150	<1	9	1 skim milk, 2 carb.
Yogurt, Fruit-On-The-Bottom Snackpack, Mixed Berry (4 oz)	110	20	1	<1	5	95	0	5	1/2 skim milk, 1/2 carb.
Yogurt, Fruit-On-The-Bottom Snackpack, Strawberry (4 oz)	110	20	1	<1	5	70	0	5	1/2 skim milk, 1/2 carb.

MILK AND YOGURT

Products	Cal.	Carb. (g)	Fat (g)	Sat. Fat (g)	Chol. (mg)	Sod. (mg)	Fib. (g)	Prot. (g)	Servings/Exchanges
Yogurt, Fruit-On-The-Bottom, Strawberry (8 oz)	210	40	2	1	10	140	<1	9	1 skim milk, 2 carb.
Yogurt, Fruit-On-The-Bottom, Strawberry Banana (8 oz)	210	40	2	1	10	140	<1	9	1 skim milk, 2 carb.
Yogurt, Light Nonfat, Banana Creme Pie (8 oz)	120	21	0	0	5	130	0	8	1 skim milk, 1/2 carb.
Yogurt, Light Nonfat, Blueberry (8 oz)	120	23	0	0	5	130	0	8	1 skim milk, 1 carb.
Yogurt, Light Nonfat, Cherry Vanilla (8 oz)	120	23	0	0	5	135	0	8	1 skim milk, 1 carb.
Yogurt, Light Nonfat Snackpack, Raspberry (4 oz)	125	11	0	0	<5	85	0	4	1/2 skim milk, 1/2 carb.
Yogurt, Light Nonfat Snackpack, Strawberry (4 oz)	113	11	0	0	<5	80	0	4	1/2 skim milk, 1/2 carb.
Yogurt, Light Nonfat, Strawberry (8 oz)	120	22	0	0	5	160	0	8	1 skim milk, 1/2 carb.
Yogurt, Light Nonfat, Cookies 'N Cream Crunch (8 oz)	160	32	<1	0	5	160	<1	NA	1 skim milk, 1 carb.
Yogurt, Strawberry Sprinkl'ins (4.1 oz)	130	25	1	1	5	85	0	5	1 skim milk, 1 carb.
Yogurt, Vanilla w/Cherry Crystals Sprinkl'ins (4.1 oz)	120	22	1	0	5	85	0	6	1 skim milk, 1/2 carb.

KRAFT

Yogurt, Light N' Lively Free Nonfat Blueberry (4.4 oz)	70	13	0	0	5	55	0	4	1 skim milk
Yogurt, Light N' Lively Free Nonfat Peach (4.4 oz)	70	12	0	0	5	65	0	4	1 skim milk
Yogurt, Light N' Lively Free Nonfat Strawberry (4.4 oz)	70	12	0	0	5	55	0	4	1 skim milk
Yogurt, Light N' Lively Low-Fat Blueberry (4.4 oz)	130	25	1	<1	10	60	0	4	1 skim milk, 1 carb.
Yogurt, Light N' Lively Low-Fat Peach (4.4 oz)	130	26	1	<1	10	65	0	4	1 skim milk, 1 carb.
Yogurt, Light N' Lively Low-Fat Pineapple (4.4 oz)	130	26	1	<1	10	60	0	4	1 skim milk, 1 carb.
Yogurt, Light N' Lively Low-Fat Red Raspberry (4.4 oz)	120	23	1	<1	10	65	0	5	1 skim milk, 1 carb.
Yogurt, Light N' Lively Low-Fat Strawberry (4.4 oz)	130	26	1	<1	10	60	0	4	1 skim milk, 1 carb.
Yogurt, Light N' Lively Low-Fat Strawberry Banana (4.4 oz)	130	25	1	<1	10	60	0	4	1 skim milk, 1 carb.

MILK AND YOGURT

Products	Cal.	Carb. (g)	Fat (g)	Sat. Fat (g)	Chol. (mg)	Sod. (mg)	Fib. (g)	Prot. (g)	Servings/Exchanges
Yogurt, Light N' Lively Low-Fat Strawberry Fruit Cup (4.4 oz)	130	25	1	<1	10	60	0	14	1 skim milk, 1 carb.
LACTAID									
Milk, Lactaid 100, Reduced-Fat (1 cup)	130	12	5	3	20	125	0	8	1 reduced-fat milk
Milk, Lactaid 100, Fat-Free (1 cup)	80	13	0	0	0	125	0	8	1 skim milk
OVALTINE									
Malted Milk Drink, Chocolate Malt (4 Tbsp)	80	18	0	0	0	115	<1	1	1 whole milk
Malted Milk Drink, Malt (4 Tbsp)	80	18	0	0	0	55	0	2	1 skim milk
Malted Milk Drink, Rich Chocolate (4 Tbsp)	80	19	0	0	0	140	0	<1	1 skim milk
PET									
Milk, Regular Evaporated (2 Tbsp)	40	3	2	2	10	30	0	2	1 fat
Milk, Skimmed Evaporated (2 Tbsp)	25	4	0	0	0	40	0	2	free
PILLSBURY									
Instant Breakfast, Chocolate (1 pkt)	130	26	<1	0	26	141	NA	6	2 carb.

Food	Cal.	Carb.	Fat	Sat. Fat	Chol.	Sod.	Fiber	Prot.	Exchanges
Instant Breakfast, Strawberry (1 pkt)	130	26	<1	NA	NA	130	NA	5	2 carb.
SLIM FAST									
Regular Slim Fast, Powder w/Skim Milk, Chocolate (1 cup)	190	32	1	1	NA	130	2	14	2 skim milk, 1/2 carb.
Regular Slim Fast, Powder w/Skim Milk, Vanilla (1 cup)	190	32	1	<1	NA	NA	2	14	2 skim milk, 1/2 carb.
Ultra Slim Fast, French Vanilla (11 oz can)	220	40	3	<1	5	220	5	10	1 1/2 skim milk, 1 1/2 carb.
Ultra Slim Fast, Orange Pineapple (11 oz can)	220	46	2	<1	10	200	5	7	1 skim milk, 2 carb.
Ultra Slim Fast, Powder w/Skim Milk, Chocolate Royale (1 cup)	200	36	2	1	5	130	5	14	2 skim milk, 1 carb.
Ultra Slim Fast, Powder w/Skim Milk, Vanilla (1 cup)	200	37	1	<1	5	130	5	14	2 skim milk, 1 carb.
Ultra Slim Fast, Rich Chocolate Royale (11 oz can)	220	38	3	1	5	220	5	10	1 1/2 slim milk, 1 carb.
SWISS MISS									
Cocoa Mix, Fat Free (1 pkt)	50	9	0	0	0	230	1	3	1 reduced-fat milk

MILK AND YOGURT

Products	Cal.	Carb. (g)	Fat (g)	Sat. Fat (g)	Chol. (mg)	Sod. (mg)	Fib. (g)	Prot. (g)	Servings/Exchanges
WEIGHT WATCHERS									
Cocoa Mix w/Marshmallows (1 pkt)	60	10	0	0	0	160	0	6	1 skim milk
Milk, Nonfat Skim (1 cup)	90	13	1	0	NA	140	0	9	1 skim milk
Yogurt, Ultimate 90, Nonfat Plain (1 cup)	90	13	1	0	5	135	0	10	1 skim milk
Yogurt, Ultimate 90, Nonfat Blueberry (1 cup)	90	13	0	0	5	120	0	10	1 skim milk
Yogurt, Ultimate 90, Nonfat Lemon (1 cup)	90	13	0	0	5	120	0	10	1 skim milk
Yogurt, Ultimate 90, Nonfat Strawberry (1 cup)	90	13	0	0	5	120	0	10	1 skim milk
YOPLAIT									
Yogurt, Custard-Style, Fruit Flavored Multi-Pack (4 oz)	120	21	2	2	10	60	0	5	1/2 skim milk, 1 carb.
Yogurt, Custard-Style, Fruit Flavors (6 oz)	190	32	4	2	15	90	0	7	1 skim milk, 1 carb.
Yogurt, Custard-Style, Vanilla (6 oz)	190	32	4	2	15	90	0	7	1 skim milk, 1 carb.
Yogurt, Go-Gurt, Fruit Flavored (2.25 oz)	70	11	2	1	5	30	0	3	1/2 skim milk, 1/2 carb.
Yogurt, Light, Fruit Flavors (6 oz)	90	15	0	0	<5	75	0	5	1 skim milk

	Cal.				C				
Yogurt, Light, Indulgent Flavors (6 oz)	90	15	0	0	<5	85	0	6	1 skim milk
Yogurt, Original 99% Fat-Free, Coconut Cream Pie (6 oz)	180	34	3	2	10	85	0	5	1 skim milk, 1 carb.
Yogurt, Original 99% Fat Free, Fruit Flavors (4 oz)	110	22	1	<1	5	55	0	4	1/2 skim milk, 1 carb.
Yogurt, Original 99% Fat-Free, Fruit Flavors (6 oz)	170	33	2	1	10	80	0	5	1 skim milk, 1 carb.
Yogurt, Original 99% Fat-Free, Lemon (6 oz)	180	36	2	1	10	80	0	5	1 skim milk, 1 1/2 carb.
Yogurt, Original 99% Fat-Free, Pina Colada (6 oz)	170	33	2	2	10	95	0	5	1 skim milk, 1 carb.
Yogurt, Trix Multi-Pack, Fruit Flavored (4 oz)	120	23	2	1	5	55	0	4	1/2 skim milk, 1 carb.

NUTS, SEEDS, AND NUT/SEED PRODUCTS

Products	Cal.	Carb. (g)	Fat (g)	Sat. Fat (g)	Chol. (mg)	Sod. (mg)	Fib. (g)	Prot. (g)	Servings/Exchanges
Almond Butter, Plain (1 Tbsp)	101	3	10	<1	0	2	<1	2	2 fat
Almond Butter, Salted (1 Tbsp)	98	3	9	<1	0	70	<1	2	2 fat
Almonds, Dried, Whole (1 oz)	165	6	15	1	0	3	4	5	1 med-fat meat, 2 fat
Almonds, Dry-Roasted (1 oz)	166	7	15	1	0	221	4	5	1 med-fat meat, 2 fat
Almonds, Dry-Roasted, Whole, Unsalted (1 oz)	166	7	15	1	0	3	4	5	1 med-fat meat, 2 fat
Almonds, Oil-Roasted (1 oz)	175	5	16	2	0	221	3	6	1 med-fat meat, 2 fat
Almonds, Toasted (1 oz)	167	7	14	1	0	3	3	6	1 med-fat meat, 2 fat
Beechnuts, Dried (1 oz)	164	10	14	2	0	11	<1	2	1/2 strch, 3 fat
Brazilnuts, Dried (1 oz)	186	4	19	5	0	<1	2	4	1 med-fat meat, 3 fat
Cashew Butter, Unsalted (1 Tbsp)	94	4	8	2	0	2	<1	3	2 fat
Cashews, Dry-Roasted (1 oz)	161	9	13	3	0	179	<1	5	1/2 strch, 3 fat
Cashews, Oil-Roasted (1 oz)	163	8	14	3	0	178	1	5	1/2 strch, 3 fat
Chinese Chestnuts, Dried (1 oz)	103	23	<1	<1	0	1	<1	2	1 1/2 strch

Food										Exchanges
Chinese Chestnuts, Roasted (1 oz)	68	15	<1	<1	0	1	<1	1		1 strch
Coconut, Dried, Shredded, Sweetened (1/4 cup)	117	11	8	7	0	61	1	<1	1	1 strch, 2 fat
Coconut, Fresh (2.5 x 2-inch piece)	159	7	15	13	0	9	4	2	2	1/2 strch, 3 fat
Coconut, Toasted (1 oz)	168	13	13	12	0	11	2	2	2	1 strch, 3 fat
Coconut Milk, Raw (1 cup)	552	13	57	51	0	36	5	6	6	1 strch, 11 fat
English Walnut Halves, Dried (1 oz)	182	5	18	2	0	3	1	4	4	1 med-fat meat, 3 fat
European Chestnuts, Roasted (1 oz)	69	15	<1	<1	0	<1	2	<1	<1	1 strch
Filberts/Hazelnuts, Dried, Whole (1 oz)	177	4	18	1	0	<1	2	4	4	1 med-fat meat, 3 fat
Filberts/Hazelnuts, Dry Roasted, Salted (1 oz)	188	5	18	1	0	221	2	3	3	3 fat
Filberts/Hazelnuts, Oil Roasted, Salted (1 oz)	187	6	18	1	0	223	2	4	4	1/2 strch, 3 fat
Hickory Nuts, Dried (1 oz)	186	5	18	2	0	<1	2	4	4	4 fat
Japanese Chestnuts, Dried (1 oz)	101	23	<1	<1	0	10	<1	2	2	1 1/2 strch
Japanese Chestnuts, Roasted (1 oz)	57	13	<1	<1	0	5	<1	<1	<1	1 strch
Macadamia Nuts (1 oz)	199	4	21	3	0	1	3	2	2	4 fat
Macadamia Nuts, Oil Roasted (1 oz)	204	4	22	3	0	74	3	2	2	4 fat
Mixed Nuts, Dry Roasted (1 oz)	168	7	15	2	0	190	3	5	5	1/2 strch, 3 fat

NUTS, SEEDS, AND NUT/SEED PRODUCTS

Products	Cal.	Carb. (g)	Fat (g)	Sat. Fat (g)	Chol. (mg)	Sod. (mg)	Fib. (g)	Prot. (g)	Servings/Exchanges
Mixed Nuts, Oil Roasted (1 oz)	175	6	16	4	0	185	3	5	1/2 strch, 3 fat
Mixed Nuts, Oil Roasted, No Peanuts (1 oz)	172	6	16	3	0	196	2	4	1/2 strch, 3 fat
Mixed Nuts, Oil Roasted, Unsalted (1 oz)	173	6	16	2	0	3	2	4	1 med-fat meat, 2 fat
Peanut Butter, Chunky (1 Tbsp)	94	4	8	2	0	78	1	4	1 med-fat meat, 1 fat
Peanut Butter, Natural, Salted (1 Tbsp)	94	3	8	1	0	40	1	4	1 med-fat meat, 1 fat
Peanut Butter, Natural, Unsalted (1 Tbsp)	94	3	8	1	0	<1	1	4	1 med-fat meat, 1 fat
Peanut Butter, Smooth (1 Tbsp)	94	3	8	2	0	77	<1	4	1 med-fat meat, 1 fat
Peanut Butter, Smooth, Salted (2 Tbsp)	190	6	16	4	0	149	2	8	1 high-fat meat, 1 fat
Peanuts, Dry-Roasted, Unsalted (1 oz)	166	6	14	2	0	2	2	7	1 med-fat meat, 2 fat
Peanuts, Oil-Roasted (1 oz)	165	5	14	2	0	123	3	8	1 med-fat meat, 2 fat
Peanuts, Spanish, Raw (1 oz)	167	5	14	2	0	6	3	8	1 med-fat meat, 2 fat
Pecans, Dried Halves	189	5	19	2	0	<1	2	2	4 fat
Pecans, Dry-Roasted (1 oz)	187	6	18	2	0	222	3	2	3 fat
Pecans, Oil-Roasted (1 oz)	194	5	20	2	0	214	2	2	4 fat

Food									Exchanges
Pine (Pignoli) Nuts, Dried (1 oz)	173	6	17	3	0	20	3	3	1 med-fat meat, 2 fat
Pistachio Nuts, Dry-Roasted (1 oz)	170	8	15	2	0	218	3	4	1/2 strch, 3 fat
Pumpkin Kernels, Roasted (1 oz)	148	4	12	2	0	163	1	9	1 med-fat meat, 1 fat
Pumpkin Seeds, Roasted (1 oz)	126	15	6	1	0	163	2	5	1 strch, 1 fat
Sesame Seeds, Dried, Whole (1 Tbsp)	52	2	5	1	0	1	1	2	1 fat
Sunflower Seeds, Dry (1 oz)	162	5	14	2	0	<1	3	7	1 med-fat meat, 2 fat
Sunflower Seeds, Dry-Roasted (1 oz)	163	7	14	2	0	<1	3	6	1 med-fat meat, 2 fat
Sunflower Seeds, Oil-Roasted (1 oz)	174	4	16	2	0	171	2	6	1 med-fat meat, 2 fat
Tahini/Sesame Butter (1 Tbsp)	91	3	9	1	0	<1	1	3	2 fat
BAKER'S									
Coconut, Angel Flake (2 Tbsp)	70	6	5	5	0	45	1	1	1/2 strch, 1 fat
Coconut, Premium Shredded (1/3 cup)	140	12	9	NA	0	85	2	1	1 strch, 2 fat
BEER NUTS									
Cashew Halves (1 oz)	170	8	13	3	0	65	NA	5	1 med-fat meat, 2 fat
Peanuts (1 oz)	170	7	14	3	0	80	2	7	1 med-fat meat, 2 fat

NUTS, SEEDS, AND NUT/SEED PRODUCTS

Products	Cal.	Carb. (g)	Fat (g)	Sat. Fat (g)	Chol. (mg)	Sod. (mg)	Fib. (g)	Prot. (g)	Servings/Exchanges
BLUE DIAMOND									
Almonds, Whole, Dry Roasted (1 oz)	166	5	15	NA	0	121	NA	6	1 med-fat meat, 2 fat
CORNNUTS									
Barbeque (1 oz)	130	20	5	<1	0	170	2	2	1 strch, 1 fat
Chili Picante (1 oz)	130	19	5	<1	0	280	2	2	1 strch, 1 fat
Nacho Cheese (1 oz)	130	20	4	1	0	190	2	2	1 strch, 1 fat
Original (1 oz)	120	20	5	<1	0	180	2	3	1 strch, 1 fat
Ranch (1 oz)	130	19	5	1	0	230	2	3	1 strch, 1 fat
ESTEE									
Peanut Butter, Creamy/Chunky (2 Tbsp)	190	7	15	3	0	0	2	7	1 high-fat meat, 1 fat
FISHER									
Cashews, Honey Roasted (1 oz)	150	7	13	3	0	NA	NA	4	1 med-fat meat, 2 fat
Mixed Nuts (1 oz)	170	7	15	2	0	125	NA	6	1 med-fat meat, 2 fat

FRITO-LAY

Cashews, Salted (1 oz)	180	7	15	3	0	190	1	5	1 med-fat meat, 2 fat
Peanuts, Honey Roasted (1.6 oz)	270	10	21	4	0	80	3	10	1/2 carb., 1 med-fat meat, 3 fat
Peanuts, Hot (1.1 oz)	190	6	16	3	0	250	2	7	1 med-fat meat, 2 fat
Peanuts, Salted (1.1 oz)	200	5	16	4	0	180	2	7	1 med-fat meat, 2 fat
Sunflower Seeds (1 oz)	180	5	15	2	0	25	2	7	1 med-fat meat, 2 fat

JIFF

Peanut Butter, Creamy (2 Tbsp)	190	7	16	3	0	150	2	8	1 high-fat meat, 2 fat
Peanut Butter, Extra Crunchy (2 Tbsp)	190	7	16	3	0	130	2	8	1 high-fat meat, 2 fat
Peanut Butter, Reduced-Fat, Creamy (2 Tbsp)	190	15	12	3	0	250	2	8	1 carb., 1 high-fat meat, 1 fat
Peanut Butter, Simply Jiff, Creamy (2 Tbsp)	190	6	16	3	0	65	2	8	1 high-fat meat, 2 fat
Peanut Butter, Smooth Sensations, Chocolate Silk (2 Tbsp)	190	14	15	3	0	115	1	5	1 carb., 1 high-fat meat, 1 fat

NUTS, SEEDS, AND NUT/SEED PRODUCTS

Products	Cal.	Carb. (g)	Fat (g)	Sat. Fat (g)	Chol. (mg)	Sod. (mg)	Fib. (g)	Prot. (g)	Servings/Exchanges
LAURA SCUDDER'S									
Peanut Butter, Nutty (2 Tbsp)	200	6	16	3	0	110	2	8	1 high-fat meat, 2 fat
Peanut Butter, Smooth (2 Tbsp)	200	6	16	3	0	110	2	8	1 high-fat meat, 2 fat
Peanut Butter, Smooth, Unsalted (2 Tbsp)	200	6	16	3	0	5	2	8	1/2 carb., 1 high-fat meat, 1 fat
PETER PAN									
Peanut Butter, Creamy (2 Tbsp)	190	6	16	4	0	150	2	8	1 high-fat meat, 2 fat
Peanut Butter, Crunchy (2 Tbsp)	190	6	16	3	0	120	2	9	1 high-fat meat, 2 fat
Peanut Butter Spread, Smart Choice , Reduced Fat (2 Tbsp)	180	14	11	3	0	180	2	8	1 carb., 1 high-fat meat, 1 fat
PLANTERS									
Cashews, Honey-Roasted (1 oz)	170	11	12	2	0	170	NA	4	1 carb., 2 fat
Nut Topping (2 Tbsp)	100	3	9	1	0	5	1	3	2 fat
Peanuts, Honey-Roasted (1 oz)	160	8	13	2	0	90	2	6	1/2 carb., 1 med-fat meat, 2 fat

Pecans, Honey-Roasted (1 oz)	200	8	18	2	0	80	NA	2	2 1/2 carb., 1 high-fat meat, 1 fat
Select Mix, Cashews, Almonds, & Macadamias (1 oz)	170	6	16	3	0	105	2	4	1 med-fat meat, 2 fat
PROGRESSO									
Pignoli Nuts (1 oz)	170	2	13	1	0	0	0	10	1 high fat meat, 1 fat
REESE'S									
Peanut Butter, Creamy (2 Tbsp)	200	8	15	2	0	140	2	7	1/2 carb., 1 high-fat meat, 2 fat
Peanut Butter, Extra Crunchy (2 Tbsp)	200	6	16	3	0	80	2	7	1 high-fat meat, 2 fat
SKIPPY									
Peanut Butter, Creamy (2 Tbsp)	190	7	16	4	3	150	2	7	1 high-fat meat, 2 fat
Peanut Butter, Creamy, Roasted Honey Nut (2 Tbsp)	190	7	17	4	0	125	2	7	1 high-fat meat, 2 fat
Peanut Butter, Reduced-Fat Creamy (2 Tbsp)	190	15	12	3	0	190	2	7	1 carb., 1 high-fat meat, 1 fat
Peanut Butter, Reduced-Fat Super Chunk (2 Tbsp)	190	14	12	3	0	170	2	7	1 carb., 1 high-fat meat, 1 fat
Peanut Butter, Super Chunk (2 Tbsp)	190	7	16	3	0	140	2	7	1 high-fat meat, 2 fat

SAUCES, CONDIMENTS, AND GRAVIES

Products	Cal.	Carb. (g)	Fat (g)	Sat. Fat (g)	Chol. (mg)	Sod. (mg)	Fib. (g)	Prot. (g)	Servings/Exchanges
Apple Butter (2 Tbsp)	65	17	<1	0	0	0	<1	<1	1 carb.
Catsup/Ketchup (1 Tbsp)	16	4	<1	0	0	182	<1	<1	free
Catsup/Ketchup, Low-Sodium (1 Tbsp)	16	4	<1	<1	0	3	<1	<1	free
Chutney (1 Tbsp)	26	7	<1	<1	0	38	<1	<1	1/2 carb.
Gravy, Au Jus, Canned (1/2 cup)	19	3	<1	<1	0	60	0	1	free
Gravy, Beef, Canned (1/2 cup)	62	6	3	1	4	652	<1	4	1/2 carb., 1 fat
Gravy, Beef, Homemade (1/2 cup)	89	7	5	2	3	767	<1	4	1/2 carb., 1 fat
Gravy, Brown, Dry Mix w/Water (1/2 cup)	38	7	<1	<1	1	538	<1	1	1/2 carb.
Gravy, Chicken, Canned (1/2 cup)	94	7	7	2	2	687	<1	2	1/2 carb., 1 fat
Gravy, Chicken Giblet, Homemade (1/2 cup)	97	6	5	1	55	683	<1	6	1/2 carb., 1 fat
Gravy, Mushroom, Canned (1/2 cup)	60	7	6	<1	0	678	<1	2	1/2 carb., 1 fat
Gravy, Sausage (1/2 cup)	206	8	16	6	33	408	<1	8	1/2 carb., 3 fat
Gravy, Turkey, Canned (1/2 cup)	61	6	3	<1	2	687	<1	3	1/2 strch, 1 fat

Guacamole w/Tomatoes (1 Tbsp)	17	1	2	<1	0	27	<1	<1	free
Honey (1 Tbsp)	64	17	0	0	0	<1	<1	<1	1 carb.
Horseradish, Prepared (1 Tbsp)	7	2	<1	<1	0	47	<1	<1	free
Jam, Cherry/Strawberry (1 Tbsp)	54	14	<1	0	0	2	<1	<1	1 carb.
Jam, Not Cherry or Strawberry (1 Tbsp)	54	14	<1	0	0	2	<1	<1	1 carb.
Jam/Marmalade, Artificially Sweetened (1 Tbsp)	2	11	<1	<1	0	0	<1	<1	free
Jam/Marmalade/Preserves, Reduced-Sugar (1 Tbsp)	36	9	<1	<1	0	5	<1	<1	1/2 carb.
Jam/Preserves (1 Tbsp)	48	13	<1	<1	0	8	<1	<1	1 carb.
Jelly (1 Tbsp)	52	14	<1	<1	0	7	<1	<1	1 carb.
Jelly, Blackberry (1 Tbsp)	50	13	0	0	0	10	0	0	1 carb.
Jelly, Dietetic (1 Tbsp)	6	11	0	0	0	<1	<1	<1	free
Jelly, Reduced-Sugar (1 Tbsp)	34	9	<1	<1	0	<1	<1	<1	1/2 carb.
Marmalade, Orange (1 Tbsp)	49	13	0	0	0	11	<1	<1	1 carb.
Mustard, Dijon (1 Tbsp)	19	2	1	<1	0	379	<1	<1	free
Mustard, Honey (1 Tbsp)	50	7	3	<1	0	91	<1	<1	1/2 carb.
Mustard, Prepared (1 Tbsp)	12	1	<1	<1	0	196	<1	<1	free

SAUCES, CONDIMENTS, AND GRAVIES

Products	Cal.	Carb. (g)	Fat (g)	Sat. Fat (g)	Chol. (mg)	Sod. (mg)	Fib. (g)	Prot. (g)	Servings/Exchanges
Olives, Green, Pitted (10)	45	<1	5	<1	0	936	<1	<1	1 fat
Olives, Small Ripe, Canned (10)	37	2	3	<1	0	279	1	<1	1 fat
Olives, Stuffed Green (10)	41	<1	5	<1	0	827	<1	<1	1 fat
Peppers, Pickled Hot Jalapeño (2)	8	2	<1	<1	0	121	<1	<1	free
Pickle, Dill (1)	12	3	<1	<1	0	833	<1	<1	free
Pickle, Dill, Low-Sodium (1)	12	3	<1	<1	0	12	<1	<1	free
Pickle, Sour (1)	4	<1	<1	<1	0	423	<1	<1	free
Pickle, Sweet (1 medium)	41	11	<1	<1	0	329	<1	<1	1/2 carb.
Pickle Slices, Dill (10)	11	3	<1	<1	0	769	<1	<1	free
Pickle Slices, Dill, Low-Sodium (10)	11	3	<1	<1	0	11	<1	<1	free
Pickle Slices, Fresh Pack (4)	22	5	<1	0	0	202	<1	<1	free
Pickle Slices, Sour (10)	8	2	<1	<1	0	846	<1	<1	free
Relish, Hot Dog (1 Tbsp)	14	4	<1	<1	0	167	<1	<1	free
Relish, Sweet Pickle (1 Tbsp)	20	5	<1	<1	0	124	<1	<1	free

Sauce, Bearnaise, Homemade (1/2 cup)	321	1	34	20	237	444	<1	2	7 fat
Sauce, Black Bean (1/2 cup)	129	14	6	1	0	1322	2	3	1 strch, 1 fat
Sauce, Cheese (1/2 cup)	221	9	16	10	36	515	<1	10	1/2 carb., 1 med-fat meat, 2 fat
Sauce, Curry (1/2 cup)	74	3	6	1	0	392	<1	3	1 fat
Sauce, Hollandaise, Dry Mix & Water (1/2 cup)	119	7	10	6	26	783	<1	2	1/2 carb., 2 fat
Sauce, Hot Chili/Red Pepper (2 Tbsp)	7	1	<1	<1	0	8	<1	<1	free
Sauce, Hot Green Chili (1 Tbsp)	6	2	<1	0	0	4	<1	<1	free
Sauce, Marinara Tomato (1/2 cup)	85	13	4	<1	0	786	1	2	1 carb., 1 fat
Sauce, Salsa/Mexican, Homemade (1/2 cup)	23	5	<1	<1	0	468	1	<1	1 vegetable
Sauce, Soy (1 Tbsp)	10	2	<1	<1	0	1028	0	<1	free
Sauce, Spanish-Style Tomato (1/2 cup)	40	9	<1	<1	0	576	2	2	1/2 carb.
Sauce, Tartar (1 Tbsp)	74	<1	8	2	7	99	<1	<1	2 fat
Sauce, Teriyaki (1 Tbsp)	15	3	0	0	0	690	<1	1	free
Sauce, White, Homemade (1/2 cup)	178	10	14	4	14	185	<1	4	1/2 strch, 3 fat
Sauce, Worcestershire (1 Tbsp)	11	3	0	0	0	167	0	0	free

SAUCES, CONDIMENTS, AND GRAVIES

Products	Cal.	Carb. (g)	Fat (g)	Sat. Fat (g)	Chol. (mg)	Sod. (mg)	Fib. (g)	Prot. (g)	Servings/Exchanges
Spaghetti Sauce, Meat, Canned (1/2 cup)	150	19	7	1	8	590	4	4	1 carb., 2 fat
Spaghetti Sauce, Meat, Homemade (1/2 cup)	145	11	8	2	23	565	2	8	2 carb., 1 med-fat meat, 1 fat
Spaghetti Sauce, Canned (1/2 cup)	136	20	6	<1	0	618	4	2	1 carb., 1 fat
Syrup, Maple (1 Tbsp)	52	13	<1	0	0	2	0	0	1 carb.
Syrup, Pancake (1 Tbsp)	57	15	0	0	0	17	0	0	1 carb.
BETTY CROCKER									
Bac-Os, Salad Topping Bits or Chips (1 1/2 Tbsp)	30	2	2	0	0	120	0	3	3 fat
CAMPBELL'S									
Spaghetti Sauce, Italian-Style (1/2 cup)	50	12	0	0	0	360	2	2	1 carb.
Spaghetti Sauce, Marinara, Homestyle (1/2 cup)	40	10	0	0	0	360	2	2	1/2 carb.
Spaghetti Sauce, Mushroom Garlic (1/2 cup)	50	11	1	0	0	330	2	2	1 carb.
Spaghetti Sauce, Mushroom (1/2 cup)	50	11	1	0	0	330	2	2	1 1/2 carb.
Spaghetti Sauce, Traditional (1/2 cup)	50	12	0	0	0	360	2	2	1 1/2 carb.
Spaghetti Sauce, Xtra Garlic Onion (1/2 cup)	50	12	1	0	0	320	2	2	1 carb.

CARY'S

Syrup, Sugar-Free (1/4 cup)	35	9	0	0	0	105	0	0	1/2 carb.

CHEF MATE

Gravy, Country Sausage (1/4 cup)	96	4	8	2	13	236	<1	3	2 fat
Sauce, Basic Cheese (1/2 cup)	82	8	5	2	6	471	0	2	1/2 carb., 1 fat
Sauce, Coney Island–Style (1/4 cup)	76	6	5	<1	2	383	1	2	1/2 carb., 1 fat
Sauce, Creole (1/4 cup)	25	4	<1	0	0	340	0	<1	free
Sauce, Golden Cheese (1/4 cup)	139	2	11	6	29	501	<1	7	1 med-fat meat, 1 fat
Sauce, Hoisin (1 Tbsp)	35	7	<1	0	0	250	0	<1	1/2 carb.
Sauce, Hot Dog Chili (1/4 cup)	69	9	2	<1	4	399	2	3	1/2 carb.
Sauce, Italian (1/4 cup)	60	11	1	<1	0	304	<1	1	1 carb.
Sauce, Lemon (2 Tbsp)	43	10	<1	0	0	3	0	<1	1/2 carb.
Sauce, Sharp Cheddar Cheese (1/4 cup)	133	2	12	5	23	473	<1	6	1 med-fat meat, 1 fat
Sauce, Sloppy Joe Barbecue (1/3 cup)	119	9	7	3	23	574	<1	7	1/2 carb., 1 fat
Sauce, Sweet & Sour Glaze (2 Tbsp)	50	12	0	0	0	229	0	<1	1 carb.
Sauce, Sweet 'n Sour (2 Tbsp)	40	8	<1	0	0	116	<1	<1	1/2 carb.

SAUCES, CONDIMENTS, AND GRAVIES

Products	Cal.	Carb. (g)	Sat. Fat (g)	Fat (g)	Chol. (mg)	Sod. (mg)	Fib. (g)	Prot. (g)	Servings/Exchanges
Sauce, Szechuan (2 Tbsp)	42	6	2	<1	0	436	0	<1	1/2 carb.
Sauce, Teriyaki (1 Tbsp)	20	4	<1	0	0	159	0	<1	free
CLAUSSEN									
Pickle Relish, Sweet (1 Tbsp)	14	3	<1	<1	0	90	NA	<1	free
Pickles, Bread'n Butter Chips (1)	7	2	0	0	0	61	NA	<1	free
Pickles, Hamburger Dill Chips (10)	<1	<1	<1	<1	0	42	<1	<1	free
Pickles, Kosher Dill Halves (1)	9	1	<1	<1	0	769	NA	<1	free
Pickles, Kosher Dill Slices (1)	1	<1	<1	<1	0	107	NA	0	free
Pickles, Kosher Dill Spears (1)	4	<1	<1	<1	0	312	<1	<1	free
Pickles, Kosher Mini Dills (1)	4	<1	<1	<1	0	300	<1	<1	free
CONTADINA									
Bolognese Sauce (5 oz)	130	0	7	1	25	500	NA	8	1 med-fat meat
Pasta Ready Tomatoes & 3-Cheeses (1/2 cup)	70	10	2	<1	4	490	2	2	1/2 carb.
Pasta Ready Tomatoes & Mushrooms (1/2 cup)	50	9	1	0	0	641	1	1	1/2 carb.

Food									
Pasta Ready Tomatoes & Olives (1/2 cup)	60	8	2	0	0	641	1	1	1/2 carb.
Pasta Ready Tomatoes & Red Pepper (1/2 cup)	60	8	2	0	0	691	1	1	1/2 carb.
Pizza Sauce, All-Purpose (1/4 cup)	25	6	0	0	0	20	1	1	1/2 carb.
Pizza Sauce, Chunky, Basic (1/4 cup)	27	4	<1	0	0	250	1	<1	1/2 carb.
Pizza Sauce, Deluxe (1/4 cup)	30	5	1	0	2	120	1	1	1/2 carb.
Pizza Sauce, Fully Prepared (1/4 cup)	25	6	0	0	0	270	1	1	1/2 carb.
Pizza Sauce & 3-Cheeses, Chunky (1/4 cup)	35	5	<1	0	0	190	1	1	1/2 carb.
Pizza Sauce & Mushrooms, Chunky (1/4 cup)	30	5	0	0	0	290	1	1	1/2 carb.
Pizza Sauce w/Basil (1/4 cup)	25	6	0	0	0	20	1	1	1/2 carb.
Pizza Sauce w/Cheese (1/4 cup)	30	4	1	0	0	350	1	1	1/2 carb.
Pizza Sauce w/Pepperoni (1/4 cup)	30	4	1	0	0	360	1	1	1/2 carb.
Pizza Sauce, Original (1/4 cup)	25	4	<1	0	0	300	1	1	1/2 carb.
Pizza Sauce, Squeeze (1/4 cup)	38	6	2	0	0	385	1	1	1/2 carb.
Pizza Sauce, Squeeze, Italian Cheese (1/4 cup)	30	4	<1	0	0	380	<1	<1	1/2 carb.
Spaghetti Sauce (1/2 cup)	90	17	2	0	0	440	NA	2	1 carb.
Spaghetti Sauce, Mushroom (1/2 cup)	90	18	2	<1	0	430	NA	2	1 carb.

SAUCES, CONDIMENTS, AND GRAVIES

Products	Cal.	Carb. (g)	Fat (g)	Sat. Fat (g)	Chol. (mg)	Sod. (mg)	Fib. (g)	Prot. (g)	Servings/Exchanges
Sauce, Marinara, Deluxe (1/2 cup)	73	9	4	<1	0	469	2	2	1/2 carb., 1 fat
Sauce, Sweet 'n Sour (2 Tbsp)	40	8	1	0	0	115	0	0	1/2 carb.
DEL MONTE									
Sloppy Joe Sauce (1/4 cup)	70	16	0	0	0	680	0	1	1 carb.
Spaghetti Sauce, Traditional (1/2 cup)	70	11	2	NA	NA	430	NA	1	1 carb.
Spaghetti Sauce w/Garlic & Onion (1/2 cup)	70	10	2	0	NA	430	NA	1	1 carb.
Spaghetti Sauce w/Meat (1/2 cup)	70	9	2	NA	NA	440	NA	2	1 carb.
Spaghetti Sauce w/Mushrooms (1/2 cup)	70	11	2	NA	NA	440	NA	1	1 carb.
DI GIORNO									
Sauce, Alfredo (1/4 cup)	180	3	18	7	25	600	0	3	4 fat
Sauce, Alfredo, Light (1/4 cup)	140	9	10	6	30	600	0	5	1/2 carb., 1 med-fat meat, 1 fat
Sauce, Basil Pesto (1/4 cup)	320	2	31	6	15	530	<1	7	1 med-fat meat, 5 fat
Sauce, Four-Cheese (1/4 cup)	160	3	15	7	30	410	0	5	1 med-fat meat, 2 fat

Sauce, Garlic Pesto (1/4 cup)	340	3	33	7	15	540	<1	7	1 med-fat meat, 6 fat
Sauce, Marinara (1/2 cup)	70	15	0	0	0	220	2	2	1 carb.
Sauce, Plum Tomato & Mushroom (1/2 cup)	60	13	0	0	0	260	2	2	1 carb.
ESTEE									
Fruit Spread, Apple Spice (1 Tbsp)	16	4	0	0	0	20	0	0	free
Fruit Spread, Grape (1 Tbsp)	16	4	0	0	0	20	0	0	free
Fruit Spread, Strawberry (1 Tbsp)	16	4	0	0	0	20	0	0	free
Ketchup (1 Tbsp)	15	5	0	0	0	190	0	0	free
Syrup, Blueberry Breakfast (1/4 cup)	80	20	0	0	0	70	0	0	1 carb.
Syrup, Maple Breakfast (1/4 cup)	80	20	0	0	0	125	0	0	1 carb.
FEATHERWEIGHT									
Syrup, Lite Pancake (1 Tbsp)	16	4	0	0	0	25	0	0	free
FRANCO-AMERICAN									
Gravy, Au Jus (1/4 cup)	10	2	0	0	0	330	0	0	free
Gravy, Beef (1/4 cup)	25	4	1	NA	NA	340	0	0	1/2 carb.
Gravy, Brown, w/Onions (1/2 cup)	25	4	1	0	5	340	0	0	1/2 carb.

SAUCES, CONDIMENTS, AND GRAVIES

Products	Cal.	Carb. (g)	Fat (g)	Sat. Fat (g)	Chol. (mg)	Sod. (mg)	Fib. (g)	Prot. (g)	Servings/Exchanges
Gravy, Chicken (1/4 cup)	45	3	4	NA	NA	240	0	0	1 fat
Gravy, Chicken Giblet (1/4 cup)	30	3	2	0	NA	310	0	1	1 fat
Gravy, Mushroom (1/4 cup)	25	3	1	NA	NA	290	0	0	free
Gravy, Pork (1/4 cup)	40	3	3	2	NA	330	0	0	1 fat
Gravy, Turkey (1/4 cup)	30	3	2	0	NA	290	0	0	1 fat
GENERAL MILLS									
Bac-Os, Salad Topping (1 Tbsp)	25	2	<1	NA	0	103	NA	3	free
GREEN GIANT									
Relish, Corn, Canned (1 Tbsp)	20	5	0	0	0	40	0	0	free
Sauce, Sloppy Joe Sandwich (1/4 cup)	50	11	<1	<1	0	423	2	2	1 carb.
GREY POUPON									
Country Dijon Mustard (1 Tbsp)	18	0	0	0	0	360	0	0	free
HEALTHY CHOICE									
BBQ Sauce, Hickory (2 Tbsp)	26	6	<1	0	0	229	<1	<1	1/2 carb.

BBQ Sauce, Hot & Spicy (2 Tbsp)	25	6	<1	0	0	220	<1	<1	1/2 carb.
BBQ Sauce, Original (2 Tbsp)	30	7	<1	0	0	220	<1	<1	1/2 carb.
Ketchup (1 Tbsp)	9	2	<1	0	2	97	<1	<1	free
Pasta Sauce, Extra Chunky Garlic & Onion (1/2 cup)	40	10	0	0	0	350	NA	2	1/2 carb.
Pasta Sauce, Extra Chunky Mushroom (1/2 cup)	45	10	0	0	0	350	NA	2	1/2 carb.
Pasta Sauce, Traditional (1/2 cup)	40	9	1	NA	0	380	NA	2	1/2 carb.
Pasta Sauce w/Garlic & Herbs (1/2 cup)	40	9	1	NA	0	350	NA	2	1/2 carb.
Spaghetti Sauce, Chunky Italian Vegetable (1/2 cup)	40	9	0	0	0	350	NA	1	1/2 carb.
Spaghetti Sauce, Chunky Mushroom (1/2 cup)	45	10	0	0	0	350	NA	2	1/2 carb.
Spaghetti Sauce w/Mushrooms (1/2 cup)	40	9	1	NA	0	390	NA	2	1/2 carb.

HUNGRY JACK

Syrup, Maple, Butter (1 Tbsp)	100	26	0	0	0	23	0	0	2 carb.
Syrup, Maple, Butter, Lite (1 Tbsp)	55	14	0	0	0	104	0	0	1 carb.
Syrup, Pancake, Regular (2 Tbsp)	100	26	0	0	0	25	0	0	2 carb.
Syrup, Pancake, Regular Lite (2 Tbsp)	50	14	0	0	0	105	0	0	1 carb.

SAUCES, CONDIMENTS, AND GRAVIES

Products	Cal.	Carb. (g)	Fat (g)	Sat. Fat (g)	Chol. (mg)	Sod. (mg)	Fib. (g)	Prot. (g)	Servings/Exchanges
HUNT'S									
BBQ Sauce, Bold Original (2 Tbsp)	46	11	<1	0	0	315	<1	<1	1 carb.
BBQ Sauce, Hickory (2 Tbsp)	40	9	0	0	0	410	1	0	1/2 carb.
BBQ Sauce, Hickory & Brown Sugar (2 Tbsp)	75	18	<1	0	0	382	1	<1	1 carb.
BBQ Sauce, Honey Mustard (2 Tbsp)	48	12	<1	0	0	450	<1	<1	1 carb.
BBQ Sauce, Hot & Spicy (2 Tbsp)	48	12	<1	0	0	450	<1	<1	1 carb.
BBQ Sauce, Light (2 Tbsp)	26	6	<1	0	0	223	<1	<1	1/2 carb.
BBQ Sauce, Mesquite (2 Tbsp)	40	9	0	0	0	360	1	1	1/2 carb.
BBQ Sauce, Mild Dijon (2 Tbsp)	39	9	<1	0	0	400	<1	<1	1/2 carb.
BBQ Sauce, Original (2 Tbsp)	40	9	0	0	0	410	1	0	1/2 carb.
BBQ Sauce, Teriyaki (2 Tbsp)	46	11	<1	0	0	351	1	<1	1 carb.
Chicken Sensations, BBQ Flavor (1 Tbsp)	35	3	3	<1	0	308	<1	<1	1 fat
Chicken Sensations, Italian Garlic (1 Tbsp)	30	1	3	<1	0	326	1	<1	1 fat
Chicken Sensations, Lemon Herb (1 Tbsp)	31	2	3	<1	0	378	<1	<1	1 fat

Food									Exchanges
Chicken Sensations, Southwestern (1 Tbsp)	27	1	3	<1	0	281	<1	<1	1 fat
Salsa, Alfresco, Medium (2 Tbsp)	10	2	<1	0	0	161	<1	<1	free
Salsa, Homestyle, Medium (2 Tbsp)	27	6	<1	0	0	236	<1	<1	1 vegetable
Sauce, Pepper, Original & Hot (1 tsp)	<1	<1	0	0	0	205	0	0	free
Sauce, Picante, Mild (2 Tbsp)	11	2	<1	0	0	256	<1	<1	free
Sauce, Steak (1 Tbsp)	10	2	<1	0	0	256	<1	<1	free
Spaghetti Sauce, Chunky (1/2 cup)	50	12	1	<1	0	470	2	1	1 carb.
Spaghetti Sauce, Home Style (1/2 cup)	60	10	2	<1	0	530	2	2	1/2 carb., 1 fat
Spaghetti Sauce, Italian-Style Vegetable (1/2 cup)	64	9	3	<1	0	616	3	3	1/2 carb., 1 fat
Spaghetti Sauce, Old Country Traditional (1/2 cup)	53	7	3	<1	0	542	3	2	1/2 carb., 1 fat
Spaghetti Sauce, Original Traditional (1/2 cup)	70	12	2	<1	0	530	2	2	1 carb.
Spaghetti Sauce Flavored w/Meat (1/2 cup)	70	12	2	<1	2	570	2	2	1 carb.
Spaghetti Sauce Flavored w/Meat, Old Country (1/2 cup)	70	10	3	NA	0	560	NA	2	1/2 carb., 1 fat
Spaghetti Sauce w/Garlic & Herbs, Old Country (1/2 cup)	80	13	2	<1	0	560	NA	2	1 carb.

SAUCES, CONDIMENTS, AND GRAVIES

Products	Cal.	Carb. (g)	Fat (g)	Sat. Fat (g)	Chol. (mg)	Sod. (mg)	Fib. (g)	Prot. (g)	Servings/Exchanges
Spaghetti Sauce w/Mushrooms, Old Country (1/2 cup)	53	7	3	<1	0	542	3	2	1/2 carb., 1 fat
Spaghetti Sauce w/Mushrooms, Original (1/2 cup)	70	12	2	<1	0	560	2	2	1 carb.
Spaghetti Sauce w/Parmesan, Classic Italian (1/2 cup)	60	8	2	<1	0	550	NA	3	1/2 carb.
Spaghetti Sauce w/Tomato & Basil, Classic Italian (1/2 cup)	50	8	2	<1	0	550	NA	1	1/2 carb.
KRAFT									
BBQ Sauce, Charcoal Grill (2 Tbsp)	60	13	0	0	0	460	0	0	1 carb.
BBQ Sauce, Hickory Smoke (2 Tbsp)	40	9	0	0	0	420	0	0	1/2 carb.
BBQ Sauce, Hickory Smoke Onion Bits (2 Tbsp)	45	11	0	0	0	360	0	0	1 carb.
BBQ Sauce, Honey (2 Tbsp)	50	13	0	0	0	360	0	0	1 carb.
BBQ Sauce, Hot (2 Tbsp)	40	9	0	0	0	520	0	0	1/2 carb.
BBQ Sauce, Honey Mustard (2 Tbsp)	60	13	0	0	0	300	0	0	1 carb.

BBQ Sauce, Hot Hickory Smoke (2 Tbsp)	40	9	0	●	0	380	0	0	1/2 carb.
BBQ Sauce, Kansas City–Style (2 Tbsp)	50	11	0	●	0	310	0	0	1 carb.
BBQ Sauce, Mesquite Smoke (2 Tbsp)	40	9	0	●	0	420	0	0	1/2 carb.
BBQ Sauce, Onion Bits (2 Tbsp)	45	11	0	0	0	360	0	0	1 cart.
BBQ Sauce, Original (2 Tbsp)	40	9	0	0	0	420	0	0	1/2 carb.
BBQ Sauce, Roasted Garlic (2 Tbsp)	50	12	0	0	0	360	0	0	1/2 carb.
BBQ Sauce, Spicy Honey (2 Tbsp)	60	14	0	0	0	360	0	0	1 carb.
BBQ Sauce, Teriyaki (2 Tbsp)	60	12	0	0	0	440	0	<1	1 carb.
BBQ Sauce, Thick'n Spicy Hickory Smoke (2 Tbsp)	50	12	0	0	0	450	0	0	1 carb.
BBQ Sauce, Thick'n Spicy Honey (2 Tbsp)	60	13	0	0	0	360	0	0	1 carb.
BBQ Sauce, Thick'n Spicy Mesquite (2 Tbsp)	50	12	0	0	0	440	0	0	1 carb.
BBQ Sauce, Thick'n Spicy Original (2 Tbsp)	50	12	0	0	0	440	0	0	1 carb.
Fruit Spread, Reduced-Calorie, Grape (1 Tbsp)	20	5	0	0	0	20	0	0	free
Fruit Spread, Reduced-Calorie, Strawberry (1 Tbsp)	20	5	0	0	0	20	0	0	free
Jam, Grape (1 Tbsp)	60	14	0	0	0	10	0	0	1 carb
Jam, Red Plum (1 Tbsp)	60	13	0	0	0	10	0	0	1 carb

SAUCES, CONDIMENTS, AND GRAVIES

Products	Cal.	Carb. (g)	Fat (g)	Sat. Fat (g)	Chol. (mg)	Sod. (mg)	Fib. (g)	Prot. (g)	Servings/Exchanges
Jam, Strawberry (1 Tbsp)	50	13	0	0	0	10	0	0	1 carb.
Jelly, Apple (1 Tbsp)	60	14	0	0	0	10	0	0	1 carb.
Jelly, Apple Strawberry (1 Tbsp)	50	13	0	0	0	10	0	0	1 carb.
Jelly, Grape (1 Tbsp)	50	14	0	0	0	10	0	0	1 carb.
Jelly, Guava (1 Tbsp)	50	13	0	0	0	10	0	0	1 carb.
Jelly, Red Currant (1 Tbsp)	50	13	0	0	0	10	0	0	1 carb.
Jelly, Strawberry (1 Tbsp)	60	14	0	0	0	10	0	0	1 carb.
Preserves, Apricot (1 Tbsp)	50	13	0	0	0	10	0	0	1 carb.
Preserves, Blackberry (1 Tbsp)	50	13	0	0	0	10	0	0	1 carb.
Preserves, Orange Marmalade (1 Tbsp)	50	14	0	0	0	10	0	0	1 carb.
Preserves, Peach (1 Tbsp)	50	14	0	0	0	10	0	0	1 carb.
Preserves, Pineapple (1 Tbsp)	50	14	0	0	0	10	0	0	1 carb.
Preserves, Red Raspberry (1 Tbsp)	50	13	0	0	0	10	0	0	1 carb.
Preserves, Strawberry (1 Tbsp)	50	13	0	0	0	10	0	0	1 carb.

Sandwich Spread & Burger Sauce (1 Tbsp)	550	3	4	<1	<5	105	0	0	1 fat
Sauce, Cocktail (1/4 cup)	60	13	<1	0	0	800	1	1	1 carb.
Sauce, Horseradish (1 tsp)	20	<1	2	0	<5	35	0	0	free
Sauce, Horseradish, Cream-Style (1 tsp)	0	0	0	0	0	50	0	0	free
Sauce, Horseradish, Mustard (1 tsp)	0	0	0	0	0	55	0	0	free
Sauce, Lemon Herb Tartar (2 Tbsp)	150	<1	16	3	15	170	0	0	3 fat
Sauce, Prepared Horseradish (1 tsp)	0	0	0	0	0	50	0	0	free
Sauce, Sauceworks Sweet & Sour (2 Tbsp)	60	14	0	0	0	125	0	0	1 carb.
Sauce, Tartar (2 Tbsp)	90	4	9	2	10	170	0	0	2 fat
Sauce, Tartar, Fat-Free (2 Tbsp)	25	5	0	0	0	200	0	0	free
LA CHOY									
Sauce, Brown Gravy (1 Tbsp)	90	24	6	0	0	90	1	6	1 1/2 carb., 1 fat
Sauce, Plum (1 oz)	45	11	<1	0	0	17	NA	<1	1 carb.
Sauce, Soy (1 Tbsp)	11	1	<1	0	0	1315	0	1	free
Sauce, Soy, Lite (1 Tbsp)	15	2	<1	0	0	505	0	1	free
Sauce, Stir-Fry Mandarin Soy (1/2 cup)	71	16	<1	0	0	851	1	2	1 carb.

SAUCES, CONDIMENTS, AND GRAVIES

Products	Cal.	Carb. (g)	Fat (g)	Sat. Fat (g)	Chol. (mg)	Sod. (mg)	Fib. (g)	Prot. (g)	Servings/Exchanges
Sauce, Stir-Fry Szechwan (1/2 cup)	73	16	<1	0	0	612	2	3	1 carb.
Sauce, Stir-Fry Teriyaki (1/2 cup)	90	21	<1	0	0	997	1	2	1 1/2 carb.
Sauce, Sweet & Sour (1 Tbsp)	26	7	<1	0	0	59	0	<1	1/2 carb.
Sauce, Teriyaki (1 Tbsp)	17	3	<1	0	0	917	0	1	free
Sauce, Teriyaki, Light (1 Tbsp)	18	4	<1	0	0	439	0	1	free
LIBBY'S									
Gravy, Country Chicken (1/4 cup)	60	3	4	<1	5	330	0	1	1 fat
Gravy, Country Sausage (1/4 cup)	90	3	7	2	5	280	0	1	2 fat
Sauce, Sloppy Joe (1/3 cup)	45	10	0	0	0	430	1	1	1/2 carb.
Sauce, Tomato (1/4 cup)	20	4	0	0	0	280	<1	0	free
MRS. BUTTERWORTH'S									
Syrup, Pancake (1 oz)	111	16	<1	<1	0	32	<1	0	1 carb.
Syrup, Pancake, Lite (1 oz)	62	8	0	0	0	63	<1	0	1/2 carb.

OCEAN SPRAY

Jellied Cranberry Sauce (1/4 cup)	110	27	0	0	0	35	1	0	2 carb.
Whole Berry Cranberry Sauce (1/4 cup)	110	28	0	0	0	35	1	0	2 carb.

OLD EL PASO

Enchilada Sauce, Green Chili (1/4 cup)	30	3	2	0	0	330	0	<1	1/2 fat
Enchilada Sauce, Mild (1/4 cup)	30	4	2	0	0	190	0	0	free
Grilling Sauce, Chile Pepper & Spice (2 Tbsp)	60	14	0	0	0	380	0	<1	1 carb.
Grilling Sauce, Sweet N Smoky (2 Tbsp)	60	14	0	0	0	380	0	<1	1 carb.
Relish, Jalapeño (1 Tbsp)	5	1	0	0	0	110	0	0	free
Salsa, Green Chili, Medium (2 Tbsp)	10	2	0	0	0	110	<1	0	free
Salsa, Homestyle, Mild (2 Tbsp)	10	1	0	0	0	220	0	0	free
Salsa, Picante, Hot (2 Tbsp)	10	2	0	0	0	160	0	0	free
Salsa, Picante, Medium (2 Tbsp)	10	2	0	0	0	140	0	0	free
Salsa, Picante, Mild (2 Tbsp)	10	2	0	0	0	130	0	0	free
Salsa, Thick 'n Chunky, Medium (2 Tbsp)	10	2	0	0	0	230	0	0	free
Salsa Verde, Medium (2 Tbsp)	10	2	0	0	0	95	0	0	free

SAUCES, CONDIMENTS, AND GRAVIES

Products	Cal.	Carb. (g)	Fat (g)	Sat. Fat (g)	Chol. (mg)	Sod. (mg)	Fib. (g)	Prot. (g)	Servings/Exchanges
Taco Sauce, Hot (1 Tbsp)	5	1	0	0	0	90	0	0	free
Taco Sauce, Medium (1 Tbsp)	5	1	0	0	0	70	0	0	free
Taco Sauce, Mild (1 Tbsp)	5	1	0	0	0	85	0	0	free
Tomatoes & Green Chilis (1/4 cup)	10	2	0	0	0	300	0	0	free
OPEN PIT									
BBQ Sauce, Hickory Flavor (2 Tbsp)	50	11	0	0	0	380	0	0	1 carb.
BBQ Sauce, Hot (2 Tbsp)	50	11	0	0	0	380	0	0	1 carb.
BBQ Sauce, Mesquite (2 Tbsp)	50	11	<1	0	0	440	0	0	1 carb
BBQ Sauce, Onion Flavor (2 Tbsp)	50	11	0	0	0	480	0	0	1 carb.
BBQ Sauce, Original Flavor (2 Tbsp)	50	11	0	0	0	450	0	0	1 carb.
BBQ Sauce, Sweet & Sour (2 Tbsp)	45	10	0	0	0	420	0	0	1/2 carb.
BBQ Sauce, Sweet Flavor (2 Tbsp)	50	12	0	0	0	300	0	0	1 carb.
BBQ Sauce, Thick Tangy Onion (2 Tbsp)	50	12	0	0	0	380	0	0	1 carb.
BBQ Sauce, Thick Tangy Hickory (2 Tbsp)	50	12	0	0	0	390	0	0	1 carb.

BBQ Sauce, Thick Tangy Honey Spice (2 Tbsp)	45	11	0	0	0	340	0	0	1 carb.

ORTEGA

Enchilada Sauce (1 oz)	12	3	0	0	0	280	0	0	free
Green Chiles, Strips (2)	10	3	0	0	0	25	<1	<1	free
Picante Sauce, Medium (1 oz)	10	2	0	0	0	300	1	0	free
Salsa, Dipping, Medium (2 Tbsp)	10	2	0	0	0	320	1	0	free
Salsa, Green Chile, Mild (1 oz)	8	2	0	0	0	180	0	0	free
Sauce, Nacho Cheese (1/4 cup)	80	4	6	3	0	360	0	3	1 med-fat meat
Sauce/Puree, Green Chile (1/4 cup)	15	3	0	0	0	0	0	1	free
Sauce/Puree, Jalapeño (1/4 cup)	15	3	0	0	0	0	0	1	free
Sauce/Puree, Red Chile (1/4 cup)	15	3	0	0	0	0	0	1	free
Sauce/Puree, Red Jalapeño (1/4 cup)	15	3	0	0	0	0	0	1	free
Taco Sauce, Thick & Smooth, Hot (1 oz)	12	3	0	0	0	210	0	0	free
Taco Sauce, Western Style (1 oz)	8	2	0	0	0	180	0	0	free
Taco Sauce, Thick & Smooth, Mild (1 oz)	12	3	0	0	0	220	0	0	free

SAUCES, CONDIMENTS, AND GRAVIES

Products	Cal.	Carb. (g)	Fat (g)	Sat. Fat (g)	Chol. (mg)	Sod. (mg)	Fib. (g)	Prot. (g)	Servings/Exchanges
ORVAL KENT									
Pimento Spread (2 Tbsp)	130	3	12	2	10	280	1	2	2 fat
Salsa w/Green Chili, Spicy (2 Tbsp)	10	2	0	0	0	180	0	0	free
OSCAR MAYER									
Bacon Bits (1 Tbsp)	20	1	1	<1	5	180	0	3	free
PANCHO VILLA									
Taco Sauce, Mild (2 Tbsp)	15	3	0	0	0	170	0	0	free
PREGO									
Pasta Sauce, Marinara (1/2 cup)	100	10	6	2	0	620	NA	1	1 carb., 1 fat
Spaghetti Sauce, Onion & Garlic (1/2 cup)	110	16	4	NA	0	510	NA	1	1 carb., 1 fat
Spaghetti Sauce, Three-Cheese (1/2 cup)	100	17	2	NA	0	410	NA	3	1 carb.
Spaghetti Sauce, Tomato & Basil (1/2 cup)	100	18	2	NA	0	370	NA	2	1 carb., 1 fat
Spaghetti Sauce, Traditional (1/2 cup)	1135	21	5	1	0	557	4	2	1 1/2 carb., 1 fat

Food									
Spaghetti Sauce, Garden Combination (1/2 cup)	80	14	2	NA	0	420	NA	2	1 carb.
Spaghetti Sauce, Xtra Chunky, Garlic Cheese (1/2 cup)	130	22	4	1	0	610	3	3	1 1/2 carb., 1 fat
Spaghetti Sauce, Xtra Chunky, Mushroom Green Pepper (1/2 cup)	100	14	4	NA	0	410	NA	2	1 carb., 1 fat
Spaghetti Sauce, Xtra Chunky, Mushroom Onion (1/2 cup)	100	13	4	NA	0	490	NA	2	1 carb., 1 fat
Spaghetti Sauce, Xtra Chunky, Mushroom Spice (1/2 cup)	100	17	3	NA	0	450	NA	2	1 carb., 1 fat
Spaghetti Sauce, Xtra Chunky, Mushroom (1/2 cup)	130	20	5	NA	0	630	NA	2	1 carb., 1 fat
Spaghetti Sauce, Xtra Chunky, Mushroom Tomato (1/2 cup)	110	14	5	NA	0	500	NA	1	1 carb., 1 fat
Spaghetti Sauce, Xtra Chunky, Sausage Green Pepper (1/2 cup)	160	19	8	NA	0	500	NA	2	1 1/2 carb., 2 fat

SAUCES, CONDIMENTS, AND GRAVIES

Products	Cal.	Carb. (g)	Fat (g)	Sat. Fat (g)	Chol. (mg)	Sod. (mg)	Fib. (g)	Prot. (g)	Servings/Exchanges
Spaghetti Sauce, Xtra Chunky, Tomato Onion Garlic (1/2 cup)	110	14	5	NA	0	490	NA	2	1 carb., 1 fat
Spaghetti Sauce Flavored w/Meat (1/2 cup)	140	21	6	2	5	500	3	3	1 1/2 carb., 1 fat
PROGRESSO									
Pasta Sauce, Meat-Flavored (1/2 cup)	100	12	5	1	5	610	3	4	1 carb., 1 fat
Pizza Sauce (1/4 cup)	20	4	0	0	0	170	1	<1	1/2 carb.
Sauce, Authentic Alfredo (1/2 cup)	200	7	15	10	50	850	1	8	1/2 carb., 1 med-fat meat, 3 fat
Sauce, Authentic Marinara (1/2 cup)	100	12	4	1	<5	590	3	4	1 carb., 1 fat
Sauce, Authentic White Clam (1/2 cup)	150	5	10	2	20	710	0	9	1 med-fat meat, 1 fat
Sauce, Creamy Clam (1/2 cup)	110	8	6	2	10	440	0	5	1/2 carb., 1 fat
Sauce, Lobster (1/2 cup)	100	6	7	1	2	430	2	3	1/2 carb., 1 fat
Sauce, Marinara (1/2 cup)	80	8	5	<1	<5	480	2	2	1/2 carb., 1 fat
Sauce, Red Clam (1/2 cup)	60	8	1	0	10	350	1	4	1/2 carb., 1 med-fat meat

									Exchanges
Sauce, White Clam (1/2 cup)	140	5	10	2	15	510	0	7	1 med-fat meat, 1 fat
Spaghetti Sauce (1/2 cup)	100	12	5	1	<5	620	2	3	1 carb., 1 fat
QUE BUENO									
Enchilada Sauce (1/2 cup)	60	8	2	0	0	320	1	2	1/2 carb.
Salsa, Chunky (1 Tbsp)	5	<1	0	0	0	70	0	0	free
Salsa w/Green Chiles (1 Tbsp)	5	<1	0	0	0	80	0	0	free
Sauce, Jalapeño Cheese (2 Tbsp)	33	3	2	<1	3	248	0	1	1/2 fat
Sauce, Nacho Cheese (1/2 cup)	63	2	5	3	15	290	<1	3	1/2 carb., 1 fat
Sauce, Picante (1 Tbsp)	5	1	0	0	0	130	0	<1	free
Taco Sauce (2 Tbsp)	15	3	0	0	0	130	<1	0	free
REGINA									
Cooking Wine, Burgundy (1/4 cup)	20	1	1	0	0	365	0	1	free
Cooking Wine, Sherry (1/4 cup)	20	5	0	0	0	70	0	1	1/2 carb.
Vinegar, Red Wine, 50-grain (1 oz)	4	0	0	0	0	0	0	0	free
Vinegar, White Wine (1 oz)	4	1	0	0	0	0	0	0	free

SAUCES, CONDIMENTS, AND GRAVIES

Products	Cal.	Carb. (g)	Fat (g)	Sat. Fat (g)	Chol. (mg)	Sod. (mg)	Fib. (g)	Prot. (g)	Servings/Exchanges
ROSARITA									
Enchilada Sauce, Mild (2.5 oz)	25	3	1	1	0	230	1	1	free
Salsa, Extra Chunky, Medium (2 Tbsp)	30	7	1	0	0	280	NA	1	1/2 carb.
Salsa, Green Chili (1 oz)	7	2	<1	0	0	167	<1	<1	free
Salsa, Green Tomatillo, Medium (2 Tbsp)	20	4	1	0	0	190	NA	1	free
Salsa, Hot Chunky (3 Tbsp)	25	6	1	0	0	300	1	1	1/2 carb.
Salsa, Roasted, Mild (1 oz)	10	2	<1	0	0	233	<1	<1	free
Salsa, Traditional, Medium (2 Tbsp)	12	3	0	0	0	350	NA	1	free
Sauce, Zesty Jalapeño Picante, Medium (2 Tbsp)	8	2	<1	0	0	246	<1	<1	free
Taco Salsa, Mild (3 Tbsp)	25	6	1	0	0	300	1	1	1/2 carb.
SIMMER CHEF									
Sauce, Creamy Mushroom Herb (1/2 cup)	110	7	9	2	5	580	0	0	1/2 carb., 2 fat
Sauce, Family-Style Stroganoff (1/2 cup)	110	8	7	5	5	760	1	2	1/2 carb., 1 fat
Sauce, Golden Honey Mustard (1/2 cup)	150	30	2	0	0	400	1	1	2 carb.

Sauce, Hearty Onion Mushroom (1/2 cup)	50	9	1	0	0	670	1	1	1/2 carb.
Sauce, Old Country Cacciatore (1/2 cup)	110	15	4	1	0	540	2	2	1 carb., 1 fat
Sauce, Oriental Sweet & Sour (1/2 cup)	110	23	1	0	0	280	0	0	1 1/2 carb.
Sauce, Zesty Tomato Mexicali (1/2 cup)	90	16	3	1	1	400	1	2	1 carb., 1 fat

TABASCO

Sauce, Pepper (1 Tbsp)	2	<1	<1	<1	0	87	<1	<1	free

TOSTITOS

Salsa, Medium (2 Tbsp)	40	5	2	<1	5	65	1	1	1/2 carb.

WEIGHT WATCHERS

Pasta Sauce w/Mushrooms (1/3 cup)	40	9	0	0	0	430	NA	1	1 carb.

SNACK FOODS

Products	Cal.	Carb. (g)	Fat (g)	Sat. Fat (g)	Chol. (mg)	Sod. (mg)	Fib. (g)	Prot. (g)	Servings/Exchanges
Chips, Bagel (5)	298	52	7	1	0	419	6	6	3 1/2 strch, 1 fat
Chips, Yogurt (1 oz)	148	16	8	2	1	13	<1	3	1 strch, 2 fat
Cracker Crumbs, Graham (1/2 cup)	254	46	6	1	0	363	2	4	3 strch, 1 fat
Crackers, Animal (8)	45	7	1	<1	0	39	<1	<1	1/2 strch
Crackers, Graham (3)	89	16	2	<1	0	127	<1	1	1 strch
Crackers, Matzoh, Plain (1 oz)	112	24	<1	<1	0	<1	<1	3	1 1/2 strch
Crackers, Matzoh, Whole-Wheat (1)	100	22	<1	<1	0	<1	3	4	1 1/2 strch
Crackers, Norwegian Flatbread (5)	106	24	<1	<1	0	77	5	2	1 1/2 strch
Crackers, Rye Crispbread (2)	59	13	<1	<1	0	150	2	2	1 strch
Crispbread, Rye (1)	37	8	<1	<1	0	26	2	<1	1/2 strch
Melba Toast (2)	39	8	<1	<1	0	83	<1	1	1/2 strch
Oriental Snack Mix (1 oz)	155	9	12	5	0	235	4	5	1/2 strch, 2 fat
Popcorn, Air-Popped (1 cup)	31	6	<1	<1	0	<1	1	<1	1/2 strch

Popcorn, Caramel (1 cup)	152	28	5	1	2	73	2	1	1 strch, 1 fat
Popcorn, Cheese (1 cup)	58	6	4	<1	1	98	1	1	1/2 strch, 1 fat
Popcorn, Oil-Popped, Salted (1 cup)	55	6	3	<1	0	97	1	4	1/2 strch, 1 fat
Popcorn Cakes (2)	76	16	<1	<1	0	58	<1	2	1 strch
Pretzel Twists, Hard, Unsalted (1 oz)	108	23	<1	<1	0	486	<1	3	1 1/2 strch
Pretzels, Whole-Wheat (1 oz)	103	23	<1	<1	0	58	2	3	1 1/2 strch
Pretzels, Yogurt-Covered (5)	96	14	4	3	<1	13	<1	2	1 strch, 1 fat
Rice Cakes, Brown, Plain (2)	70	15	<1	<1	0	59	<1	2	1 strch
Rice Cakes, Brown, Sesame Seed (2 cakes)	71	15	<1	<1	0	41	<1	1	1 strch
Trail Mix (1/4 cup)	173	17	11	2	0	86	2	5	1 strch, 2 fat
BETTY CROCKER									
Bugles (1 1/2 cups)	160	18	9	8	0	310	<1	1	1 strch, 2 fat
Bugles, Baked, Cheddar Cheese (1 1/2 cups)	130	22	4	<1	0	440	0	2	1 1/2 strch, 1 fat
Bugles, Baked, Original (1 1/2 cups)	130	23	4	<1	0	380	0	2	1 1/2 strch, 1 fat
Bugles, Nacho Cheese (1 1/3 cups)	160	18	9	7	0	300	0	2	1 strch, 2 fat
Bugles, Smokin BBQ (1 1/3 cups)	150	19	8	7	0	330	0	1	1 strch, 2 fat

SNACK FOODS

Products	Cal.	Carb. (g)	Fat (g)	Sat. Fat (g)	Chol. (mg)	Sod. (mg)	Fib. (g)	Prot. (g)	Servings/Exchanges
Chex Mix, Bold Party Blend (1/2 cup)	140	20	6	1	0	390	2	3	1 strch, 1 fat
Chex Mix, Cheddar Cheese (1/2 cup)	140	21	5	1	0	330	2	3	1 1/2 strch, 1 fat
Chex Mix, Hot 'n Spicy (2/3 cup)	130	21	5	1	0	390	2	2	1 1/2 strch, 1 fat
Chex Mix, Nacho Fiesta (2/3 cup)	120	22	4	<1	0	350	1	2	1 1/2 strch, 1 fat
Chex Mix, Peanut Lovers (1/2 Cup)	140	19	6	1	0	350	1	3	1 strch, 1 fat
Chex Mix, Traditional (2/3 cup)	130	22	4	<1	0	410	2	2	1 1/2 strch, 1 fat
Dunk Aroos (1 tray)	120	21	4	1	0	55	0	0	1 1/2 carb., 1 fat
Fruit By The Foot (1 roll)	80	17	2	<1	0	50	0	0	1 carb.
Fruit Gushers (1 pouch)	90	20	1	0	0	45	0	0	1 carb.
Fruit Roll-Ups, Cherry (1)	50	12	<1	0	0	55	0	0	1 carb.
Fruit String Ling (1 pouch)	80	17	1	0	0	45	0	0	1 carb.
Golden Grahams Treats, Peanut Butter Chocolate (1)	90	15	4	1	0	105	0	1	1 carb., 1 fat

Golden Grahams Treats, S'Mores Chocolate Chunk (1)	90	17	3	<1	0	100	0	1	1 carb., 1 fat
Pop-Secret Popcorn, 94% Fat Free Butter (1 cup)	20	4	0	0	0	40	<1	<1	free
Pop-Secret Popcorn, Butter (1 cup)	35	4	3	<1	0	50	<1	<1	1 fat
Pop-Secret Popcorn, Cheddar Cheese (1 cup)	30	3	2	<1	0	45	<1	<1	1 fat
Pop-Secret Popcorn, Homestyle (1 cup)	35	4	3	<1	0	25	<1	<1	1 fat
Pop-Secret Popcorn, Light Butter (1 cup)	20	4	1	0	0	50	<1	<1	free
Pop-Secret Popcorn, Light Natural (1 cup)	25	4	1	0	0	45	<1	<1	free
Pop-Secret Popcorn, Movie Theater Butter (1 cup)	40	3	3	<1	0	55	<1	<1	1 fat
Pop-Secret Popcorn, Natural (1 cup)	35	4	3	<1	0	65	<1	<1	1 fat
Sweet Rewards Fat Free Bars, Blueberry w/Drizzle (1)	120	29	0	0	0	80	<1	1	2 carb.
Sweet Rewards Fat Free Bars, Double Fudge Supreme (1)	100	25	0	0	0	90	1	2	1 1/2 carb.

CLINICAL PRODUCTS

Extend Bar, Peanut Butter Crunch (1)	160	30	3	0	0	85	0	4	2 carb., 1 fat

SNACK FOODS

Products	Cal.	Carb. (g)	Fat (g)	Sat. Fat (g)	Chol. (mg)	Sod. (mg)	Fib. (g)	Prot. (g)	Servings/Exchanges
CRACKER JACK									
Fat-Free Butter Toffee (3/4 cup)	110	26	0	0	0	85	1	1	2 carb.
Fat Free Caramel (3/4 cup)	110	26	0	0	0	70	1	<1	2 carb.
Original (1/2 cup)	120	23	2	0	0	70	1	2	1 1/2 carb.
DEL MONTE									
Trail Mix, Sierra (1/4 cup)	150	20	8	3	0	65	3	4	1 strch, 1 high-fat meat
Yogurt Raisins, Strawberry (0.9-oz bag)	110	20	3	3	0	40	0	2	1 carb., 1 fat
Yogurt Raisins, Vanilla (0.9-oz bag)	110	20	3	3	0	40	0	2	1 carb., 1 fat
ESTEE									
Caramel Popcorn (1 cup)	120	26	2	0	0	90	1	<1	2 carb.
Cracked Pepper Crackers (18)	120	24	2	0	0	200	1	3	1 1/2 strch
Fruit & Nut Mix (1/4 cup)	210	19	12	7	<5	45	2	6	1 fruit, 1 high-fat meat, 1 fat
Golden Crakers (10)	130	28	2	0	0	200	1	3	2 strch
Graham Crackers, Sugar Free, Chocolate (2)	110	27	2	0	0	110	3	3	2 strch

Food								
Graham Crackers, Sugar Free, Cinnamon (2)	90	18	2	0	0	90	2	3	1 strch
Graham Crackers, Sugar Free, Old Fashioned (2)	90	17	2	0	0	115	2	3	1 strch
Mini Rice Cakes, Sugar-Free, Banana Nut (5)	60	14	<1	0	0	30	0	1	1 carb.
Mini Rice Cakes, Sugar-Free, Cinnamon Spice (5)	60	14	0	0	0	5	0	1	1 carb.
Mini Rice Cakes, Sugar-Free, Mixed Berry (5)	60	14	0	0	0	20	9	1	1 carb.
Mini Rice Cakes, Sugar-Free, Peanut Butter Crunch (5)	60	13	1	0	0	80	<1	1	1 carb.
Pretzels, Dutch (2)	130	26	1	0	0	40	1	3	2 strch
Pretzels, Unsalted (23)	120	25	1	0	0	30	1	3	1 1/2 strch
Rice Crunchie Bars, Chocolate (1)	50	15	0	0	0	40	<1	1	1 carb.
Rice Crunchie Bars, Peanut Butter (1)	60	15	1	0	0	35	0	1	1 carb.
Rice Crunchie Bars, Vanilla (1)	60	14	0	0	0	35	0	1	1 carb.
Wheat Crackers (17)	100	18	2	0	0	200	2	3	1 strch
FRANKLIN									
Crunch 'N Munch (2/3 cup)	150	22	6	2	5	170	<1	2	1 1/2 carb., 1 fat
Crunch 'N Munch, Toffee Pretzels (12)	120	25	1	0	0	200	0	1	1 1/2 carb.

SNACK FOODS

Products	Cal.	Carb. (g)	Fat (g)	Sat. Fat (g)	Chol. (mg)	Sod. (mg)	Fib. (g)	Prot. (g)	Servings/Exchanges
FRITO-LAY									
Baken-ets Fried Pork Rind, BBQ (9)	70	<1	5	2	10	400	<1	7	1 med-fat meat
Baken-ets Fried Pork Rind, Hot N' Spicy (7)	70	<1	5	2	20	440	<1	8	1 med-fat meat
Baken-ets Fried Pork Rind, Hot N' Spicy Cracklins (8)	80	<1	5	2	20	320	<1	7	1 med-fat meat
Baken-ets Fried Pork Rind, Regular (9)	80	<1	5	3	20	330	<1	8	1 med-fat meat
Baken-ets Fried Pork Rind, Regular Cracklins (8)	40	<1	6	2	15	550	<1	7	1 med-fat meat
Cheetos, Bacon Cheddar Crackers (1 pkg)	190	25	9	3	<5	410	1	3	1 1/2 strch, 2 fat
Cheetos, Cheddar Cheese Crackers (1 pkg)	210	23	11	3	<5	340	1	3	1 1/2 strch, 2 fat
Cheetos, Crunchy (1 oz)	160	15	10	3	0	290	<1	2	1 strch, 2 fat
Cheetos, Curls (1 oz)	150	15	10	3	0	290	1	20	1 strch, 2 fat
Cheetos, Flamin' Hot (1 oz)	160	15	10	2	0	280	<1	2	1 strch, 2 fat
Cheetos, Golden Toast Crackers (1 pkg)	240	25	14	4	5	440	1	4	1 1/2 strch, 3 fat
Cheetos, Nacho Cheese (1 oz)	160	15	10	3	0	260	<1	2	1 strch, 2 fat

Food	Cal.	Carb.	Fat	Sat. Fat	Chol.	Sod.	Fiber	Prot.	Exchanges
Cheetos, Puffed Balls (1 oz)	150	15	10	3	0	300	<1	2	1 strch, 2 fat
Cheetos, Puffs (1 oz)	160	15	10	3	0	370	<1	2	1 strch, 2 fat
Cheetos, Zig Zags (1 oz)	170	17	11	3	<5	370	<1	2	1 strch, 2 fat
Chester's Butter Popcorn (3 cups)	160	15	12	2	0	330	3	2	1 strch 2 fat
Chester's Caramel Craze Popcorn (3/4 cup)	130	27	2	0	0	220	1	1	2 strch
Chester's Cheddar Cheese Popcorn (3 cups)	190	17	13	3	0	300	3	3	1 strch, 3 fat
Chester's Microwave Butter Popcorn (5 cups)	200	22	12	2	0	300	4	3	1 1/2 strch, 2 fat
Cracker Snacks, Cheddars (1 pkg)	200	27	10	3	<5	530	1	5	2 strch, 2 fat
Crackers, Doritos Jalapeño Cheese (1 pkg)	230	26	14	4	<5	450	1	3	1/2 strch, 3 fat
Crackers, Peter Pan Cheese Peanut Butter (1 pkg)	210	23	10	3	0	350	1	5	1 1/2 strch, 2 fat
Crackers, Peter Pan Toast Peanut Butter (1 pkg)	210	23	11	3	0	280	<1	5	1 1/2 strch, 2 fat
Doritos, 3D's Cooler Ranch (1 oz)	140	18	6	2	<5	350	1	2	1 strch, 1 fat
Doritos, 3D's Nacho Cheesier (1 oz)	140	17	7	2	<5	360	1	2	1 strch, 1 fat
Doritos, Cooler Ranch (1 oz)	140	18	7	2	0	170	1	2	1 strch, 1 fat
Doritos, Flamin Hot (1 oz)	140	17	7	2	0	210	1	2	1 strch, 2 fat
Doritos, Nacho Cheesier (1 oz)	140	17	7	1	0	200	1	2	1 strch, 1 fat

SNACK FOODS

Products	Cal.	Carb. (g)	Fat (g)	Sat. Fat (g)	Chol. (mg)	Sod. (mg)	Fib. (g)	Prot. (g)	Servings/Exchanges
Doritos, Nacho Cheesier Crackers (1 pkg)	240	25	14	3	<5	340	1	4	1 1/2 strch, 3 fat
Doritos, Salsa Verde (1 oz)	150	20	7	2	0	210	1	2	1strch, 1 fat
Doritos, Smokey Red (1 oz)	150	21	7	2	0	210	1	2	1 1/2 strch, 1 fat
Doritos, Spicy Nacho (1 oz)	140	18	6	2	0	210	1	2	1 strch, 1 fat
Doritos, Toasted Corn (1 oz)	140	10	7	2	0	120	1	2	1 strch, 1 fat
Doritos, WOW Nacho Cheesier (1 oz)	90	18	1	0	0	240	1	2	1 strch
Fritos, BBQ (1 oz)	150	16	9	1	0	290	1	2	1 strch, 2 fat
Fritos, Chili Cheese (1 oz)	160	16	10	2	0	240	1	2	1 strch, 2 fat
Fritos, King Size (1 oz)	160	16	10	2	0	150	1	2	1 strch, 2 fat
Fritos, Original (1 oz)	160	15	10	2	0	170	1	2	1 strch, 2 fat
Fritos, Sabrositas Flamin' Hot (1 oz)	150	16	9	2	0	180	1	2	1 strch, 2 fat
Fritos, Sabrositas Lime 'N Chili (1 oz)	150	17	9	2	0	240	1	2	1 strch, 2 fat
Fritos, Scoops (1 oz)	160	17	10	1	0	105	1	2	1 strch, 2 fat

Food									Exchanges
Fritos, Texas Grill Honey BBQ (1 oz)	150	16	9	2	0	200	1	2	1 strch, 2 fat
Fritos, Wild N' Mild Ranch (1 oz)	160	15	10	2	0	160	1	2	1 strch, 2 fat
Funyuns (1 oz)	140	18	7	2	0	270	<1	2	1 strch, 1 fat
Lay's, Adobadas Potato Chips (1 oz)	170	18	10	3	0	240	1	2	1 strch, 2 fat
Lay's, Baked KC Masterpiece BBQ Potato Chips (1 oz)	120	22	3	0	0	210	2	2	1 1/2 strch, 1 fat
Lay's, Baked Original Potato Chips (1 oz)	110	23	2	0	0	150	2	2	1 1/2 strch
Lay's, Baked Roasted Herb Potato Chips (1 oz)	130	25	3	<1	0	190	2	2	1 1/2 strch, 1 fat
Lay's, Baked Sour Cream & Onion Potato Chips (1 oz)	120	21	3	0	0	210	2	2	1 1/2 strch, 1 fat
Lay's, Classic Potato Chips (1 oz)	150	15	10	3	0	180	1	2	1 strch, 2 fat
Lay's, Deli Style Original Potato Chips (1 oz)	150	16	10	3	0	180	1	1	1 strch, 2 fat
Lay's, Deli Style Salt & Vinegar (1 oz)	150	16	10	3	0	380	1	1	1 strch, 2 fat
Lay's, Flamin' Hot Potato Chips (1 oz)	150	16	10	3	0	180	1	2	1 strch, 2 fat
Lay's, KC Masterpiece BBQ Potato Chips (1 oz)	150	15	10	3	0	200	1	2	1 strch, 2 fat
Lay's, Onion & Garlic Potato Chips (1 oz)	150	16	9	3	0	200	1	2	1 strch, 2 fat

SNACK FOODS

Products	Cal.	Carb. (g)	Fat (g)	Sat. Fat (g)	Chol. (mg)	Sod. (mg)	Fib. (g)	Prot. (g)	Servings/Exchanges
Lay's, Salt & Vinegar Potato Chips (1 oz)	150	15	10	3	0	300	1	2	1 strch, 2 fat
Lay's, Sour Cream & Onion Potato Chips (1 oz)	160	12	11	3	<5	200	1	2	1 strch, 2 fat
Lay's, Toasted Onion & Cheese Potato Chips (1 oz)	160	14	10	3	0	240	1	2	1 strch, 2 fat
Lay's, Wavy Original Potato Chips (1 oz)	160	15	10	3	0	210	1	2	1 strch, 2 fat
Lay's, Wavy Ranch Potato Chips (1 oz)	160	14	11	3	0	150	1	2	1 strch, 2 fat
Lay's, Wavy Au Gratin Potato Chips (1 oz)	150	14	10	3	<5	200	1	2	1 strch, 2 fat
Lay's, WOW Mesquite BBQ Potato Chips (1 oz)	75	17	0	0	0	250	1	2	1 strch
Lay's, WOW Original Potato Chips (1 oz)	75	18	0	0	0	200	1	2	1 strch
Lay's, WOW Sour Cream & Chive Potato Chips (1 oz)	80	17	0	0	0	230	1	2	1 strch
Munchos (1 oz)	160	16	10	2	0	230	1	1	1 strch, 2 fat
Munchos, BBQ (1 oz)	160	15	10	2	0	250	1	1	1 strch, 2 fat
Rold Gold, Crispy's Thins Pretzels (1 oz)	110	22	2	0	670	0	1	3	1 1/2 strch
Rold Gold, Fat-Free Cheddar Cheese Pretzels (1 oz)	110	23	0	0	0	440	1	3	1 1/2 strch
Rold Gold, Fat-Free Honey Mustard Pretzels (1 oz)	110	23	0	0	0	380	1	3	1 1/2 strch

Rold Gold, Fat-Free Pretzel Thins (1 oz)	110	24	0	0	0	520	1	2	1 1/2 strch
Rold Gold, Fat-Free Sticks Pretzels (1 oz)	110	23	0	0	0	530	1	3	1 1/2 strch
Rold Gold, Fat-Free Tiny Twists Pretzels (1 oz)	100	23	0	0	0	420	1	3	1 1/2 strch
Rold Gold, Rods Pretzels (1 oz)	110	22	1	0	0	610	1	3	1 1/2 strch
Rold Gold, Sour Dough Nuggets (1 oz)	110	24	0	0	0	330	1	2	1 1/2 strch
Ruffles, Cheddar & Sour Cream Potato Chips (1 oz)	160	14	10	3	0	190	1	2	1 strch, 2 fat
Ruffles, French Onion Potato Chips (1 oz)	150	15	10	3	0	190	1	2	1 strch, 2 fat
Ruffles, KC Masterpiece Mesquite BBQ Potato Chips (1 oz)	150	15	10	3	0	190	1	1	1 strch, 2 fat
Ruffles, Original Potato Chips (1 oz)	150	14	10	3	0	180	1	2	1 strch, 2 fat
Ruffles, Ranch Potato Chips (1 oz)	150	15	9	3	0	280	1	2	1 strch, 2 fat
Ruffles, Reduced-Fat Regular Potato Chips (1 oz)	130	18	7	1	0	160	1	2	1 strch, 1 fat
Santitas 100% White Corn Tortilla Chips (1 oz)	130	19	6	1	0	110	1	2	1 strch, 1 fat
Santitas Restaurant-Style Tortilla Strips (1 oz)	130	19	6	1	0	110	1	2	1 strch, 1 fat
Smartfood Butter Popcorn (3 cup)	150	15	9	2	5	240	1	2	1 strch, 2 fat

SNACK FOODS

Products	Cal.	Carb. (g)	Fat (g)	Sat. Fat (g)	Chol. (mg)	Sod. (mg)	Fib. (g)	Prot. (g)	Servings/Exchanges
Smartfood Butter Popcorn, Reduced-Fat (3 1/3 cups)	130	21	4	<1	0	410	4	3	1 1/2 strch, 1 fat
Smartfood Toffee Crunch Popcorn, Low-Fat (3/4 cup)	110	25	1	0	0	220	1	1	2 strch
Smartfood White Cheddar Cheese Popcorn (2 cups)	190	17	12	3	5	310	2	3	1 strch, 2 fat
Smartfood White Cheddar Cheese Popcorn, Reduced-Fat (3 cups)	140	19	6	2	<5	280	3	4	1 strch, 1 fat
Sunchips, French Onion (1 oz)	140	18	7	1	0	115	2	2	1 strch, 1 fat
Sunchips, Harvest Cheddar (1 oz)	140	19	6	1	0	115	2	2	1 strch, 1 fat
Sunchips, Original (1 oz)	140	19	6	1	0	115	2	2	1 strch, 1 fat
Tostitos, Baked Bite Size (1 oz)	110	24	1	0	0	200	2	3	1 1/2 strch
Tostitos, Baked Bite Size Salsa & Cream Cheese (1 oz)	120	21	3	<1	0	190	1	2	1 1/2 strch, 1 fat

	Cal.	Carb. (g)	Fat (g)	Sat. Fat (g)		Sod. (mg)			Exchanges
Tostitos, Baked Original (1 oz)	110	21	1	0	3	200	1	3	1 1/2 strch
Tostitos, Bite Size (1 oz)	140	17	8	1	0	110	1	2	1 strch, 2 fat
Tostitos, Crispy Rounds (1 oz)	150	17	8	1	0	85	1	2	1 strch, 2 fat
Tostitos, Nacho Style (1 oz)	140	19	6	1	0	100	1	2	1 strch, 1 fat
Tostitos, Restaurant-Style (1 oz)	140	19	6	1	0	110	1	2	1 strch, 1 fat
Tostitos, Restaurant-Style, Hint of Lime (1 oz)	140	19	6	1	0	160	1	2	1 strch, 1 fat
Tostitos, Sante Fe Gold (1 oz)	140	19	6	1	0	80	1	2	1 strch, 1 fat
Tostitos, WOW Original Tortilla Chips (1 oz)	90	20	1	0	0	105	1	2	1 strch
GARDETTO'S									
Snack Mix, Chips & Twists, Sour Cream & Chive (1/2 cup)	130	21	4	<1	0	310	2	3	1 1/2 strch, 1 fat
Snack Mix, Snak-ens, Original (1/2 cup)	160	19	8	2	0	300	1	3	1 strch, 2 fat
Snack Mix, Snak-ens, Reduced Fat (1/2 cup)	140	20	5	1	0	320	1	3	1 strch, 1 fat
HEALTH VALLEY									
Caramel Corn Puffs, Fat-Free (1 oz)	100	21	0	0	0	45	<1	3	1 1/2 carb.

SNACK FOODS

Products	Cal.	Carb. (g)	Fat (g)	Sat. Fat (g)	Chol. (mg)	Sod. (mg)	Fib. (g)	Prot. (g)	Servings/Exchanges
Caramel Corn Puffs, Fat-Free Apple Cinnamon (1 oz)	100	21	0	0	0	50	<1	3	1 1/2 carb.
Caramel Corn Puffs, Peanut Flavor (1 oz)	100	21	0	0	0	65	<1	3	1 1/2 carb.
Cheese Flavor Puffs, w/Green Onion (1 oz)	100	21	0	0	0	75	<1	3	1 1/2 strch
Cheese Flavor Puffs, Fat-Free (1 oz)	100	21	0	0	0	75	<1	3	1 1/2 strch
Cheese Flavor Puffs, Fat-Free Zesty Chili (1 oz)	100	21	0	0	0	75	<1	3	1 1/2 strch
Crackers, Fat-Free Amaranth Graham (8)	100	23	0	0	0	30	3	4	1 1/2 strch
Crackers, Fat-Free Fire, Hot 3-Chili Cheese (6)	50	11	0	0	0	80	2	2	1 strch
Crackers, Fat-Free Fire, Medium Jalapeño Cheese (6)	50	11	0	0	0	80	2	2	1 strch
Crackers, Fat-Free Fire, Mild Chili Cheese (6)	50	11	0	0	0	80	2	2	1 strch
Crackers, Fat-Free Healthy Pizza, Cheese (6)	50	11	0	0	0	140	2	2	1 strch
Crackers, Fat-Free Healthy Pizza, Garlic (6)	50	11	0	0	0	140	2	2	1 strch
Crackers, Fat-Free Oat Bran Graham (8)	100	23	0	0	0	30	3	4	1 1/2 strch
Crackers, Fat-Free Whole-Wheat (5)	50	11	0	0	0	80	2	2	1 strch

	Cal.	Carb.	Fat	Sat. Fat	Chol.	Sod.	Fiber	Prot.	Exchanges
Crackers, Fat-Free Whole-Wheat, Cheese (5)	50	11	0	0	0	80	2	2	1 strch
Crackers, Fat-Free Whole-Wheat, Herb (5)	50	11	0	0	0	80	2	2	1 strch
Granola Bar, Fat-Free Blueberry Apple (1)	140	33	0	0	0	10	4	3	2 carb.
Granola Bar, Fat-Free Date Almcnd (1)	140	33	0	0	0	10	4	3	2 carb.
Granola Bar, Fat-Free Raspberry (1)	140	33	0	0	0	10	4	3	2 carb.
Snack Bar, Apple (1)	100	16	3	0	0	27	3	2	1 cart.
Snack Bar, Date (1)	100	16	3	0	0	25	3	3	1 carb., 1 fat
Snack Bar, Fruit (1)	200	39	3	0	0	234	5	4	2 1/2 carb., 1 fat
KEEBLER									
Chocolate Grahams (8)	130	23	4	1	0	115	0	2	1 1/2 carb., 1 fat
Cinnamon Crisps (8)	130	24	3	1	0	230	<1	1	1 1/2 carb., 1 fat
Cinnamon Crisps, Low-Fat (8)	110	23	2	<1	0	160	1	2	1 1/2 strch
Cracker Sandwiches, Cheese & Peanut Butter (1 pkg)	190	22	9	2	<5	420	<1	6	1 1/2 strch, 2 fat
Cracker Sandwiches, Club & Cheddar (1 pkg)	190	20	11	3	10	320	<1	3	1 strch, 2 fat

SNACK FOODS

Products	Cal.	Carb. (g)	Fat (g)	Sat. Fat (g)	Chol. (mg)	Sod. (mg)	Fib. (g)	Prot. (g)	Servings/Exchanges
Cracker Sandwiches, Toast & Peanut Butter (1 pkg)	190	23	9	2	30	300	1	5	1 1/2 strch, 2 fat
Cracker Sandwiches, Wheat & Cheddar (1 pkg)	180	17	10	3	5	300	0	2	1 strch, 2 fat
Crackers, Club, 33% Reduced-Fat (5)	70	12	2	0	0	200	0	1	1 strch
Crackers, Club, 50% Reduced-Sodium (4)	70	9	3	1	0	80	0	1	1/2 strch, 1 fat
Crackers, Club, Original (4)	70	9	3	1	0	1600	0	1	1/2 strch, 1 fat
Crackers, Toasteds, Buttercrisp (5)	80	10	4	1	0	150	0	1	1/2 strch, 1 fat
Crackers, Toasteds, Onion (5)	80	10	3	<1	0	230	0	1	1 strch, 1 fat
Crackers, Toasteds, Reduced-Fat Wheat (5)	60	10	2	0	0	160	<1	1	1/2 strch, 1 fat
Crackers, Toasteds, Sesame (5)	80	10	4	<1	0	160	<1	1	1 strch, 1 fat
Crackers, Toasteds, Wheat (5)	80	11	3	<1	0	160	0	1	1 strch, 1 fat
Crackers, Town House (5)	80	9	5	1	0	150	<1	1	1/2 strch, 1 fat
Crackers, Town House, 50% Reduced-Fat (6)	70	11	2	<1	0	180	<1	1	1 strch
Crackers, Town House, 50% Reduced-Sodium (5)	80	10	5	1	0	75	<1	1	1/2 strch, 1 fat

Crackers, Zesta Saltines, 50% Reduced-Sodium (5)	70	11	2	<1	0	95	<1	1	1 strch
Crackers, Zesta Saltines, Fat-Free (5)	50	11	0	0	0	150	0	1	1 strch
Crackers, Zesta Saltines, Original (5)	60	10	2	<1	0	190	<1	1	1 strch
Crackers, Zesta Saltines, Unsalted Tops (5)	70	10	2	<1	0	90	<1	1	1 strch
Crackers, Zesta Soup & Oyster (45)	70	9	3	1	0	220	0	1	1/2 strch, 1 fat
Honey Grahams (8)	140	23	5	1	0	170	0	2	1 1/2 carb., 1 fat
Honey Grahams, Low Fat (9)	120	25	2	<1	0	210	1	2	1 1/2 carb.
Munch'ems, Seasoned Original (41)	140	21	5	1	0	220	1	2	1 strch, 1 fat
Original Grahams (8)	130	23	3	1	0	135	<1	2	1 1/2 carb., 1 fat
Snackin' Cinnamon Crisp Grahams (21)	130	23	3	1	0	210	1	2	1 1/2 carb., 1 fat
Snackin' Honey Grahams (23)	130	22	4	1	0	120	<1	2	1 1/2 carb., 1 fat
Wheatables, 33% Reduced-Fat (13)	130	21	4	1	0	230	2	2	1 1/2 strch, 1 fat
Wheatables, Original (12)	140	19	6	2	0	210	1	2	1 strch, 1 fat
KELLOGG'S									
Nutri-Grain Bar, Apple Cinnamon (1)	140	27	3	<1	0	110	1	2	2 carb., 1 fat
Nutri-Grain Bar, Blueberry (1)	140	27	3	<1	0	110	1	2	2 carb., 1 fat

SNACK FOODS

Products	Cal.	Carb. (g)	Fat (g)	Sat. Fat (g)	Chol. (mg)	Sod. (mg)	Fib. (g)	Prot. (g)	Servings/Exchanges
Nutri-Grain Bar, Cherry (1)	140	27	3	<1	0	110	1	2	2 carb., 1 fat
Nutri-Grain Bar, Mixed Berry (1)	140	27	3	<1	0	110	1	2	2 carb., 1 fat
Nutri-Grain Bar, Peach (1)	140	27	3	<1	0	110	1	2	2 carb., 1 fat
Nutri-Grain Bar, Raspberry (1)	140	27	3	<1	0	110	1	2	2 carb., 1 fat
Nutri-Grain Bar, Strawberry (1)	140	27	3	<1	0	110	1	2	1 1/2 carb., 1 fat
Nutri-Grain Fruit-full Squares, Apple (1)	180	35	4	<1	0	95	1	3	2 carb., 1 fat
Nutri-Grain Fruit-full Squares, Banana (1)	190	35	5	<1	0	100	1	3	2 carb., 1 fat
Nutri-Grain Fruit-full Squares, Cinnamon Raisin (1)	180	35	4	<1	0	95	1	3	2 carb., 1 fat
Nutri-Grain Twists Cereal Bar, Apple Cinnamon (1)	140	27	3	<1	0	105	1	1	2 carb., 1 fat
Nutri-Grain Twists Cereal Bar, Banana & Strawberry (1)	140	26	3	<1	0	100	1	1	2 carb., 1 fat
Nutri-Grain Twists Cereal Bar, Strawberry & Blueberry (1)	140	27	3	<1	0	110	1	1	2 carb., 1 fat

Nutri-Grain Twists Cereal Bar, Strawberry & Crème (1)	140	26	3	<1	0	125	1	2	2 carb., 1 fat
Pop-Tarts Pastry Swirls, Apple Cinnamon (1)	260	37	11	3	0	190	1	3	2 1/2 carb., 2 fat
Pop-Tarts Pastry Swirls, Cheese (1)	260	36	11	3	0	180	0	3	2 1/2 carb., 2 fat
Pop-Tarts Pastry Swirls, Strawberry (1)	260	37	11	3	0	170	1	3	2 1/2 carb., 2 fat
Pop-Tarts Snack-Stix, Frosted Berry (1)	190	37	4	1	37	240	1	2	2 1/2 carb., 1 fat
Pop-Tarts Snack-Stix, Frosted Strawberry (1)	190	37	4	1	0	240	1	2	2 1/2 carb., 1 fat
Rice Krispies Treats, Cocoa (1)	100	16	4	1	0	105	0	1	1 carb., 1 fat
Rice Krispies Treats, Original (1)	90	18	2	<1	0	100	0	1	1 carb.
Rice Krispies Treats, Peanut Butter Chocolate (1)	110	16	4	1	0	100	0	2	1 carb., 1 fat
Snack 'Ums, Big Boomin' Pops (1 cup)	120	27	0	0	0	135	0	2	2 carb.
Snack 'Ums, Big Rollin' Froot Loops (1 1/4 cup)	120	28	1	<1	0	150	1	2	2 carb.
Snack 'Ums, Rice Krispies Treats Krunch (1 cup)	130	26	2	<1	0	10	0	2	2 carb
KRAFT									
Handi-Snacks, Cheez 'n Breadsticks (1 pkg)	120	12	6	3	15	320	0	4	1 strch, 1 fat
Handi-Snacks, Cheez 'n Crackers (1 pkg)	110	9	7	3	15	300	0	3	1/2 strch, 1 fat

SNACK FOODS

Products	Cal.	Carb. (g)	Fat (g)	Sat. Fat (g)	Chol. (mg)	Sod. (mg)	Fib. (g)	Prot. (g)	Servings/Exchanges
Handi-Snacks, Cheez 'n Pretzels (1 pkg)	100	11	5	3	15	410	<1	4	1 strch, 1 fat
Handi-Snacks, Mozzarella String Cheese (1 pkg)	80	0	6	4	0	240	0	7	1 med-fat meat
Handi-Snacks, Nacho Stix'n Cheez (1)	110	11	6	3	15	320	0	4	1 strch, 1 fat
M & M MARS									
Granola Bars, Kudos Chocolate Chip (1)	120	20	5	3	0	70	1	2	1 carb., 1 fat
Granola Bars, Kudos Peanut Butter (1)	130	19	5	2	0	85	1	2	1 carb., 1 fat
MEAD JOHNSON									
Choice DM Bar, Fudge Brownie (1)	140	19	5	3	<5	80	3	6	1 carb., 1 fat
Choice DM Bar, Peanutty Chocolate (1)	140	19	5	3	<5	80	3	6	1 carb., 1 fat
MEDICAL FOODS									
Nite Bite, Chocolate Fudge (1)	100	15	4	1	5	40	0	3	1 carb., 1/2 fat
Nite Bite, Peanut Butter (1)	100	15	4	1	5	80	0	3	1 carb., 1/2 fat
NABISCO									
Air Crisps, Cheese Nips (32)	130	21	4	1	<5	300	<1	3	1 1/2 strch, 1 fat

Food	Cal	Carb		Fat		Sod	Fib		Exchanges
Air Crisps, Ritz Original (24)	140	22	5	1	0	240	<1	2	1 1/2 strch, 1 fat
Air Crisps, Wheat Thins (24)	130	21	5	1	0	290	1	2	1 1/2 strch, 1 fat
Better Cheddars (22)	150	17	8	2	<5	290	<1	4	1 strch, 2 fat
Better Cheddars, Reduced-Fat (24)	140	19	6	2	<5	350	<1	4	1 strch, 1 fat
Cereal Bar, Snackwell's Apple Cinnamon (1)	130	26	3	<1	0	70	1	1	1 1/2 carb., 1 fat
Cereal Bar, Snackwell's Blueberry (1)	120	28	0	0	0	85	1	1	2 carb.
Cereal Bar, Snackwell's Mixed Berry	130	26	3	<1	0	95	1	1	2 carb., 1 fat
Cereal Bar, Snackwell's Strawberry (1)	120	28	0	0	0	115	1	1	2 carb.
Cheese Nips (27)	140	19	6	2	<5	350	<1	3	1 strch, 1 fat
Cheese Nips, Reduced-Fat (31)	130	21	4	1	0	310	<1	3	1 strch, 1 fat
Chicken-In-A-Biskit (12)	160	17	9	2	0	270	<1	2	1 strch, 2 fat
Crackers, Barnum's Animal (10)	120	22	4	<1	0	140	NA	NA	1 1/2 strch, 1 fat
Crackers, Harvest Crisps, 5-Grain (13)	130	23	4	<1	0	270	1	3	1 1/2 strch, 1 fat
Crackers, Honey Maid Chocolate Graham (8)	120	22	3	<1	0	170	1	2	1 1/2 carb., 1 fat
Crackers, Honey Maid Graham, Low-Fat (8)	110	23	2	0	0	200	<1	2	1 strch
Crackers, Honey Maid Honey Graham (8)	120	22	3	0	0	180	1	2	1 1/2 carb., 1 fat

SNACK FOODS

Products	Cal.	Carb. (g)	Fat (g)	Sat. Fat (g)	Chol. (mg)	Sod. (mg)	Fib. (g)	Prot. (g)	Servings/Exchanges
Crackers, Honey Maid Low-Fat Cinnamon Graham (8)	110	23	2	0	0	170	<1	2	1 1/2 strch
Crackers, Premium Saltine (5)	60	10	2	<1	0	180	0	1	1/2 strch
Crackers, Premium Saltine, Unsalted Tops (5)	60	10	2	0	0	105	0	1	1/2 strch
Crackers, Ritz (5)	80	10	4	<1	10	135	0	1	1/2 strch, 2 fat
Crackers, Ritz Bits, Cheese (14)	170	17	10	3	5	300	0	3	1 strch, 2 fat
Crackers, Ritz Bits, Peanut Butter (14)	150	18	8	2	0	200	1	3	1 strch, 2 fat
Crackers, Ritz, Reduced Fat (5)	70	11	2	0	0	140	0	1	1 strch
Crackers, Snackwell's Fat-Free Cracked Pepper (5)	60	10	2	0	0	115	0	1	1/2 strch
Crackers, Snackwell's French Onion (28)	130	23	3	<1	0	270	<1	2	1 1/2 strch, 1 fat
Crackers, Snackwell's Wheat (5)	70	11	2	0	0	150	<1	1	1 strch
Crackers, Snackwell's Zesty Cheese (38)	130	23	3	<1	0	320	<1	2	1 1/2 strch, 1 fat
Crackers, Swiss Cheese (15)	140	18	7	2	0	350	<1	2	1 strch, 1 fat
Crackers, Triscuits (7)	140	22	5	1	0	170	4	3	1 1/2 strch, 1 fat

Crackers, Triscuits, Reduced Fat (8)	130	24	3	<1	0	170	4	3	1 1/2 strch, 1 fat
Crackers, Triscuit Thin Crisps (15)	130	21	5	1	0	170	3	3	1 1/2 strch, 1 fat
Crackers, Wheatsworth, Wheat Crackers (5)	80	10	4	<1	0	170	1	2	1/2 strch, 1 fat
Crackers, Wheat Thins, Original (16)	140	19	6	1	0	260	1	2	1 strch, 1 fat
Crackers, Wheat Thins, Reduced-Fat (18)	120	21	4	<1	0	270	1	3	1 1/2 strch, 1 fat
Crackers, Vegetable Thins (14)	160	19	9	2	0	310	1	2	1 strch, 2 fat
Twigs Snack Sticks (15)	150	17	7	2	0	300	<1	4	1 strch, 1 fat
Sociables (7)	80	9	4	<1	0	150	0	1	1/2 strch, 1 fat

NATURE VALLEY

Granola Bars, Crunchy, Oats N' Honey (2)	180	29	6	<1	0	160	2	4	2 carb., 1 fat
Granola Bars, Chewy, Low-Fat (1)	110	21	2	0	0	65	1	2	1 1/2 strch

NESTLE

Snack Bar, Sweet Success Chocolate Brownie (1)	120	18	4	2	0	35	3	2	1 carb., 1 fat
Snack Bar, Sweet Success Chocolate Chip (1)	120	18	4	2	0	35	3	2	1 carb., 1 fat
Snack Bar, Sweet Success Chocolate Peanut Butter (1)	120	18	4	2	0	35	3	2	1 carb., 1 fat

SNACK FOODS

Products	Cal.	Carb. (g)	Fat (g)	Sat. Fat (g)	Chol. (mg)	Sod. (mg)	Fib. (g)	Prot. (g)	Servings/Exchanges
OCEAN SPRAY									
Craisins (1/3 cup)	130	33	0	0	0	0	2	0	2 carb.
Cran Fruit (1/4 cup)	120	29	0	0	0	35	2	0	2 carb.
OLD EL PASO									
Tortilla Chips, Nachips (1 oz = 9 chips)	150	17	8	2	0	85	2	3	1 strch, 2 fat
Tortilla Chips, White Corn (1 oz = 11 chips)	140	16	8	1	0	60	1	2	1 strch, 2 fat
ORVILLE REDENBACHER'S									
Mini Popcorn Cake, Caramel (6)	60	13	0	0	0	35	1	1	1 carb.
Mini Popcorn Cake, Chocolate Peanut Crunch (6)	60	12	<1	0	0	25	2	2	1 carb.
Mini Popcorn Cake, Chocolate Peanut Crunch, Low-Fat (6)	60	12	1	0	0	20	1	2	1 carb.
Mini Popcorn Cake, Peanut Caramel Crunch (6)	60	13	<1	0	0	35	1	1	1 carb.
Popcorn Cake, Caramel (1)	34	8	<1	0	0	16	<1	1	1/2 carb.

Popcorn Cake, White Cheddar Cheese (2)	63	13	<1	<1	0	83	2	1	1 carb.

PEPPERIDGE FARM

Chips, Three Cheese Bagel (1 oz)	250	28	12	2	10	425	<1	7	2 strch, 2 fat
Cracker Trio (4)	70	10	3	0	0	100	1	1	1/2 strch, 1 fat
Crackers, Butter-Flavored Thins (4)	70	10	3	1	10	95	0	1	1/2 strch, 1 fat
Crackers, Cracked Wheat (3)	105	14	4	2	0	225	<1	2	1 strch, 1 fat
Crackers, Hearty Wheat, Distinctive Assortment (3)	80	10	4	0	0	90	1	2	1/2 strch, 1 fat
Crackers, Goldfish, Cheddar, LoSalt (60)	150	18	6	2	10	175	<1	3	1 strch, 1 fat
Crackers, Goldfish, Original (55)	140	19	6	2	10	250	<1	4	1 strch, 1 fat
Crackers, Goldfish, Parmesan Cheese (60)	140	19	5	2	0	300	1	4	1 strch, 1 fat
Crackers, Goldfish, Pizza Flavor (55)	140	19	6	2	0	160	1	3	1 strch, 1 fat
Crackers, Goldfish, Pretzel Flavor (55)	140	19	6	2	0	160	1	3	1 strch, 1 fat
Crackers, Goldfish, White Cheddar Cheese (55)	150	18	7	2	<5	270	<1	3	1 strch, 1 fat
Crackers, Hearty Wheat (3)	80	10	4	0	0	100	1	2	1/2 strch, 1 fat
Crackers, Pretzel Distinctive (9)	130	23	3	0	?	440	?	?	1 1/2 strch, 1 fat

SNACK FOODS

Products	Cal.	Carb. (g)	Fat (g)	Sat. Fat (g)	Chol. (mg)	Sod. (mg)	Fib. (g)	Prot. (g)	Servings/Exchanges
Snack Mix, Goldfish, Cheddar (1/2 cup)	160	19	7	2	<5	370	1	3	1 strch, 1 fat
Snack Mix, Goldfish, Fat-Free Pretzel (1/2 cup)	100	21	0	0	0	400	<1	3	1 1/2 strch
Snack Mix, Goldfish, Garlic w/Bagel Chips (1/2 cup)	140	22	5	<1	0	360	1	3	1 1/2 strch, 1 fat
Snack Mix, Goldfish, Original (1/2 cup)	170	19	8	2	<5	380	2	5	1 strch, 2 fat
Snack Mix, Goldfish, Savory (1/2 cup)	150	20	7	1	0	380	1	3	1 strch, 1 fat
Snack Sticks, Sesame (9)	140	19	5	1	0	280	1	4	1 strch, 1 fat
PLANTERS									
Fiddle Faddle (3/4 cup)	150	20	7	3	10	180	1	2	1 carb., 1 fat
Fiddle Faddle, Fat-Free (1 cup)	110	28	0	0	0	210	NA	2	2 carb.
QUAKER									
Chewy Granola Bars, Apple & Cinnamon (1)	110	21	2	1	0	70	1	1	1 1/2 carb.
Chewy Granola Bars, Apple Berry (1)	110	23	2	<1	0	80	1	1	1 1/2 carb.
Chewy Granola Bars, Chocolate Chip (1)	120	21	4	2	0	70	1	2	1 1/2 carb., 1 fat

Food									
Chewy Granola Bars, Chocolate Chip Graham Slam (1)	10	22	2	<1	0	80	1	2	1 1/2 carb.
Chewy Granola Bars, Chocolate Chunk (1)	110	22	2	<1	0	80	1	2	1 1/2 carb.
Chewy Granola Bars, Cookies'n Cream (1)	110	22	3	<1	0	80	1	2	1 1/2 carb., 1 fat
Chewy Granola Bars, Oatmeal Raisin (1)	110	22	2	<1	0	70	1	1	1 1/2 carb.
Chewy Granola Bars, Peanut Butter & Chocolate Chunk (1)	120	20	3	1	0	105	1	2	1 carb., 1 fat
Chewy Granola Bars, Peanut Butter Graham Slam (1)	110	22	2	0	0	80	1	2	1 1/2 carb.
Chewy Granola Bars, S'mores (1)	110	22	2	<1	0	80	1	1	1 1/2 carb.
Crispy Mini's Rice Snacks, BBQ (10)	70	12	2	0	0	140	0	1	1 carb.
Crispy Mini's Rice Snacks, Honey Nut (8)	60	15	0	0	0	90	0	1	1 carb.
Fruit & Oatmeal Cereal Bars, Apple Cinnamon (1)	140	26	3	0	0	85	1	2	2 carb., 1 fat
Fruit & Oatmeal Cereal Bars, Blueberry (1)	140	26	3	0	0	120	1	2	2 carb., 1 fat
Fruit & Oatmeal Cereal Bars, Cherry Cobbler (1)	140	26	3	0	0	95	1	2	2 carb., 1 fat
Fruit & Oatmeal Cereal Bars, Strawberry (1)	140	26	3	0	0	125	1	1	2 carb., 1 fat

SNACK FOODS

Products	Cal.	Carb. (g)	Fat (g)	Sat. Fat (g)	Chol. (mg)	Sod. (mg)	Fib. (g)	Prot. (g)	Servings/Exchanges
Fruit & Oatmeal Cereal Bars, Very Berry (1)	140	27	3	0	0	80	1	2	2 carb., 1 fat
Mini Rice Cakes, Apple Cinnamon (8)	60	15	0	0	0	50	0	1	1 carb.
Mini Rice Cakes, Banana Nut (8)	60	15	0	0	0	85	0	1	1 carb.
Mini Rice Cakes, Caramel Corn (7)	60	13	0	0	0	150	0	1	1 carb.
Mini Rice Cakes, Chocolate Crunch (7)	60	13	1	0	0	45	0	1	1 carb.
Mini Rice Cakes, Honey Nut (8)	60	0	0	0	0	90	0	1	1 carb.
Mini Rice Cakes, Cheddar Cheese (9)	70	11	3	3	NA	210	0	1	1 carb.
Rice Cakes, Apple Cinnamon (1)	50	11	0	0	0	0	0	1	1/2 carb.
Rice Cakes, Banana Nut (1)	50	11	0	0	0	45	0	1	1 carb.
Rice Cakes, Blueberry Crunch (1)	50	11	0	0	0	0	0	1	1 carb.
Rice Cakes, Butter Popped Corn (1)	35	7	0	0	0	45	0	1	1/2 carb.
Rice Cakes, Caramel Apple (1)	60	12	<1	0	0	50	0	1	1 carb.
Rice Cakes, Caramel Chocolate Chip (1)	60	13	1	0	0	20	0	1	1 carb.
Rice Cakes, Caramel Corn (1)	50	12	0	0	0	30	0	1	1 carb.

Food									
Rice Cakes, Chocolate Crunch (1)	60	12	0	0	0	35	0	1	1 carb.
Rice Cakes, Cinnamon Streusel (1)	60	12	1	0	0	20	0	1	1 carb.
Rice Cakes, Monterey Jack Corn (1)	40	8	0	0	0	80	0	1	1/2 carb.
Rice Cakes, Peanut Butter (1)	60	12	1	0	0	60	0	1	1 carb.
Rice Cakes, Salt Free (1)	35	7	0	0	0	0	0	1	1 carb.
Rice Cakes, Salted (1)	35	7	0	0	0	15	0	1	1/2 carb.
Rice Cakes, Strawberry Crunch (1)	50	11	0	0	0	0	0	1	1 carb.
Rice Cakes, White Cheddar Corn (1)	45	8	<1	0	0	130	0	1	1/2 carb.
ROSS									
Ensure Glucerna Bar, Chocolate Graham (1)	140	24	4	1	<5	100	4	5	1 1/2 carb., 1 fat
RY KRISP									
Crackers, Seasoned Rye (2)	60	10	2	0	0	90	3	1	1/2 strch
Crackers, Sesame Rye (2)	60	11	2	0	0	80	3	2	1/2 strch
SLIM FAST									
Breakfast/Lunch Bars, Dutch Chocolate (1)	140	20	5	3	5	80	2	5	1 carb., 1 fat
Breakfast/Lunch Bars, Peanut Butter (1)	150	19	5	3	5	80	2	6	1 carb., 1 fat

SNACK FOODS

Products	Cal.	Carb. (g)	Fat (g)	Sat. Fat (g)	Chol. (mg)	Sod. (mg)	Fib. (g)	Prot. (g)	Servings/Exchanges
Energy Snack Bars, Peanut Butter Crunch (1)	130	21	4	2	<5	80	<1	1	1 1/2 carb., 1 fat
Energy Snack Bars, Rich Chewy Caramel (1)	120	22	4	3	<5	80	2	<1	1 1/2 carb., 1 fat
Meal-On-The-Go Bars, Oatmeal Raisin (1)	220	36	5	4	<5	110	2	8	2 1/2 carb., 1 med-fat meat
Meal-On-The-Go Bars, Rich Chocolate Brownie (1)	220	34	5	3	<5	110	2	8	2 carb., 1 med-fat meat
SUNSHINE									
Big Cheez It (13)	150	16	8	2	0	230	<1	4	1 strch, 2 fat
Big Cheez It, Reduced Fat (15)	140	20	5	1	0	280	<1	4	1 strch, 1 fat
Cheez It, Heads and Tails (37)	140	18	6	2	0	330	1	3	1 strch, 1 fat
Cheez-It, Original (27)	160	16	8	2	0	240	<1	4	1 strch, 2 fat
Cheez It, Party Mix (1/2 cup)	140	19	5	1	0	270	1	4	1 strch, 1 fat
Cheez It, Reduced Fat (29)	140	20	5	1	0	280	<1	4	1 strch, 1 fat
Cheez It, Reduced Fat Party Mix (1/2 cup)	130	21	3	<1	0	300	1	4	1 1/2 strch, 1 fat
Cheez It, Snack Mix (1/2 cup)	130	21	5	1	0	330	2	3	1 1/2 strch, 1 fat
Cheez It, Snack Mix, Big Crunch (3/4 cup)	110	20	6	1	0	360	<1	3	1 strch, 1 fat

Cheez It, Snack Mix, Double Cheese (3/4 cup)	110	19	5	1	0	450	<1	3	1 strch, 1 fat
Cheez It, White Cheddar (26)	150	18	7	2	<5	280	<1	3	1 strch, 1 fat
Crackers, Hi Ho (4)	70	8	4	1	0	130	<1	1	1/2 strch, 1 fat
Hi Ho, Reduced Fat (5)	70	10	3	<1	0	140	<1	1	1/2 strch, 1 fat
Krispy Saltines, Fat Free (5)	50	11	0	0	0	150	0	1	1 strch
Krispy Saltines, Original (5)	60	10	2	0	0	180	<1	2	1/2 strch

SOUPS AND STEWS

BANQUET

Products	Cal.	Carb. (g)	Fat (g)	Sat. Fat (g)	Chol. (mg)	Sod. (mg)	Fib. (g)	Prot. (g)	Servings/Exchanges
Beef Stew (1 cup)	160	17	4	2	25	1110	4	14	1 strch, 1 med-fat meat
CAMPBELL'S, READY-TO-SERVE									
Chunky Beef (10.8 oz)	180	20	6	2	20	1090	4	13	1 strch, 1 med-fat meat
Chunky Beef Pasta (10.8 oz)	190	23	4	1	20	1200	3	16	1 1/2 strch, 2 lean meat
Chunky Beef w/Country Vegetable (10.8 oz)	200	22	5	2	NA	1130	4	16	1 1/2 strch, 2 lean meat
Chunky Chicken Broccoli Cheese (10.8 oz)	250	17	15	6	30	1400	1	11	1 strch, 1 med-fat meat, 2 fat
Chunky Chicken Corn Chowder (10.8 oz)	310	22	19	9	30	1080	4	12	1 1/2 strch, 1 med-fat meat, 3 fat
Chunky Chicken Mushroom Chowder (1 cup)	210	15	12	4	10	970	3	10	1 strch, 1 med-fat meat, 1 fat
Chunky Chicken Noodle (1 cup)	160	20	4	1	25	1310	3	12	1 strch, 1 med-fat meat
Chunky Chicken Noodle w/Mushroom (10.8 oz)	150	13	5	2	30	1150	1	14	1 strch, 1 med-fat meat
Chunky Chicken Rice (1 cup)	140	18	3	1	18	840	2	25	1 strch, 3 lean meat

Chunky Chicken Vegetable (1 cup)	130	12	3	2	20	950	3	9	1 strch, 1 lean meat
Chunky Chili Beef w/Beans (11 oz)	300	38	7	2	20	1080	9	21	2 1/2 strch, 2 lean meat
Chunky Manhattan Clam Chowder (1 cup)	130	20	4	1	5	900	3	6	1 strch, 1 fat
Chunky Minestrone (1 cup)	140	22	5	2	5	800	2	5	1 1/2 strch, 1 fat
Chunky New England Clam Chowder (10.8 oz)	300	26	18	7	15	1210	3	9	2 strch, 4 fat
Chunky Pepper Steak (1 cup)	140	18	3	1	20	830	3	11	1 strch, 1 lean meat
Chunky Potato Ham Chowder (10.8 oz)	270	20	18	9	25	1050	3	7	1 strch, 1 med-fat meat, 3 fat
Chunky Sirloin Burger w/Vegetables (10.8 oz)	230	25	11	5	25	1160	5	12	1 1/2 strch, 1 med-fat meat, 1 fat
Chunky Split Pea n'Ham (10.8 oz)	240	33	4	2	20	1400	4	18	2 strch, 2 lean meat
Chunky Steak Potato (10.8 oz)	200	24	5	2	25	1100	4	15	1 1/2 strch, 2 lean meat
Chunky Stroganoff Beef (10.3 oz)	310	28	16	6	45	1180	4	16	2 strch, 2 med-fat meat, 1 fat
Chunky Tortellini w/Chicken & Vegetable (1 cup)	110	18	2	<1	10	910	2	6	1 strch, 1 fat
Chunky Vegetable (10.8 oz)	160	28	4	1	0	1090	5	4	2 strch, 1 fat
CAMPBELL'S CONDENSED (PREPARED W/WATER)									
Beef Consomme (1 cup)	25	2	0	0	5	820	0	4	1 very lean meat

SOUPS AND STEWS

Products	Cal.	Carb. (g)	Fat (g)	Sat. Fat (g)	Chol. (mg)	Sod. (mg)	Fib. (g)	Prot. (g)	Servings/Exchanges
Black Bean (1 cup)	120	19	2	<1	0	1030	5	6	1 strch
Broccoli Cheese (1 cup)	110	9	7	3	10	860	2	3	1/2 strch, 1 fat
Cheddar Cheese (1 cup)	90	10	4	3	10	950	1	15	1/2 strch, 1 fat
Chicken & Stars (1 cup)	70	9	2	<1	1	1010	1	3	1/2 strch
Chicken Alphabet w/Vegetable (1 cup)	80	11	2	<1	10	880	1	4	1 strch
Chicken Dumpling (1 cup)	80	10	3	<1	125	1049	2	4	1/2 strch, 1 fat
Chicken Gumbo (1 cup)	60	9	2	<1	10	990	1	2	1/2 strch
Chicken Noodle (1 cup)	70	9	2	1	15	980	1	3	1/2 strch, 1 fat
Chicken Vegetable (1 cup)	80	12	2	<1	10	940	2	3	1 strch
Chicken w/Rice (1 cup)	70	9	3	<1	3	940	0	3	1/2 strch, 1 fat
Chicken w/Wild Rice (1 cup)	70	9	2	<1	10	900	1	3	1 strch
Chicken Won Ton (1 cup)	45	5	<1	0	15	940	1	4	1 very lean meat
Chili Beef w/Bean (1 cup)	170	24	5	3	15	910	4	7	1 1/2 strch, 1 fat
Cream of Asparagus (1 cup)	90	11	4	1	5	860	1	3	1 strch, 1 fat

Cream of Broccoli (1 cup)	100	9	6	3	3	770	1	2	1/2 strch, 1 fat
Cream of Broccoli, 98% Fat-Free (1 cup)	80	12	3	1	3	730	1	2	1 strch, 1 fat
Cream of Celery (1 cup)	110	9	7	3	3	900	1	2	1/2 strch, 1 fat
Cream of Celery, 98% Fat-Free (1 cup)	70	9	3	1	3	850	1	2	1/2 strch, 1 fat
Cream of Chicken (1 cup)	130	11	8	3	10	890	1	3	1 strch, 2 fat
Cream of Chicken, 98% Fat-Free (1 cup)	80	10	3	2	10	830	0	3	1 strch, 1 fat
Cream of Chicken Broccoli (1 cup)	120	9	8	3	15	860	1	4	1/2 strch, 2 fat
Cream of Chicken Mushroom (1 cup)	130	9	9	3	15	1000	1	3	1/2 strch, 2 fat
Cream of Chicken Noodle (1 cup)	130	12	7	2	15	800	2	5	1 strch, 1 fat
Cream of Mexican Pepper (1 cup)	110	10	7	2	3	860	2	2	1/2 strch, 1 fat
Cream of Mushroom (1 cup)	110	9	7	3	3	870	1	2	1/2 strch, 1 fat
Cream of Mushroom, 98% Fat-Free (1 cup)	70	9	3	1	3	830	0	1	1/2 strch, 1 fat
Cream of Potato (1 cup)	90	14	3	2	10	890	1	2	1 strch, 1 fat
Cream of Shrimp (1 cup)	100	8	7	2	20	890	1	2	1/2 strch, 1 fat
Creamy Onion (1 cup)	110	13	6	2	20	910	1	2	1 strch, 1 fat
Curly Noodle & Chicken Broth (1 cup)	80	12	3	<1	15	840	1	3	1 strch, 1 fat

SOUPS AND STEWS

Products	Cal.	Carb. (g)	Fat (g)	Sat. Fat (g)	Chol. (mg)	Sod. (mg)	Fib. (g)	Prot. (g)	Servings/Exchanges
Double Noodle & Chicken Broth (1 cup)	100	15	3	<1	15	810	2	4	1 strch, 1 fat
Fiesta Tomato (1 cup)	70	16	0	0	0	860	1	1	1 strch
French Onion w/Beef Stock (1 cup)	70	10	3	0	3	980	1	2	1/2 strch, 1 fat
Golden Corn (1 cup)	120	20	4	1	3	730	2	2	1 strch, 1 fat
Golden Mushroom (1 cup)	80	10	3	1	5	930	1	2	1/2 strch, 1 fat
Green Pea (1 cup)	180	29	3	<1	5	890	5	9	2 strch, 1 fat
Hearty Vegetable w/Pasta (1 cup)	90	18	<1	0	0	830	2	2	1 strch
Italian Tomato Basil/Oregano (1 cup)	100	23	<1	0	0	820	2	2	1 1/2 strch
Manhattan Clam Chowder (1 cup)	70	12	2	<1	3	910	2	2	1 strch
Minestrone (1 cup)	100	16	2	<1	0	960	4	5	1 strch
Nacho Cheese Soup/Dip (1 cup)	140	11	8	4	15	810	2	5	1 strch, 2 fat
New England Clam Chowder (1 cup)	100	15	3	1	3	980	1	4	1 strch, 1 fat
Noodles & Ground Beef (1 cup)	100	11	4	2	25	900	2	5	1 strch, 1 fat
Old-Fashioned Tomato Rice (1 cup)	120	23	2	<1	5	790	1	2	1 1/2 strch

Old-Fashioned Vegetable (1 cup)	70	10	3	<1	3	950	2	2	1/2 strch, 1 fat
Oyster Stew (1 cup)	90	6	6	4	20	940	0	2	1/2 strch, 1 fat
Scotch Broth (1 cup)	80	9	3	2	10	870	1	4	1/2 strch, 1 fat
Split Pea, Ham, & Bacon (1 cup)	180	28	4	2	3	860	5	10	2 strch, 1 fat
Tomato (1 cup)	100	18	2	0	0	730	2	2	1 strch
Tomato Bisque (1 cup)	130	24	3	2	5	900	2	2	1 1/2 strch, 1 fat
Turkey Noodle (1 cup)	80	10	3	<1	15	970	1	4	1/2 strch, 1 fat
Turkey Vegetable (1 cup)	80	11	3	<1	10	840	2	3	1 strch, 1 fat
Vegetable (1 cup)	80	14	2	<1	3	920	2	3	1 strch
Vegetable Beef (1 cup)	80	10	2	<1	10	810	2	5	1/2 strch
Vegetarian Vegetable (1 cup)	70	14	<1	0	0	770	2	2	1 strch
CAMPBELL'S HEALTHY REQUEST									
Chicken Broth (1 cup)	20	1	0	0	0	480	0	3	free
Chicken Noodle (1 cup)	160	25	3	1	20	480	2	9	1 1/2 strch, 1 fat
Chicken Vegetable (1 cup)	120	18	2	<1	20	480	2	7	1 strch, 1 lean meat
Chicken w/Rice (1 cup)	100	15	2	<1	40	480	1	6	1 strch

SOUPS AND STEWS

Products	Cal.	Carb. (g)	Fat (g)	Sat. Fat (g)	Chol. (mg)	Sod. (mg)	Fib. (g)	Prot. (g)	Servings/Exchanges
Minestrone (1 cup)	120	24	2	<1	3	480	3	4	1 1/2 strch
Hearty Vegetable (1 cup)	100	20	1	0	0	470	2	3	1 strch
Penne Pasta, Zesty (1 cup)	90	17	<1	0	5	470	2	4	1 strch
Southwest-Style Vegetable (1 cup)	140	28	1	<1	0	480	5	5	2 strch
Split Pea w/Ham (1 cup)	170	27	3	1	15	480	4	9	2 strch, 1 fat
Tomato Vegetable (1 cup)	120	22	2	<1	5	480	3	4	1 1/2 strch
Turkey Vegetable Rice (1 cup)	120	17	3	1	15	480	2	7	1 strch, 1 lean meat
Vegetable Beef (1 cup)	140	20	3	1	20	480	3	9	1 strch, 1 fat
CAMPBELL'S HOME COOKIN'									
Chicken Noodle (1 cup)	130	24	3	<1	0	750	4	3	1 1/2 strch, 1 fat
Country Vegetable (10.8 oz)	130	26	2	0	5	940	2	4	2 strch
Hearty Lentil (1 cup)	130	24	<1	<1	0	860	5	7	1 1/2 strch
Italian Vegetable (1 cup)	100	14	4	2	5	860	2	3	1 strch, 1 fat
Minestrone (1 cup)	120	19	2	1	5	990	3	4	1 strch

Potato w/Roasted Garlic (1 cup)	180	21	9	3	21	800	2	5	1 1/2 strch, 2 fat
Split Pea w/Ham (1 cup)	170	30	2	<1	5	880	6	10	2 strch, 1 lean meat
Tomato Garden (10.8 oz)	150	27	4	2	5	900	4	5	2 strch, 1 fat
CHEF MATE									
Beef Stew (1 cup)	192	19	6	2	33	1190	3	15	1 strch, 2 med-fat meat
Chili w/Beans (1 cup)	412	29	25	11	56	1171	11	18	2 strch, 2 med-fat meat, 3 fat
Chili w/o Beans (1 cup)	430	18	32	14	85	1588	3	19	1 strch, 2 med-fat meat, 5 fat
Spice Chili (1 cup)	423	33	24	11	56	1485	4	17	2 strch, 2 med-fat meat, 3 fat
HEALTH VALLEY									
5-Bean Vegetable (7.5 oz)	100	14	0	0	0	260	3	8	1 strch
14-Garden Vegetable (7.5 oz)	50	9	0	0	0	260	3	4	1/2 strch
Beef Broth (7.5 oz)	17	2	1	0	1	420	0	1	free
Black Bean w/Vegetable (7.5 oz)	70	9	0	0	0	248	17	9	1/2 strch, 1 very lean meat
Chicken Broth (1 cup)	35	1	2	NA	2	410	0	4	free
Country Corn & Vegetable (7.5 oz)	70	13	0	0	0	290	3	4	1 strch
Country Corn & Vegetable (1 cup)	80	17	0	0	0	240	5	6	1 strch

SOUPS AND STEWS

Products	Cal.	Carb. (g)	Fat (g)	Sat. Fat (g)	Chol. (mg)	Sod. (mg)	Fib. (g)	Prot. (g)	Servings/Exchanges
Fat-Free Italian Minestrone (7.5 oz)	80	12	0	0	0	290	4	8	1 strch, 1 very lean meat
Fat-Free Pasta Cacciatore (1 cup)	90	19	0	0	0	210	NA	6	1 strch
Fat-Free Pasta Primavera (1 cup)	80	21	0	0	0	210	11	8	1 1/2 strch, 1 very lean meat
Fat-Free Pasta Romano (1 cup)	140	32	0	0	0	250	13	10	2 strch, 1 very lean meat
Rotini Vegetable Pasta (1 cup)	100	20	0	0	0	290	4	4	1 strch
Lentil (7.5 oz)	170	28	2	0	0	435	17	9	2 strch, 1 very lean meat
Lentil & Carrot (7.5 oz)	84	23	0	0	0	206	13	9	1 1/2 strch
Pasta Italiano (1 cup)	280	62	0	0	0	720	6	10	4 strch
Country Corn & Vegetable (1 cup)	80	17	0	0	0	240	5	6	1 strch
Split Pea & Carrot (7.5 oz)	80	17	0	0	0	290	13	9	1 strch, 1 very lean meat
Tomato Vegetable (7.5 oz)	75	16	0	0	0	225	5	6	1 strch
Vegetable Barley (7.5 oz)	84	18	0	0	0	186	4	6	1 strch
HEALTHY CHOICE									
Bean & Ham (1 cup)	166	31	1	<1	4	979	7	9	2 strch, 1 lean meat

Beef & Potato (1 cup)	116	16	1	<1	5	452	<1	11	1 strch, 1 lean meat
Broccoli Cheddar (1 cup)	116	22	2	1	4	304	2	4	1 1/2 strch
Chicken Alfredo w/Pasta (1 cup)	132	17	2	1	10	333	2	2	1 strch, 1 lean meat
Chicken Corn Chowder (1 cup)	176	30	3	1	8	466	2	8	2 strch, 1 fat
Chicken Pasta (1 cup)	119	18	3	1	6	493	1	7	1 strch, 1 lean meat
Chicken w/Rice (1 cup)	119	19	2	<1	6	324	3	9	1 strch, 1 lean meat
Chili Beef (1 cup)	189	32	2	<1	12	441	5	15	2 strch, 1 very lean meat
Clam Chowder (1 cup)	123	23	1	<1	12	481	2	7	1 1/2 strch
Country Vegetable (1 cup)	112	24	1	<1	0	453	3	5	1 1/2 strch
Cream of Chicken w/Mushroom (1 cup)	77	14	<1	<1	0	450	<1	4	1 strch, 1 lean meat
Cream of Mushroom (1 cup)	56	13	<1	<1	2	478	3	<1	1 strch
Garden Vegetable (1 cup)	108	22	1	<1	0	454	6	5	1 1/2 strch
Lentil (1 cup)	135	28	<1	<1	0	472	5	10	2 strch
Minestrone (1 cup)	107	24	1	<1	1	370	5	5	1 1/2 strch
Old-Fashioned Chicken Noodle (1 cup)	137	19	3	1	9	402	<1	9	1 strch, 1 lean meat
Split Pea & Ham (1 cup)	164	26	2	<1	7	468	5	11	2 strch, 1 lean meat

SOUPS AND STEWS

Products	Cal.	Carb. (g)	Fat (g)	Sat. Fat (g)	Chol. (mg)	Sod. (mg)	Fib. (g)	Prot. (g)	Servings/Exchanges
Tomato Garden (1 cup)	80	18	1	<1	0	298	3	2	1 strch
Turkey w/Wild Rice (1 cup)	72	9	1	<1	3	407	3	9	1/2 strch, 1 very lean meat
LIBBY'S									
Chili, No Beans (7.5 oz)	390	11	30	NA	NA	800	NA	18	1 strch, 2 med-fat meat, 4 fat
Chili & Beans (7.5 oz)	270	25	13	NA	NA	390	NA	13	1 1/2 strch, 1 med-fat meat, 2 fat
LIPTON CUP-A-SOUP									
Chicken Broth (6 oz)	20	3	1	0	0	440	0	1	free
Chicken Noodle (6 oz)	50	8	1	NA	10	540	0	2	1/2 strch
Chicken Vegetable (6 oz)	50	10	1	0	10	520	0	1	1/2 strch
Cream of Chicken (6 oz)	70	3	2	0	NA	640	0	12	1/2 strch, 1 fat
Cream of Mushroom (6 oz)	60	10	2	0	NA	610	0	1	1/2 strch
Creamy Broccoli & Cheese (6 oz)	70	9	3	2	NA	540	1	2	1/2 strch, 1 fat
Creamy Chicken-Flavored Vegetable (6 oz)	80	10	4	2	0	590	NA	2	1/2 strch, 1 fat

Green Pea (6 oz)	80	12	1	0	0	520	3	4	1 strch, 1 fat
Hearty Chicken Supreme (6 oz)	60	10	1	0	15	590	0	3	1/2 strch
Ring Noodle (6 oz)	50	9	1	0	10	560	0	2	1/2 strch
Spring Vegetable (6 oz)	45	8	1	0	10	500	NA	2	1/2 strch
Tomato (6 oz)	90	20	1	NA	0	510	NA	2	1 strch
OLD EL PASO									
Black Bean w/Bacon (1 cup)	160	26	2	<1	5	960	7	11	1 1/2 strch, 1 lean meat
Chicken Vegetable (1 cup)	110	13	3	<1	15	620	0	9	1 strch, 1 lean meat
Chicken w/Rice (1 cup)	90	10	3	<1	15	680	0	8	1/2 strch, 1 lean meat
Chili w/Beans (1 cup)	217	17	10	NA	32	480	6	15	1 strch, 2 med-fat meat
Garden Vegetable (1 cup)	110	17	3	<1	0	710	0	5	1 strch, 1 fat
Hearty Beef (1 cup)	120	14	3	2	25	690	0	10	1 strch, 1 lean meat
Hearty Chicken Noodle (1 cup)	110	10	3	1	25	NA	0	9	1/2 strch, 1 lean meat
PROGRESSO									
Basil Rotini Tomato (1 cup)	120	22	2	0	<5	890	2	5	1 1/2 strch
Bean & Ham (1 cup)	160	25	2	<1	10	870	8	10	1 1/2 strch, 1 lean meat

SOUPS AND STEWS

Products	Cal.	Carb. (g)	Fat (g)	Sat. Fat (g)	Chol. (mg)	Sod. (mg)	Fib. (g)	Prot. (g)	Servings/Exchanges
Beef Barley (1 cup)	130	13	4	2	25	780	3	10	1 strch, 1 med-fat meat
Beef Barley, 99% Fat-Free (1 cup)	140	20	2	1	20	470	3	11	1 strch, 1 lean meat
Beef Minestrone (1 cup)	140	18	3	1	10	970	3	10	1 strch, 1 med-fat meat
Beef Noodle (1 cup)	140	15	4	2	30	950	1	13	1 strch, 1 med-fat meat
Beef Vegetable & Rotini (1 cup)	130	14	3	1	25	780	4	13	1 strch, 1 med-fat meat
Chickarina (1 cup)	130	12	5	2	20	1010	<1	8	1 strch, 1 med-fat meat
Chicken & Wild Rice (1 cup)	100	15	2	0	15	850	1	7	1 strch
Chicken Barley (1 cup)	110	16	2	0	15	850	3	8	1 strch, 1 lean meat
Chicken Broth (1 cup)	20	1	2	0	0	920	0	1	free
Chicken Minestrone (1 cup)	110	15	2	0	15	890	2	9	1 strch, 1 lean meat
Chicken Noodle (1 cup)	90	9	2	0	25	950	<1	9	1/2 strch, 1 lean meat
Chicken Noodle, 99% Fat Free (1 cup)	90	13	2	0	20	950	1	7	1 strch, 1 lean meat
Chicken Rice & Vegetables (1 cup)	90	13	2	0	10	890	1	6	1 strch, 1 lean meat
Chicken Rice w/Vegetables, 99% Fat Free (1 cup)	110	16	2	0	10	780	1	7	1 strch, 1 lean meat

Item									Exchanges
Chicken Vegetable (1 cup)	90	13	2	0	15	820	2	7	1 strch, 1 lean meat
Clam & Rotini Chowder (1 cup)	190	21	9	2	10	800	0	7	1 1/2 strch, 2 fat
Creamy Mushroom Chicken, 99% Fat Free (1 cup)	90	12	2	<1	10	840	1	7	1 strch, 1 lean meat
Escarole in Chicken Broth (1 cup)	25	3	1	0	<5	930	1	1	free
Green Split Pea (1 cup)	170	25	3	1	5	870	5	10	1 1/2 strch, 1 fat
Hearty Black Bean, 99% Fat Free (1 cup)	170	30	2	0	<5	730	10	8	2 strch
Hearty Chicken and Rotini (1 cup)	90	12	2	0	15	970	<1	8	1 strch, 1 very lean meat
Hearty Penne/Chicken Broth (1 cup)	80	14	1	0	0	1020	<1	4	1 strch
Hearty Tomato (1 cup)	100	19	2	0	0	800	1	2	1 strch
Homestyle Chicken & Vegetable (1 cup)	90	11	2	0	15	900	<1	7	1 strch, 1 lean meat
Lentil, 99% Fat Free (1 cup)	130	20	2	0	0	440	6	8	1 strch, 1 lean meat
Lentil (1 cup)	140	22	2	0	0	750	7	9	1 1/2 strch, 1 lean meat
Macaroni & Bean (1 cup)	160	23	4	1	<5	800	6	7	1 1/2 strch, 1 fat
Manhattan Clam Chowder (1 cup)	110	11	2	0	3	710	3	12	1 strch, 1 lean meat
Meatballs & Pasta Pearls (1 cup)	140	13	7	3	15	700	0	7	1 strch, 1 med-fat meat
Minestrone (1 cup)	120	21	2	0	0	960	5	5	1 1/2 strch

SOUPS AND STEWS

Products	Cal.	Carb. (g)	Fat (g)	Sat. Fat (g)	Chol. (mg)	Sod. (mg)	Fib. (g)	Prot. (g)	Servings/Exchanges
Minestrone, 99% Fat Free (1 cup)	130	23	2	0	0	710	4	7	1 1/2 strch
Minestrone Parmesan (1 cup)	100	16	3	<1	0	29	3	3	1 strch, 1 fat
New England Clam Chowder (1 cup)	190	20	10	3	15	920	1	6	1 strch, 1 med-fat meat, 1 fat
New England Clam Chowder, 99% Fat Free (1 cup)	130	22	2	0	5	700	1	5	1 strch
Oregano Enee Italian Style Vegetable (1 cup)	90	15	2	0	0	960	1	3	1 strch
Peppercorn Penne Vegetable (1 cup)	100	20	1	0	0	920	2	3	1 strch
Potato Broccoli & Cheese (1 cup)	160	21	6	2	<5	960	1	5	1 1/2 strch, 1 fat
Roasted Garlic Pasta Lentil (1 cup)	120	20	2	0	0	960	5	7	1 strch, 1 lean meat
Rotisserie Seasoned Chicken (1 cup)	100	15	2	0	15	920	2	7	1 strch, 1 lean meat
Split Pea, 99% Fat Free (1 cup)	170	29	2	0	0	620	5	10	2 strch, 1 lean meat
Tomato Garden Vegetable, 99% Fat Free (1 cup)	100	19	2	0	0	660	2	3	1 strch
Turkey Rice w/Vegetables (1 cup)	110	18	1	0	15	1040	1	7	1 strch, 1 very lean meat
Vegetable, 99% Fat Free (1 cup)	70	13	1	0	0	870	2	20	1 strch
Spicy Chicken & Penne (1 cup)	110	14	2	0	5	950	1	9	1 strch, 1 lean meat

Split Pea w/Ham (1 cup)	150	20	4	2	15	830	5	9	1 strch, 1 med-fat meat
Tomato (1 cup)	100	19	2	0	0	790	1	2	1 strch
Tomato Basil (1 cup)	100	19	2	0	0	790	1	2	1 strch
Tomato Vegetable (1 cup)	90	15	2	0	0	990	4	3	1 strch
Tortellini/Chicken Broth (1 cup)	70	10	2	<1	10	970	2	3	1/2 strch
Vegetable (1 cup)	90	15	2	<1	<5	810	2	3	1 strch
UNCLE BEN'S									
Club Black Bean & Rice Soup (1 cup)	150	28	2	0	0	430	6	7	2 strch
WEIGHT WATCHERS									
Chicken & Noodle (10 1/2 oz)	80	9	2	0	NA	1230	NA	6	1/2 strch
Mushroom (10 1/2 oz)	90	14	2	0	NA	1250	NA	3	1 strch
Vegetable (10 1/2 oz)	90	13	2	0	NA	1370	NA	4	1 strch

VEGETABLES AND VEGETABLE JUICES

Products	Cal.	Carb. (g)	Fat (g)	Sat. Fat (g)	Chol. (mg)	Sod. (mg)	Fib. (g)	Prot. (g)	Servings/Exchanges
Alfalfa Sprouts (1 cup)	10	1	<1	<1	0	2	<1	1	free
Artichoke Hearts (1/2 cup)	36	7	<1	0	0	42	<1	3	1 vegetable
Artichokes, Cooked (1/2)	30	7	<1	0	0	57	3	2	1 vegetable
Asparagus, Frozen (1/2 cup)	23	4	<1	<1	0	3	3	2	1 vegetable
Asparagus, Spears, Canned (1/2 cup)	23	3	<1	<1	0	472	2	3	1 vegetable
Bamboo Shoots, Canned (1 cup)	25	4	<1	<1	0	9	2	2	1 vegetable
Bamboo Shoots, Sliced, Cooked (1 cup)	14	2	<1	<1	0	5	1	2	free
Bamboo Shoots, Sliced, Raw (1 cup)	41	8	<1	<1	0	6	3	4	1 vegetable
Bean Sprouts (1 cup)	31	6	<1	<1	0	6	2	3	1 vegetable
Beans, Green or Wax, Canned (1/2 cup)	14	3	<1	0	0	171	1	<1	1 vegetable
Beans, Green, Frozen (1/2 cup)	18	4	<1	0	0	9	2	<1	1 vegetable
Beets, Canned (1/2 cup)	26	6	<1	0	0	233	2	<1	1 vegetable
Beets, Harvard, Diced (1/2 cup)	136	25	4	<1	0	287	2	<1	1 carb, 1 vegetable, 1 fat

Food									
Beets, Pickled (1/2 cup)	74	19	<1	<1	C	301	1	<1	1 carb., 1 vegetable
Broccoli, Cooked w/Cheese Sauce (1/2 cup)	110	6	7	4	15	365	2	6	1 vegetable, 1 fat
Broccoli, Cooked w/Cream Sauce (1/2 cup)	93	8	6	2	3	346	2	4	1 vegetable, 1 fat
Broccoli, Raw, Chopped (1 cup)	25	5	<1	<1	0	24	3	3	1 vegetable
Broccoli, Spears, Frozen (1/2 cup)	26	5	<1	0	0	22	3	3	1 vegetable
Brussel Sprouts, Frozen, Cooked (1/2 cup)	33	7	<1	<1	0	18	3	3	1 vegetable
Cabbage, Bok Choy, Cooked (1 cup)	20	3	<1	<1	0	58	3	3	1 vegetable
Cabbage, Chinese, Raw (1 cup)	12	3	<1	0	0	7	<1	<1	1 vegetable
Cabbage, Fresh, Cooked (1/2 cup)	16	3	<1	0	0	6	2	<1	1 vegetable
Cabbage, Raw, Green (1 cup)	18	4	<1	0	0	13	2	1	1 vegetable
Cabbage, Red, Cooked (1/2 cup)	16	4	<1	<1	0	6	2	<1	1 vegetable
Carrot Juice, Canned (1/2 cup)	47	11	<1	<1	0	34	<1	1	2 vegetable
Carrots, Canned (1/2 cup)	17	4	<1	0	0	176	1	<1	1 vegetable
Carrots, Fresh, Cooked (1/2 cup)	35	8	<1	0	0	52	3	<1	1 vegetable
Carrots, Raw (1 cup)	47	11	<1	0	0	38	3	1	2 vegetable
Cauliflower, Frozen, Cooked (1/2 cup)	17	3	<1	0	0	16	2	1	1 vegetable

VEGETABLES AND VEGETABLE JUICES

Products	Cal.	Carb. (g)	Fat (g)	Sat. Fat (g)	Chol. (mg)	Sod. (mg)	Fib. (g)	Prot. (g)	Servings/Exchanges
Cauliflower, Raw (1 cup)	25	5	<1	0	0	30	3	2	1 vegetable
Celery, Fresh, Cooked (1/2 cup)	14	3	<1	0	0	68	1	<1	1 vegetable
Celery, Raw (1 cup)	19	4	<1	0	0	104	2	<1	1 vegetable
Coleslaw (1/2 cup)	97	9	7	1	3	178	1	<1	1 vegetable, 1 fat
Collard Greens, Fresh, Cooked (1/2 cup)	17	4	<1	0	0	10	1	<1	1 vegetable
Corn, Canned (1/2 cup)	83	20	<1	<1	0	286	6	3	1 strch
Corn, Cream-Style, Canned (1/2 cup)	92	23	<1	<1	0	365	2	2	1 1/2 strch
Corn, Frozen, Cooked (1/2 cup)	66	17	<1	0	0	4	2	3	1 strch
Corn on the Cob, Cooked, (1 medium)	83	19	1	<1	0	13	2	3	1 strch
Corn on the Cob, Frozen (1, 3-inch)	70	14	<1	NA	0	5	1	2	1 strch
Cucumber, Raw (1 cup)	14	3	<1	0	0	2	<1	<1	1 vegetable
Cucumber Salad, Marinated in Vinegar (1 cup)	48	13	<1	<1	0	350	1	<1	1/2 carb, 1 vegetable
Eggplant, Fresh, Cooked (1/2 cup)	13	3	<1	0	0	1	1	<1	1 vegetable
Endive/Escarole, Raw (1 cup)	9	2	<1	0	0	11	2	<1	1 vegetable

French Fries, Frozen, Oven-Heated (10)	167	20	9	3	0	307	2	2	1 strch, 2 fat
Hominy, Yellow, Canned (1/2 cup)	58	12	<1	<1	0	168	2	1	1 strch
Jicama (1 cup)	46	11	<1	<1	0	5	6	1	2 vegetable
Kale, Fresh, Cooked (1/2 cup)	21	4	<1	0	0	15	1	1	1 vegetable
Kohlrabi, Cooked (1/2 cup)	24	6	<1	0	0	17	<1	2	1 vegetable
Leeks, Cooked (1/2 cup)	16	4	<1	0	0	6	1	<1	1 vegetable
Lettuce, Iceburg, Raw (1 cup)	7	1	<1	0	0	5	<1	<1	1 vegetable
Lettuce, Romaine, Chopped (1 cup)	9	1	<1	<1	0	5	1	<1	free
Lettuce, Romaine, Raw (1 cup)	9	1	<1	0	0	5	1	<1	1 vegetable
Lima Beans, Frozen, Cooked (1/2 cup)	95	18	<1	0	0	26	7	7	1 strch
Mixed Vegetables, No Corn, Peas, or Pasta (1/2 cup)	20	3	0	0	0	15	1	1	1 vegetable
Mixed Vegetables w/Corn (1 cup)	80	18	0	0	0	80	4	4	1 strch
Mixed Vegetables w/Pasta (1 cup)	80	15	0	0	0	85	5	3	1 strch
Mushrooms, Canned (1/2 cup)	19	4	<1	0	0	331	2	2	1 vegetable
Mushrooms, Fresh, Cooked (1/2 cup)	21	4	<1	<1	0	2	2	2	1 vegetable

VEGETABLES AND VEGETABLE JUICES

Products	Cal.	Carb. (g)	Fat (g)	Sat. Fat (g)	Chol. (mg)	Sod. (mg)	Fib. (g)	Prot. (g)	Servings/Exchanges
Mushrooms, Raw (1 cup)	18	3	<1	0	0	3	<1	2	1 vegetable
Mustard Greens, Fresh, Cooked (1/2 cup)	10	2	<1	0	0	11	1	2	1 vegetable
Okra, Batter-Fried (1/2 cup)	88	6	7	1	8	67	1	1	1 vegetable, 1 fat
Okra, Frozen, Cooked (1/2 cup)	34	8	<1	<1	0	3	3	2	1 vegetable
Onions, Creamed (1/2 cup)	100	11	6	2	5	334	1	3	2 vegetable, 1 fat
Onions, Fresh, Cooked (1/2 cup)	46	11	<1	0	0	3	2	1	2 vegetable
Onions, Green, Raw (1 cup)	32	7	<1	0	0	16	3	2	1 vegetable
Onions, Raw (1 cup)	61	14	<1	0	0	5	3	2	2 vegetable
Palm Hearts, Cooked (1/2 cup)	75	20	<1	<1	0	10	1	2	1 strch
Parsnips, Raw Slices (1/2 cup)	50	12	<1	<1	0	7	3	<1	2 vegetable
Pea Pods, Fresh, Cooked (1/2 cup)	34	6	<1	0	0	3	2	3	1 vegetable
Pea Pods, Raw (1 cup)	61	11	<1	<1	0	6	4	4	2 vegetable
Peas, Green, Canned (1/2 cup)	59	11	<1	<1	0	186	4	4	1 strch
Peas, Green, Fresh, Cooked (1/2 cup)	67	13	<1	0	0	2	4	4	1 strch

Food	Cal	Carb	Fat	Sat Fat	Chol	Sod	Fiber	Prot	Exchanges
Peas, Green, Frozen, Cooked (1/2 cup)	62	11	<1	0	0	70	4	4	1 strch
Peppers, Green, Fresh, Cooked (1/2 cup)	19	5	<1	0	0	1	<1	<1	1 vegetable
Peppers, Green, Raw (1 cup)	27	6	<1	0	0	2	2	<1	1 vegetable
Peppers, Hot Green Chili, Raw (1 cup)	60	14	<1	0	0	10	2	3	2 vegetable
Peppers, Jalapeño, Canned (1/2 cup)	16	3	<1	<1	0	995	1	<1	1 vegetable
Peppers, Sweet, Red, Cooked (1/2 cup)	19	5	<1	<1	0	1	<1	<1	1 vegetable
Plantain, Cooked (1/2 cup)	89	24	<1	0	0	4	2	<1	1 strch
Potatoes, Baked w/Skin (3 oz)	93	22	<1	0	0	7	2	2	1 1/2 strch
Potatoes, Cooked, Peeled (3 oz)	73	17	<1	0	0	4	2	2	1 strch
Potatoes, Hash Brown, Frozen Cooked (1/2 cup)	170	22	9	4	0	27	2	3	1 1/2 strch, 2 fat
Potatoes, Mashed, Flakes, Milk/Fat Added (1/2 cup)	119	16	6	4	0	349	2	2	1 strch, 1 fat
Potatoes, Scalloped (1 cup)	211	27	9	3	15	821	5	7	2 strch, 2 fat
Potatoes, Sweet, Canned (1/2 cup)	92	22	<1	0	0	53	3	2	1 1/2 strch
Potatoes Au Gratin, Homemade w/Margarine (1 cup)	323	28	19	10	37	1060	4	13	2 strch, 4 fat
Radishes (1 cup)	20	4	<1	0	0	28	2	<1	1 vegetable
Sauerkraut, Canned (1/2 cup)	22	5	<1	0	0	780	3	1	1 vegetable

VEGETABLES AND VEGETABLE JUICES

Products	Cal.	Carb. (g)	Fat (g)	Sat. Fat (g)	Chol. (mg)	Sod. (mg)	Fib. (g)	Prot. (g)	Servings/Exchanges
Spinach, Canned (1/2 cup)	25	4	<1		0	29	3	3	1 vegetable
Spinach, Frozen, Cooked (1/2 cup)	27	5	<1	0	0	82	3	3	1 vegetable
Spinach, Raw (1 cup)	12	2	<1	0	0	44	3	2	1 vegetable
Spinach Salad, No Dressing (1 cup)	89	10	4	<1	0	157	2	4	2 vegetable, 1 fat
Squash, Spaghetti, Cooked (1/2 cup)	23	5	<1	<1	0	14	1	<1	1 vegetable
Squash, Summer, Fresh, Cooked (1/2 cup)	18	4	<1	<1	0	1	1	<1	1 vegetable
Squash, Summer, Raw (1 cup)	26	6	<1	<1	0	3	3	2	1 vegetable
Squash, Winter (1 cup)	83	22	<1	0	0	8	7	2	1 1/2 strch
Succotash, Canned (1/2 cup)	81	18	<1	<1	0	282	3	3	1 strch
Succotash, Cooked (1/2 cup)	111	24	<1	<1	0	16	4	5	1 1/2 strch
Tater Tots, Frozen, Oven-Heated (3 oz)	146	21	8	2	0	345	2	2	1 1/2 strch, 2 fat
Tomato Juice (1/2 cup)	21	5	<1	0	0	440	<1	<1	1 vegetable
Tomato Paste, Canned (1/2 cup)	110	25	1	<1	0	1034	6	5	1 strch, 1 vegetable
Tomato Sauce (1/2 cup)	37	9	<1	0	0	738	2	2	1 vegetable

Tomatoes, Canned (1/2 cup)	24	5	<1	0	0	196	1	1	1 vegetable
Tomatoes, Raw (1 cup)	38	8	<1	0	0	16	2	2	1 vegetable
Tossed Green Salad (3/4 cup)	19	4	<1	0	0	11	1	<1	1 vegetable
Turnip Greens, Fresh, Cooked (1/2 cup)	14	3	<1	0	0	21	2	<1	1 vegetable
Turnips, Fresh, Cooked (1/2 cup)	14	4	<1	0	0	39	2	<1	1 vegetable
Vegetable Juice (1/2 cup)	23	6	<1	0	0	442	1	<1	1 vegetable
Vegetable Juice Cocktail (1/2 cup)	23	6	<1	<1	0	442	1	<1	1 vegetable
Water Chestnuts (1/2 cup)	35	9	0	0	0	6	2	<1	1 vegetable
Watercress, Raw (1 cup)	4	<1	0	0	0	14	<1	<1	1 vegetable
Yam, Plain (1/2 cup)	79	19	<1	0	0	6	2	1	1 strch
Zucchini Squash, Fresh, Cooked (1/2 cup)	14	4	0	0	0	3	1	<1	1 vegetable
Zucchini, Raw (1 cup)	18	4	<1	0	0	4	2	2	1 vegetable
BETTY CROCKER									
Mashed Potatoes & Gravy, Hearty Beef (3/4 cup)	170	24	7	2	0	720	1	3	1 1/2 strch, 1 fat
Mashed Potatoes & Gravy, Roasted Chicken (3/4 cup)	180	25	7	2	<5	680	1	3	1 1/2 strch, 1 fat

VEGETABLES AND VEGETABLE JUICES

Products	Cal.	Carb. (g)	Fat (g)	Sat. Fat (g)	Chol. (mg)	Sod. (mg)	Fib. (g)	Prot. (g)	Servings/Exchanges
Mashed Potatoes, Butter & Herb (1/2 cup)	160	20	8	2	5	470	1	3	1 strch, 2 fat
Mashed Potatoes, Chicken & Herb (1/2 cup)	150	21	7	2	<5	520	1	3	1 1/2 strch, 1 fat
Mashed Potatoes, Four Cheese (1/2 cup)	150	20	7	2	<5	570	2	3	1 strch, 1 fat
Mashed Potatoes, Potato Buds (2/3 cup)	160	19	8	2	<5	460	1	3	1 strch, 2 fat
Mashed Potatoes, Roasted Garlic (1/2 cup)	150	19	8	2	<5	400	2	3	1 strch, 2 fat
Mashed Potatoes, Sour Cream & Chives (1/2 cup)	150	21	7	2	5	440	1	3	1 1/2 strch, 1 fat
Potatoes, Au Gratin (1/2 cup)	150	22	6	2	5	600	1	3	1 1/2 strch, 1 fat
Potatoes, Broccoli Au Gratin, Homestyle (1/2 cup)	140	21	6	2	<5	530	2	3	1 1/2 strch, 1 fat
Potatoes, Cheddar & Bacon (1/2 cup)	150	21	6	2	<5	650	1	3	1 1/2 strch, 1 fat
Potatoes, Cheddar & Sour Cream (1/2 cup)	130	25	3	1	<5	570	1	3	1 1/2 strch, 1 fat
Potatoes, Cheddar Cheese, Homestyle (1/2 cup)	120	21	3	1	<5	600	1	4	1 1/2 strch, 1 fat
Potatoes, Cheesy Scalloped, Homestyle (1/2 cup)	140	21	6	2	<5	540	3	3	1 1/2 strch, 1 fat
Potatoes, Chicken & Vegetable (2/3 cup)	160	24	6	2	<5	560	2	4	1 1/2 strch, 1 fat
Potatoes, Hash Browns (1/2 cup)	190	30	8	2	0	620	3	3	2 strch, 2 fat

Potatoes, Julienne (1/2 cup)	150	21	6	2	<5	630	1	3	1 1/2 strch, 1 fat
Potatoes, Ranch (1/2 cup)	160	25	6	2	<5	610	2	3	1 1/2 strch, 1 fat
Potatoes, Scalloped (1/2 cup)	160	23	6	2	<5	610	1	3	1 1/2 strch, 1 fat
Potatoes, Sour Cream 'n Chive (1/2 cup)	160	22	7	2	5	600	2	3	1 1/2 strch, 1 fat
Potatoes, Three Cheese (1/2 cup)	150	23	6	2	<5	600	2	3	1 1/2 strch, 1 fat
Potatoes, Twice Baked Cheddar & Bacon (2/3 cup)	210	22	11	3	85	580	1	6	1 1/2 strch, 2 fat
BIRD'S EYE									
Artichoke Hearts, Deluxe (1/2 cup)	38	8	<1	<1	0	47	6	3	1 vegetable
Japanese-Style Vegetables (1/2 cup)	78	8	5	2	12	320	2	2	1 vegetable, 1 fat
Spinach, Creamed (1/2 cup)	111	7	8	5	22	565	1	4	1 vegetable, 2 fat
Stir-Fry Vegetables, Broccoli (3/4 cup)	45	9	<1	0	0	34	4	3	2 vegetable
Stir-Fry, Vegetables, Cauliflower & Carrots (2/3 cup)	38	8	<1	0	0	33	3	2	1 vegetable
Stir-Fry Vegetables, Chinese (1/2 cup)	36	8	<1	0	0	540	2	2	2 vegetable
Stir-Fry Vegetables, Japanese (1/2 cup)	30	7	<1	0	0	516	NA	2	1 vegetable
Stir-Fry Vegetables, Pepper (3/4 cup)	29	6	<1	0	0	21	3	3	1 vegetable

VEGETABLES AND VEGETABLE JUICES

Products	Cal.	Carb. (g)	Fat (g)	Sat. Fat (g)	Chol. (mg)	Sod. (mg)	Fib. (g)	Prot. (g)	Servings/Exchanges
CAMPBELL'S									
Tomato Juice (1 cup)	50	9	0	0	9	860	1	2	2 vegetable
V8 100% Vegetable Juice (1 cup)	50	10	0	0	0	620	1	1	2 vegetable
V8 Light Tangy 100% Vegetable Juice (1 cup)	60	11	0	0	0	340	1	2	2 vegetable
V8 Picante Vegetable Juice (1 cup)	50	10	0	0	0	680	1	2	2 vegetable
V8 Spicy Hot 100% Vegetable Juice (1 cup)	50	10	0	0	0	780	1	2	2 vegetable
CONTADINA									
Tomato Paste (2 Tbsp)	30	6	0	0	0	20	1	2	1/2 strch
Tomato Paste, Italian (2 Tbsp)	35	7	<1	0	0	290	1	1	1/2 strch
Tomato Puree (1/4 cup)	20	4	0	0	0	15	<1	<1	1 vegetable
Tomato Sauce (1/4 cup)	15	3	0	0	0	280	<1	<1	1 vegetable
Tomato Sauce, Italian (1/4 cup)	15	4	0	0	0	320	1	<1	1 vegetable
Tomato Sauce, Thick & Zesty (1/4 cup)	20	3	0	0	0	340	1	1	1 vegetable
Tomatoes, Crushed, in Puree (1/2 cup)	30	6	1	0	0	350	1	1	1 vegetable

Tomatoes, Italian (Pear) (1/2 cup)	25	4	0	0	0	220	1	1	1 vegetable
Tomatoes, Italian Stewed (1/2 cup)	50	8	1	0	0	260	1	1	1 vegetable
Tomatoes, Mexican Stewed (1/2 cup)	50	10	1	0	0	290	1	1	2 vegetable
Tomatoes, Recipe-Ready (1/2 cup)	25	5	<1	<1	0	570	1	1	1 vegetable
Tomatoes, Stewed (1/2 cup)	50	9	1	0	1	220	1	1	2 vegetable
Tomatoes, Whole Peeled (1/2 cup)	25	4	0	0	0	218	1	1	1 vegetable
GREEN GIANT									
Baby Peas in Butter Sauce, LeSueur (3/4 cup)	100	16	2	2	<5	370	16	5	1 strch
Beets, Harvard, Canned (1/3 cup)	60	15	0	0	0	270	2	<1	1/2 carb., 1 vegetable
Broccoli in Cheese Sauce (2/3 cup)	70	9	3	1	<5	520	2	3	2 vegetable, 1 fat
Broccoli Spears in Butter Sauce (1/2 cup)	50	7	2	1	<5	330	2	2	1 vegetable
Broccoli, Cauliflower, Carrots in Butter Sauce (3/4 cup)	60	8	2	2	<5	300	2	2	1 vegetable
Broccoli, Pasta, Sweet Peas in Butter Sauce (3/4 cup)	70	11	2	2	<5	280	2	3	1/2 strch, 1 vegetable
Corn, Shoepeg White, in Butter Sauce (3/4 cup)	120	21	3	2	1	320	3	3	1 1/2 strch, 1 fat

VEGETABLES AND VEGETABLE JUICES

Products	Cal.	Carb. (g)	Fat (g)	Sat. Fat (g)	Chol. (mg)	Sod. (mg)	Fib. (g)	Prot. (g)	Servings/Exchanges
Corn Niblets in Butter Sauce (2/3 cup)	130	23	3	2	<5	350	3	3	1 1/2 strch, 1 fat
Cream Style Corn (1/2 cup)	110	23	1	0	0	330	2	2	1 1/2 strch
Green Bean Casserole (2/3 cup)	130	10	9	5	15	510	2	2	2 vegetable, 2 fat
Honey Glazed Carrots (1 cup)	90	13	4	<1	0	140	2	<1	1/2 carb., 1 vegetable, 1 fat
Mixed Vegetables in Butter Sauce (3/4 cup)	70	11	2	1	<5	240	3	2	2 vegetable
Pasta Accents Vegetables, Alfredo (2 cups)	210	25	8	3	5	480	4	9	1 1/2 strch, 1 vegetable, 2 fat
Pasta Accents Vegetables, Creamy Cheddar (2 1/3 cup)	250	36	8	3	5	700	5	9	2 strch, 1 vegetable, 1 fat
Pasta Accents Vegetables, Florentine (2 cup)	310	44	9	3	7	910	5	13	2 strch, 2 vegetable, 2 fat
Pasta Accents Vegetables, Garlic (2 cups)	260	36	10	5	15	640	12	7	2 1/2 strch, 2 fat
Pasta Accents Vegetables, Oriental (2 1/2 cup)	260	35	9	4	20	580	4	8	2 strch, 1 vegetable, 2 fat
Pasta Accents Vegetables, Primavera (2 1/4 cup)	290	39	9	3	5	530	4	12	2 strch, 2 vegetable, 2 fat
Pasta Accents Vegetables, White Cheddar (1 3/4 cup)	270	37	9	3	10	750	3	9	2 strch, 1 vegetable, 2 fat

Select American Mixtures, Broccoli/Waterchestnut Stir-Fry (2/3 cup)	25	5	0	0	0	30	2	1	1 vegetable
Select American Mixtures, Broccoli/Carrots Skillet (2/3 cup)	25	4	0	0	0	30	2	2	1 vegetable
Southwestern Style Corn (3/4 cup)	90	18	1	0	0	130	1	3	1 strch
Sweet Peas in Butter Sauce (3/4 cup)	100	16	2	2	<5	400	5	4	1 strch
Three-Bean Salad, Canned (1/2 cup)	90	20	0	0	20	490	4	3	1 strch
Vegetables Alfredo (3/4 cup)	80	9	3	2	5	450	3	4	2 vegetable, 1 fat
Vegetables, Teriyaki (1 1/4 cup)	100	7	7	1	0	510	2	2	1 vegetable, 1 fat

LIBBY'S

Pumpkin, Solid Pack, Canned (1/2 cup)	40	9	<1	0	0	5	5	2	2 vegetable

MRS. PAUL'S

Onion Rings, Old-Fashioned (2.5 oz)	200	24	10	NA	NA	367	NA	3	1 1/2 strch, 2 fat
Sweet Potatoes, Candied (1/2 cup)	276	67	1	<1	0	109	2	<1	1 strch, 3 1/2 carb.

ORE IDA

Baked Potato, Topped, Broccoli & Cheese (1/2)	300	48	8	3	20	410	8	10	3 strch, 2 fat

VEGETABLES AND VEGETABLE JUICES

Products	Cal.	Carb. (g)	Fat (g)	Sat. Fat (g)	Chol. (mg)	Sod. (mg)	Fib. (g)	Prot. (g)	Servings/Exchanges
Baked Potato, Twice, Cheddar Cheese (1)	228	28	11	7	6	565	NA	6	2 strch, 2 fat
Cheddar Browns (1 patty)	85	14	2	1	3	365	NA	3	1 strch
Cottage Fries (3 oz or 13 fries)	125	20	4	<1	0	17	NA	2	1 strch, 1 fat
Country Fries (3 oz or 15 fries)	111	19	3	<1	0	10	NA	2	1 strch, 1 fat
Crinkle Cuts, Lite (3 oz)	89	16	2	<1	0	22	NA	2	1 strch
Crispers (3 oz or 15 fries)	231	25	14	3	0	471	NA	2	1 1/2 strch, 3 fat
Crispy Crowns (3 oz or 12 pieces)	172	20	9	2	0	412	NA	2	1 strch, 2 fat
Crispy Crunchies (3 oz or 12 fries)	162	18	9	2	0	310	2	2	1 strch, 2 fat
Fast Fries (3 oz or 23 fries)	142	20	6	2	0	232	2	2	1 strch, 1 fat
Golden Crinkles (3 oz or 14 fries)	155	22	7	1	0	18	NA	2	1 1/2 strch, 1 fat
Golden Fries (3 oz or 15 fries)	123	20	4	<1	0	17	NA	2	1 strch, 1 fat
Golden Patties (1 patty)	163	19	9	2	0	275	NA	2	1 strch, 2 fat
Golden Twirls (3 oz or 10 fries)	162	22	7	1	0	25	2	2	1 1/2 strch, 1 fat
Hash Browns, Microwave (2 oz)	117	13	7	1	0	133	NA	1	1 strch, 1 fat

Hash Browns, Shredded (3 oz)	68	15	0	0	0	27	NA	2	1 strch
Hash Browns, Southern-Style (3 oz)	70	16	0	0	0	20	NA	2	1 strch
Hash Browns, Toaster (1 patties)	99	12	6	3	3	173	NA	1	1 strch, 1 fat
Hot Tots (3 oz or 9 pieces)	152	21	6	1	0	385	2	2	1 strch, 1 fat
Onion Ringers (2 oz)	142	18	7	1	0	129	NA	2	1 strch, 1 fat
Pixie Crinkles (3 oz or 32 fries)	142	21	5	1	0	30	NA	2	1 1/2 strch, 1 fat
Potato Wedges w/Skin, Homestyle (3 oz or 7 fries)	109	19	3	<1	0	16	NA	2	1 strch, 1 fat
Potatoes, Mashed (2/3 cup)	106	18	3	<1	3	185	<1	3	1 strch, 1 fat
Potatoes O'Brien (3 oz)	62	14	0	0	0	17	NA	1	1 strch
Shoestrings (3 oz or 39 fries)	149	22	6	1	0	16	NA	2	1 1/2 strch, 1 fat
Snackin' Fries (1 pkg)	340	36	20	4	0	590	3	4	2 1/2 strch, 4 fat
Stew Vegetables (2 oz)	33	7	0	0	0	45	<1	<1	1/2 strch
Tater Tots (3 oz or 9 pieces)	146	20	7	1	0	401	NA	2	1 strch, 1 fat
Tater Tots, Microwave (1 pkg)	204	29	9	2	0	352	NA	2	2 strch, 2 fat
Tater Tots, Onion (3 oz or 9 pieces)	145	16	7	1	0	518	NA	2	1 strch, 1 fat
Texas Crispers (3 oz or 7 pieces)	172	19	10	3	0	280	2	2	1 strch, 2 fat

VEGETABLES AND VEGETABLE JUICES

Products	Cal.	Carb. (g)	Fat (g)	Sat. Fat (g)	Chol. (mg)	Sod. (mg)	Fib. (g)	Prot. (g)	Servings/Exchanges
Waffle Fries (3 oz or 9 fries)	142	22	5	2	0	35	2	2	1 1/2 strch, 1 fat
Zesties (3 oz or 12 fries)	162	21	9	2	0	374	1	2	1 1/2 strch, 2 fat
PROGRESSO									
Artichoke Hearts, Marinated (2 pieces)	50	2	5	1	0	110	0	0	1 fat
Zucchini, Italian-Style (1/2 cup)	50	7	2	0	0	400	2	2	1 vegetable
STOUFFER'S									
Green Bean Mushroom Casserole, Side Dish (1)	130	13	8.2	2	10	530	2	3	1/2 strch, 1 vegetable, 2 fat
Spinach, Cream, Side Dish (1)	150	8	12	4	15	380	2	4	1 vegetable, 2 fat

VEGETARIAN FOODS

Products	Cal.	Carb. (g)	Fat (g)	Sat. Fat (g)	Chol. (mg)	Sodium (mg)	Fiber (g)	Pro. (g)	Exchanges
Miso (1/2 cup)	284	39	8	1	0	5032	8	17	2 1/2 strch, 1 med-fat meat, 1 fat
Miso Sauce (1/2 cup)	191	36	3	<1	0	2008	3	7	2 1/2 strch, 1 fat
Tempeh (1/2 cup)	165	14	6	<1	0	5	5	16	1 strch, 2 lean meat
Tofu, Firm, Raw (1/2 cup)	183	5	11	2	0	18	3	20	3 lean meat
Tofu, Regular (1/2 cup)	94	2	6	<1	0	9	2	10	1 med-fat meat
Tofu Yogurt (1 cup)	254	43	5	<1	0	92	<1	9	3 strch, 1 fat
Vegetarian Bacon Strips (3 strips)	47	<1	4	<1	0	220	<1	2	1 fat
Vegetarian Breakfast Links (1 link)	64	3	5	<1	0	222	<1	5	1 med-fat meat
Vegetarian Breakfast Patties (1)	97	4	7	1	0	337	1	7	1 med-fat meat
Vegetarian Chicken Slices (2)	132	4	8	1	0	474	3	10	1 med-fat meat, 1 fat
Vegetarian Chicken, Breaded, Fried (1 slice)	97	3	7	1	0	228	3	6	1 med-fat meat

VEGETARIAN FOODS

Products	Cal.	Carb. (g)	Fat (g)	Sat. Fat (g)	Chol. (mg)	Sod. (mg)	Fib. (g)	Prot. (g)	Servings/Exchanges
Vegetarian Chili (1 cup)	282	30	4	<1	0	1052	8	38	2 strch, 4 very lean meat
Vegetarian Fillets (1)	136	4	9	1	0	230	3	11	2 med-fat meat
Vegetarian Fish Sticks (2)	165	5	10	2	0	279	4	13	2 med-fat meat
Vegetarian Frankfurter (1)	102	4	5	<1	0	219	2	10	1 med-fat meat
Vegetarian Luncheon Meat (1 slice)	188	6	11	2	0	576	3	17	1/2 strch, 2 med-fat meat
Vegetarian Meat Patties (1)	142	6	6	1	0	391	3	15	1/2 strch, 2 lean meat
Vegetarian Meatballs (7)	140	6	6	<1	0	385	3	15	1/2 strch, 2 lean meat
Vegetarian Pot Pie (1)	524	41	34	10	20	538	5	15	3 strch, 1 med-fat meat, 6 fat
Vegetarian Sandwich Spread (3 Tbsp)	72	4	4	<1	0	302	2	4	1 med-fat meat
Vegetarian Scallops, Breaded & Fried (1/2 cup)	257	8	16	3	0	434	5	20	1/2 strch, 3 med-fat meat
Vegetarian Soyburger (1)	142	6	6	1	0	391	3	15	1/2 strch, 2 lean meat
GREEN GIANT									
Harvest Burger, Italian (1)	140	8	5	2	0	370	5	17	1/2 strch, 2 lean meat

Harvest Burger, Original (1)	140	8	4	2	0	370	5	18	1/2 strch, 2 lean meat
Harvest Burger, Southwestern-Style (1)	140	9	4	2	0	370	5	16	1/2 strch, 2 lean meat
HEALTH VALLEY									
Soy Moo Milk, Fat-Free (1 cup)	110	19	0	0	0	25	0	7	1 carb.
LIFE LITE									
Soft Serve Tofutti, Chocolate (1/2 cup)	90	20	1	NA	0	80	NA	2	1 carb.
Soft Serve Tofutti, Vanilla (1/2 cup)	90	20	1	NA	0	80	NA	2	1 carb.
Tofutti, All Flavors (1/2 cup)	200	20	1	NA	0	80	NA	2	1 1/2 carb., 2 fat
Tofutti, Better Than Cheese Cake (1 slice)	160	16	10	4	0	110	NA	2	1 carb., 2 fat
Tofutti, Better Than Cream Cheese (2 Tbsp)	80	1	8	3	0	200	NA	1	2 fat
Tofutti, Egg Watchers (1/4 cup)	50	2	2	<1	0	100	NA	7	1 lean meat
LOMA LINDA									
Big Franks (1)	110	2	7	1	0	240	2	10	1 med-fat meat
Big Franks, Low Fat (1)	80	3	3	<1	0	220	2	11	2 very lean meat
Chicken Supreme Dry Mix (1/3 cup)	90	6	1	0	0	720	4	15	1/2 strch, 2 very lean meat
Chik Nuggets (5)	240	13	16	3	0	710	5	12	1 strch, 1 med-fat meat, 2 fat

VEGETARIAN FOODS

Products	Cal.	Carb. (g)	Fat (g)	Sat. Fat (g)	Chol. (mg)	Sod. (mg)	Fib. (g)	Prot. (g)	Servings/Exchanges
Corn Dogs (1)	150	22	4	<1	0	500	3	7	1 1/2 strch, 1 med-fat meat
Dinner Cuts (2 slices)	90	3	2	1	0	500	2	17	2 very lean meat
Fried Chik'n (2 pieces)	160	4	10	2	0	440	2	12	2 med-fat meat
Linketts (1)	70	1	5	<1	0	160	1	7	1 med-fat meat
Little Links (2)	90	2	6	1	0	230	2	8	1 med-fat meat
Nuteena (3/8-inch slice)	160	6	13	5	0	120	2	6	1/2 strch, 1 med-fat meat, 2 fat
Ocean Platter Dry Mix (1/3 cup)	90	8	1	0	0	450	4	14	1/2 strch, 2 very lean meat
Patty Dry Mix (1/3 cup)	90	7	1	0	0	480	5	14	1/2 strch, 2 very lean meat
Redi-Burger (5/8-inch slice)	120	7	3	<1	0	450	4	18	1/2 strch, 2 very lean meat
Sandwich Spread Dry Mix (1/4 cup)	80	7	5	1	0	260	3	4	1/2 strch, 1 fat
Savory Dinner Loaf Dry Mix (1/3 cup)	90	7	2	0	0	560	5	14	1/2 strch, 2 very lean meat
Soyagen All Purpose (1/3 cup)	130	12	6	1	0	150	3	6	1 strch, 1 med-fat meat
Soyagen Carob (1/3 cup)	130	13	6	1	0	170	2	6	1 strch, 1 med-fat meat

Food								Exchanges
Soyagen No Sucrose (1/3 cup)	130	12	6	1	0	160	3	6	1 strch, 1 med-fat meat
Swiss Stake (1)	120	8	6	1	0	430	4	9	1/2 strch, 1 med-fat meat
Tender Bits (6)	110	7	5	<1	0	440	3	11	1/2 strch, 1 med-fat meat
Tender Rounds (8)	120	5	5	1	0	330	3	14	2 lean meat
Vege-Burger (1/4 cup)	70	2	2	<1	0	115	2	11	1 lean meat
Vita-Burger Chunks (1/4 cup)	70	6	1	0	0	350	3	10	1/2 strch, 1 very lean meat
Vita-Burger Granules (3 Tbsp)	70	6	1	0	0	350	3	10	1/2 strch, 1 very lean meat
MORNINGSTAR FARMS									
America'a Original Veggie Dog (1)	80	6	<1	0	0	580	1	11	1/2 strch, 1 very lean meat
Better'n Burgers (1)	80	6	0	0	0	360	3	13	1/2 strch, 1 very lean meat
Better'n Eggs (1/4 cup)	20	0	0	0	0	90	0	5	1 very lean meat
Breakfast Links (2)	60	2	2	<1	0	340	2	8	1 lean meat
Breakfast Patties (1)	80	3	3	<1	0	270	2	10	1 lean meat
Breakfast Sandwich w/Scramblers/Pattie/Cheese (1)	280	12	3	<1	10	1000	5	28	1 strch, 4 very lean meat
Breakfast Strips (2)	60	2	5	<1	0	220	<1	2	1 fat

VEGETARIAN FOODS

Products	Cal.	Carb. (g)	Fat (g)	Sat. Fat (g)	Chol. (mg)	Sod. (mg)	Fib. (g)	Prot. (g)	Servings/Exchanges
Chik Nuggets (4)	160	17	4	<1	0	670	5	13	1 strch, 1 medium fat meat
Chik Patties (1)	150	15	6	1	0	570	2	9	1 strch, 1 med-fat meat, 1 fat
Deli Franks (1)	110	3	7	1	2	524	3	10	1 med-fat meat
Garden Grille Pattie (1)	120	18	3	1	<5	280	4	6	1 strch, 1 lean meat
Garden Veggie Pattie (1)	100	9	3	<1	0	350	4	10	1/2 strch, 1 lean meat
Grillers (1)	140	5	6	1	0	260	2	15	2 lean meat
Ground Meatless (1/2 cup)	60	4	0	0	0	260	2	10	1 very lean meat
Harvest Burger Original (1)	140	8	4	2	0	370	5	18	1/2 strch, 2 lean meat
Homestyle Noodles (2 oz)	156	32	<1	0	0	10	3	6	2 strch
MeatFree Corn Dog (1)	150	22	4	<1	0	500	3	7	1 1/2 strch, 1 medium fat meat
Meatless Buffalo Wings (5)	200	16	9	2	0	730	3	13	1 strch, 1 medium fat meat, 1 fat
Quarter Prime Patties (1)	140	6	2	0	0	370	3	24	1/2 strch, 3 very lean meat

Scramblers (1/4 cup)	35	2	0	0	0	95	0	6	1 very lean meat
Spicy Black Bean Burger (1)	110	16	1	0	0	470	5	11	1 strch, 1 very lean meat
Stuffed Sandwich, Ham/Cheese Style (1)	300	45	7	3	10	520	1	15	3 strch, 1 medium fat meat
Stuffed Sandwich, Pepperoni Pizza Style (1)	280	42	7	3	5	420	5	12	3 strch, 1 medium fat meat

NATURAL TOUCH

Dinner Entree (1)	220	2	15	3	0	380	2	19	3 med-fat meat
Garden Vege Pattie (1)	110	8	3	<1	0	280	3	10	1/2 strch, 1 med-fat meat
Lentil Rice Loaf (1-inch slice)	170	14	9	3	0	370	4	8	1 strch, 1 med-fat meat, 1 fat
Nine Bean Loaf (1-inch slice)	160	13	8	2	<5	350	5	8	1 strch, 1 med-fat meat, 1 fat
Okara Patty (1)	110	4	5	1	0	360	3	11	2 lean meat
Spicy Black Bean Burger (1)	100	15	1	0	0	330	5	11	1 strch, 1 very lean meat
Toaster Squares, Blueberry (1)	180	33	2	<1	0	65	6	6	2 strch
Toaster Squares, Date Walnut (1)	200	36	3	<1	0	50	8	6	2 1/2 strch, 1 fat
Vegan Burger (1)	70	6	0	0	0	370	3	11	1/2 strch, 1 very lean meat
Vegan Burger Crumbles (1/2 cup)	60	4	0	0	0	260	2	10	1 very lean meat
Vegan Sausage Crumbles (1/2 cup)	60	4	0	0	0	300	2	10	1 very lean meat

VEGETARIAN FOODS

Products	Cal.	Carb. (g)	Fat (g)	Sat. Fat (g)	Chol. (mg)	Sod. (mg)	Fib. (g)	Prot. (g)	Servings/Exchanges
Vege Frank (1)	100	2	6	1	0	470	2	10	1 med-fat meat
Vegetarian Chili (1 cup)	170	21	1	0	0	870	11	18	1 1/2 strch, 2 very lean meat
WORTHINGTON									
Beef-Style Meatless (3/8-inch slice)	110	4	7	1	0	620	3	9	1 med-fat meat
Bolono (3 slices)	80	2	4	1	0	720	2	10	1 med-fat meat
Chic-ketts (2 3/8-inch slices)	120	2	7	1	0	390	2	13	2 lean meat
Chicken, Sliced or Roll (2)	80	1	5	1	0	370	2	9	1 med-fat meat
Chik, Diced (1/4 cup)	40	1	0	0	0	270	1	7	1 very lean meat
Chik, Sliced (3)	70	2	<1	0	0	430	2	14	2 very lean meat
ChikStiks (1)	110	3	7	1	0	360	2	9	1 med-fat meat
Chili (1 cup)	290	21	15	3	0	1130	9	19	1 1/2 strch, 2 med-fat meat, 1 fat
Chili, Low Fat (1 cup)	170	21	1	0	0	870	11	18	1 1/2 strch, 2 very lean meat
Choplets (2 slices)	90	3	2	1	0	500	2	17	2 very lean meat

Food									Exchanges
Corned Beef, Meatless (4 slices)	140	5	9	1	0	520	2	10	1 med-fat meat, 1 fat
Country Stew (1 cup)	210	20	9	1	0	830	5	13	1 strch, 1 med-fat meat, 1 fat
CrispyChik Patties (1)	150	15	6	1	0	600	2	8	1 strch, 1 med-fat meat
Cutlets (1 slice)	70	3	1	0	0	340	2	11	2 very lean meat
Dinner Roast (3/4-inch slice)	180	5	12	2	0	580	3	12	2 med-fat meat
Fillets (2)	180	8	10	2	0	750	4	16	1/2 strch, 2 med-fat meat
FriChik (2)	120	1	8	1	0	430	1	10	1 med-fat meat, 1 fat
FriPats (1)	130	4	6	1	0	320	3	14	2 lean meat
Golden Croquettes (4)	210	14	10	2	0	600	3	14	1 strch, 2 med-fat meat
Granburger (3 Tbsp)	60	3	<1	0	0	410	2	10	1 very lean meat
Leanies (1 link)	100	2	7	1	0	430	1	7	1 med-fat meat
Multigrain Cutlet (2 slices)	100	5	2	<1	0	390	4	15	2 very lean meat
Numete (3/8-inch slice)	130	5	10	3	0	270	3	6	1 med-fat meat, 1 fat
Prime Stakes (1)	120	4	7	1	0	440	4	10	1 med-fat meat
Prosage Links (2)	60	2	3	<1	0	340	2	8	1 lean meat
Prosage Patties (1)	80	3	3	<1	0	300	2	9	1 lean meat

VEGETARIAN FOODS

Products	Cal.	Carb. (g)	Fat (g)	Sat. Fat (g)	Chol. (mg)	Sod. (mg)	Fib. (g)	Prot. (g)	Servings/Exchanges
Prosage Roll (5/8-inch slice)	140	2	10	1	0	390	2	10	1 med-fat meat, 1 fat
Protose (3/8-inch slice)	130	5	7	1	0	280	3	13	2 lean meat
Salami, Meatless (3 slices)	130	2	8	1	0	800	2	12	2 med-fat meat
Saucettes (1 link)	90	1	6	1	0	200	1	6	1 med-fat meat
Savorex, Dry (1 tsp)	10	1	0	0	0	300	0	1	free
Savory Slices (3)	150	6	9	4	0	540	3	10	1/2 strch, 1 med-fat meat, 1 fat
Smoked Beef, Meatless (6 slices)	120	6	6	1	0	730	3	11	1/2 strch, 1 med-fat meat
Smoked Turkey, Meatless (3 slices)	140	3	10	2	0	620	2	10	1 med-fat meat, 1 fat
Stakelets (1)	140	6	8	1	0	480	2	12	1/2 strch, 2 med-fat meat
Stripples (2 strips)	60	2	5	<1	0	220	<1	2	1 fat
Super-Links (1)	110	2	8	1	0	350	1	7	1 med-fat meat, 1 fat
Tuno, Drained (1/3 cup)	80	4	4	<1	0	380	1	7	1 med-fat meat
Tuno, Drained (1/2 cup)	80	2	6	1	0	290	1	6	1 med-fat meat

Food									
Turkee Slices (3 slices)	170	3	12	2	0	580	2	13	2 med-fat meat, 1 fat
Vegetable Scallops (1/2 cup)	90	3	2	<1	0	410	3	15	2 very lean meat
Vegetable Steaks (2)	80	3	2	<1	0	300	3	15	2 very lean meat
Vegetarian Burger (1/4 cup)	60	2	2	0	0	270	1	9	1 lean meat
Vegetarian Egg Rolls (1)	180	20	8	2	0	380	2	6	1 strch, 2 fat
Veja-Links (1)	50	1	3	<1	0	190	0	5	1 lean meat
Veja Links, Low Fat (1)	40	1	2	0	0	190	0	5	1 lean meat
Wham (2 slices)	80	1	5	1	0	430	0	7	1 med-fat meat

About The American Dietetic Association

The American Dietetic Association is the world's largest organization of food and nutrition professionals. Founded in 1917, The American Dietetic Association promotes optimal nutrition to improve public health and well-being. The Association has nearly 70,000 members, of whom approximately 75 percent are registered dietitians (RD). The membership also includes dietetic technicians (DTR) and others holding advanced degrees in nutrition and dietetics. As the public education center of the Association, the National Center for Nutrition and Dietetics provides programs and services to inform and educate the public about food and nutrition issues. The Center and The American Dietetic Association are located at 216 W. Jackson Boulevard, Chicago, IL 60606.

Registered dietitians offer preventive and therapeutic nutrition services in a variety of settings, including health care, business, research, and educational organizations, as well as private practice. Registered dietitians working in the health care field serve as vital members of medical teams providing medical nutrition therapy to treat illnesses, injuries, and chronic conditions such as diabetes.

The credentials "RD" signify that a practitioner has completed a rigorous program of education and training. The registered dietitian must have at least a baccalaureate degree in an approved program of dietetics or related field from an accredited U.S. college or university. In addition, he or she must complete an internship or similar experience and pass a national credentialing exam. To retain RD status, dietitians must fulfill continuing education requirements to update and enhance their knowledge and skills.

To find a registered dietitian, the expert in diet, health, and nutrition, ask your physician or call your local hospital. You can also access The American Dietetic Association's toll-free dietitian referral service by calling 800/366-1655 or visiting the web site at www.eatright.org.

About the American Diabetes Association

The American Diabetes Association is the nation's leading voluntary health organization supporting diabetes research, information, and advocacy. Its mission is to prevent and cure diabetes and to improve the lives of all people affected by diabetes. The American Diabetes Association is the leading publisher of comprehensive diabetes information. Its huge library of practical and authoritative books for people with diabetes covers every aspect of self-care—cooking and nutrition, fitness, weight control, medications, complications, emotional issues, and general self-care.

To order American Diabetes Association books:
Call 1-800-ADA-ORDER (800-232-6733).
http://store.diabetes.org [Note: there is no need to use www when typing this particular Web address]

To join the American Diabetes Association:
Call 1-800-806-7801. www.diabetes.org/membership

For more information about diabetes or ADA programs and services: Call 1-800-DIABETES (800-342-2383). E-mail: Customerservice@diabetes.org www.diabetes.org

To locate an ADA/NCQA Recognized Provider of quality diabetes care in your area: www.ncqa.org/dprp/

To find an ADA Recognized Education Program in your area: Call 1-888-232-0822.
www.diabetes.org/recognition/education.asp

To join the fight to increase funding for diabetes research, end discrimination, and improve insurance coverage: Call 1-800-DIABETES (800-342-2383).
www.diabetes.org/advocacy

To find out how you can get involved with the programs in your community: Call 1-800-DIABETES (800-342-2383). See below for program Web addresses.

- *American Diabetes Month:* Educational activities aimed at those diagnosed with diabetes—month of November. www.diabetes.org/ADM
- *American Diabetes Alert:* Annual public awareness campaign to find the undiagnosed—held the fourth Tuesday in March. www.diabetes.org/alert
- *The Diabetes Assistance & Resources Program (DAR):* diabetes awareness program targeted to the Latino community. www.diabetes.org/DAR
- *African American Program:* diabetes awareness program targeted to the African American community. www.diabetes.org/africanamerican
- *Awakening the Spirit:* Pathways to Diabetes Prevention & Control: diabetes awareness program targeted to the Native American community. www.diabetes.org/awakening

To find out about an important research project regarding type 2 diabetes: www.diabetes.org/ada/research.asp

To obtain information on making a planned gift or charitable bequest: Call 1-888-700-7029. www.diabetes.org/ada/plan.asp

To make a donation or memorial contribution: Call 1-800-DIABETES (800-342-2383). www.diabetes.org/ada/cont.asp

1400 to 1500 Cal per day
Cal from fat 360
fat grams per day 40
fat grams pr 13

3 meal per day